INNOVATIVE THERAPEUTIC APPROACHES BY CRISPR/CAS9 IN CANCER THERAPY

Other World Scientific Titles by the Editors

Autophagy, Apoptosis and Ferroptosis in Oncology: Cell Death and Cancer
ISBN: 978-981-12-9931-5

INNOVATIVE THERAPEUTIC APPROACHES BY CRISPR/CAS9 IN CANCER THERAPY

Editors

Kiavash Hushmandi
University of Tehran, Iran

Alan Prem Kumar
National University of Singapore, Singapore

World Scientific

NEW JERSEY • LONDON • SINGAPORE • BEIJING • SHANGHAI • HONG KONG • TAIPEI • CHENNAI • TOKYO

Published by

World Scientific Publishing Co. Pte. Ltd.
5 Toh Tuck Link, Singapore 596224
USA office: 27 Warren Street, Suite 401-402, Hackensack, NJ 07601
UK office: 57 Shelton Street, Covent Garden, London WC2H 9HE

Library of Congress Control Number: 2026001668

British Library Cataloguing-in-Publication Data
A catalogue record for this book is available from the British Library.

INNOVATIVE THERAPEUTIC APPROACHES BY CRISPR/CAS9 IN CANCER THERAPY

ISBN 978-981-98-2674-2 (hardcover)
ISBN 978-981-98-2675-9 (ebook for institutions)
ISBN 978-981-98-2676-6 (ebook for individuals)

For any available supplementary material, please visit
https://www.worldscientific.com/worldscibooks/10.1142/14690#t=suppl

Desk Editor: Shaun Tan Yi Jie

Typeset by Stallion Press
Email: enquiries@stallionpress.com

https://doi.org/10.1142/9789819826759_fmatter

Preface

The landscape of cancer research and treatment has been fundamentally transformed by the advent of genome editing technologies, and among these, CRISPR/Cas9 stands as one of the most revolutionary scientific breakthroughs of our time. This book, *Innovative Therapeutic Approaches by CRISPR/Cas9 in Cancer Therapy*, seeks to provide a comprehensive exploration of how this remarkable molecular tool is reshaping our understanding of cancer biology and offering unprecedented opportunities for therapeutic intervention.

CRISPR/Cas9, originally discovered as a bacterial immune defense mechanism, has evolved into a precise genome editing platform capable of targeting oncogenic mutations, disrupting tumor suppressor genes, and modulating cellular pathways with extraordinary accuracy. In the context of oncology, this technology addresses one of medicine's most persistent challenges: cancer's ability to evolve, resist treatment, and evade the immune system. Traditional therapies, chemotherapy, radiation, and surgery, while lifesaving for many, often face limitations due to drug resistance, systemic toxicity, and tumor heterogeneity. CRISPR/Cas9 offers a fundamentally different approach by enabling permanent, targeted modifications at the genomic level.

This book examines CRISPR/Cas9 applications across diverse malignancies, including prostate, bladder, cervical, ovarian, breast, lung, hepatocellular, and colorectal cancers, as well as bone sarcomas. Each chapter is designed to guide readers through the intricate mechanisms by which genome editing identifies novel therapeutic targets, overcomes multidrug resistance, enhances chemotherapy sensitivity, and potentiates immunotherapy. Special emphasis is placed on genome-wide screening technologies that systematically reveal cancer vulnerabilities and resistance mechanisms, providing actionable insights for combination therapy strategies.

Beyond the editing mechanism itself, this volume addresses the critical challenge of delivery, the major bottleneck preventing clinical translation. Comprehensive coverage of lipid nanoparticles, polymeric carriers, inorganic nanoparticles, and exosome-based systems demonstrates how nanotechnology is bridging the gap between laboratory discovery and clinical application. These innovations are essential for achieving targeted tumor delivery while minimizing off-target effects and systemic toxicity.

The integration of CRISPR/Cas9 with immunotherapy represents one of the most exciting frontiers in precision oncology. By engineering immune cells to bypass checkpoint inhibition, overcome exhaustion, and recognize tumor antigens with enhanced specificity, CRISPR-edited CAR-T cells and tumor-infiltrating lymphocytes are showing remarkable promise in clinical trials. The recent FDA approval of Casgevy, the first CRISPR-based medicine, marks a watershed moment that validates the therapeutic potential of genome editing and paves the way for oncological applications.

To the researcher, clinician, biomedical engineer, or student engaging with this text, our hope is to provide not only a comprehensive understanding of CRISPR/Cas9 technology but also to inspire innovation in translating these discoveries into treatments that improve patient outcomes. By synthesizing current knowledge with future perspectives, this book aims to contribute meaningfully to the ongoing battle against cancer, offering evidence-based pathways toward more effective, personalized, and durable therapeutic responses.

We extend our deepest gratitude to the scientists, physicians, and scholars whose pioneering works form the foundation of this volume. Your intellectual rigor, creative problem solving, and unwavering commitment to advancing human health continue to push the boundaries of what is possible in cancer medicine. To the patients and families affected by cancer, your courage inspires us to persist in this quest for better treatments and, ultimately, cures.

As we stand at the intersection of genomics, nanotechnology, immunology, and oncology, the potential for transformative impact has never been greater. This book invites you to explore the cutting edge of cancer therapeutics and join the global community working toward a future where genome editing becomes a cornerstone of precision medicine.

https://doi.org/10.1142/9789819826759_fmatter

About the Editors

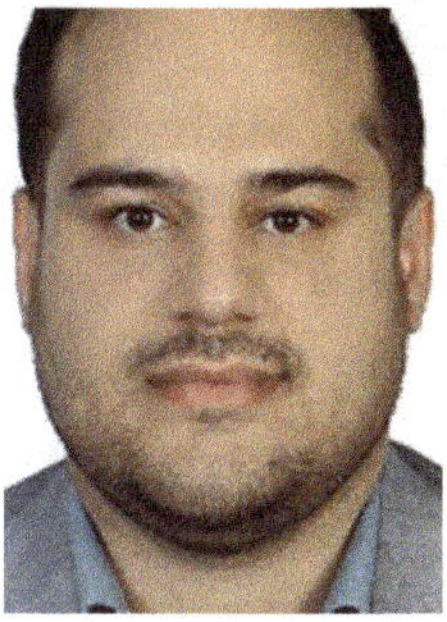

Dr. Kiavash Hushmandi is currently an Adjunct Assistant Professor at the Department of Epidemiology, University of Tehran, Iran. He received his PhD in Epidemiology from the University of Tehran. His research interests relate to molecular genetics, cancer biology, molecular epidemiology, cellular signaling, and public health. He has been among Top 2% of Scientists Worldwide by Stanford University for three consecutive years (2023–2025), and among the top 1% scientists in the Islamic World.

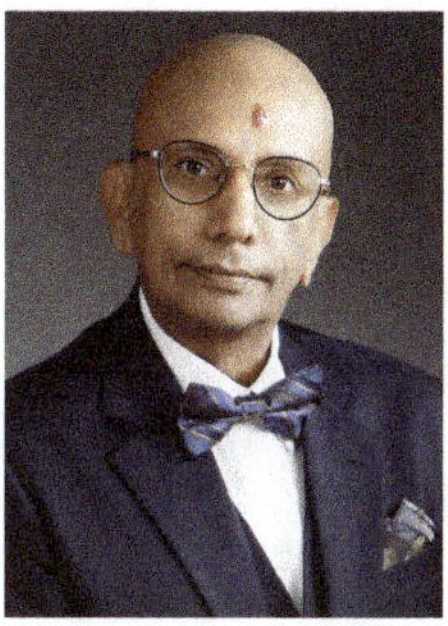

Dr. Alan Prem Kumar is an internationally recognized cancer biologist and academic leader at the Yong Loo Lin School of Medicine, National University of Singapore (NUS), Singapore where he serves as Assistant Professor in the Department of Pharmacology, Assistant Dean (Graduate Studies), and Director of the Office of Postdoctoral Affairs. His research is at the forefront of translational oncology, focusing on uncovering the molecular drivers of metastasis in female reproductive cancers and advancing precision-guided therapeutic strategies. His pioneering contributions have been recognized globally. He is a Clarivate Highly Cited Researcher (World's Top 1%) for four consecutive years (2020–2023) and among the World's Top 2% Scientists as listed by Stanford University (2022–2025). A passionate mentor and educator, he is a three-time recipient of the NUS Graduate Mentor of the Year Award (2017, 2021, 2025), reflecting his deep commitment to nurturing the next generation of biomedical scientists. Beyond academia, he contributes his expertise to scientific advisory boards including the Sansad Mobile Swasthya Seva (Parliament of India), The Sparks Foundation (Singapore) and AUM Biosciences (Singapore). He maintains dynamic industry collaborations with leading pharmaceutical and biotech partners such as Davos Life Sciences, Daiichi Sankyo, Rexahn Pharmaceuticals, and DotBio, driving innovation in targeted drug discovery and protective cancer therapeutics. His work exemplifies the powerful intersection of academic excellence, translational science, and societal impact.

https://doi.org/10.1142/9789819826759_fmatter

Contents

https://doi.org/10.1142/9789819826759_0001

CHAPTER 1

CRISPR/Cas9 in the Treatment of Lung Cancer

Mehrdad Hashemi[1,2], *Alireza Khosravinejad*[1,3], *Mina Alimohammadi*[4], *Reza Mohajer Shirazi*[1,3], *Behdokht Jamali*[5], *Kimia Sadat Esfahani*[1,3], *Ali Shirazi*[1,3], *Rojin Ghannad Zadeh*[1,6], *Faranak Jamshidian*[1,7], *Neda Zali*[3], *Najma Farahani*[1,*], *Afshin Taheriazam*[1,8,*], *Payman Rahimzadeh*[9,*], *Maliheh Entezari*[1,2,*]

[1]Farhikhtegan Medical Convergent Sciences Research Center, Farhikhtegan Hospital, Faculty of Medicine, TeMs. C., Islamic Azad University, Tehran, Iran
[2]Department of Genetics, Faculty of Advanced Sciences and Technology, TeMs. C, Islamic Azad University, Tehran, Iran
[3]Basic and Molecular Epidemiology of Gastrointestinal Disorders Research Center, Research Institute for Gastroenterology and Liver Diseases, Shahid Beheshti University of Medical Sciences, Tehran, Iran
[4]Department of Immunology, School of Medicine, Shahid Beheshti University of Medical Sciences, Tehran, Iran
[5]Department of Microbiology and Genetics, Kherad Institute of Higher Education, Bushehr, Iran
[6]Department of Art & Sciences, Faculty of Biology, University of North Florida, Jacksonville, Florida, USA

* **Corresponding authors:** Najmafarahani@gmail.com (N.F.); a.taheriazam@iautmu.ac.ir (A.T.); P.rahimzadeh76@gmail.com (P.R.); mentezari@iautmu.ac.ir (M.E.)

[7]Department of Biology, ET.C., Islamic Azad University, Tehran, Iran
[8]Department of Orthopedics, Faculty of Medicine, TeMs. C, Islamic Azad University, Tehran, Iran
[9]Surgical Research Society (SRS), Students' Scientific Research Center, Tehran University of Medical Sciences, Tehran, Iran

Abstract

CRISPR/Cas9, an RNA-guided endonuclease system derived from prokaryotic adaptive immunity, has rapidly evolved into a precise, programmable platform for editing, regulating, and interrogating mammalian genomes, with compelling implications for lung cancer therapy. By leveraging Cas9 and single-guide RNAs to induce site-specific double-strand breaks, the technology enables correction or disruption of oncogenic drivers, insertion of therapeutic sequences, and functional dissection of pathways underpinning tumorigenesis and drug resistance. In non-small-cell lung cancer, CRISPR/Cas9 has been deployed to model patient-relevant mutations (e.g., EGFR, KRAS, ALK), map resistance mechanisms to targeted agents, and uncover synthetic lethal interactions that inform rational drug combinations. Beyond gene knockout, nuclease-deactivated Cas9 effectors expand the toolkit to transcriptional modulation and epigenome editing, while emerging delivery strategies (viral and non-viral) are broadening translational feasibility. Despite these advances, challenges remain, including off-target edits, p53-dependent DNA damage responses, delivery barriers, and ethical and regulatory considerations. This article synthesizes current applications of CRISPR/Cas9 to lung cancer biology and treatment, outlines opportunities for overcoming therapy resistance, and highlights priority directions, high-fidelity editors, refined guide design, and clinically scalable delivery, for translating genome editing into durable, personalized interventions in lung cancer.

Keywords: lung neoplasms; CRISPR-Cas systems; CRISPR-associated protein 9; gene editing; precision medicine

1.1 Introduction

CRISPR-Cas9, which stands for Clustered Regularly Interspaced Short Palindromic Repeats and its associated proteins, represents a groundbreaking genome editing technology [1]. This biological defense mechanism, found predominantly in prokaryotic organisms (bacteria and archaea), serves as their natural immune system against viral invaders like bacteriophages [2]. As an RNA-guided endonuclease platform, it enables precise genetic modifications [3, 4] and holds significant potential in cancer treatment applications.

This innovative system enables scientists to address genetic mutations and introduce therapeutic genes at specific locations within human cells, potentially alleviating disease symptoms and rectifying genetic abnormalities. Its capabilities extend to investigating the molecular basis of blood-related cancers. The precision of CRISPR-Cas9 in gene editing makes it a promising therapeutic tool, particularly for diseases that have traditionally been challenging to treat [5]. The system functions through the coordination of two key components: the Cas9 endonuclease protein and single-guide RNA (sgRNA), which together enable precise genetic targeting and modification [1]. This mechanism has revolutionized genetic manipulation by allowing researchers to create specific DNA matches and perform controlled double-strand breaks [6].

Furthermore, CRISPR-Cas9 shows particular promise in addressing drug resistance issues in breast cancer treatment and is expected to play a crucial role in advancing personalized medicine approaches [7]. As a revolutionary method for modifying nucleic acids [8], ongoing refinements to this system may lead to enhanced therapeutic strategies for various genetic disorders affecting multiple body tissues [9].

The CRISPR-Cas9 system has transformed genetic research, making gene function studies more accessible while creating new therapeutic possibilities for various conditions, including cancer [10]. This groundbreaking approach provides researchers with an efficient and straightforward method for targeting specific DNA sequences [11]. The system's functionality relies on two crucial elements: the Cas9 enzyme, which performs the genetic cutting, and the sgRNA, which identifies and guides the system to the targeted genetic sequence [12].

Scientists have refined this technology to enable precise genetic regulation, modification, and editing, establishing it as the preferred method among researchers for addressing disease-causing mutations. This advancement has particularly enhanced the potential for clinical gene therapy applications [13].

The CRISPR-Cas9 system encompasses six distinct types (I through VI), with types IV–VI being more recent discoveries [14]. Each type exhibits unique characteristics in their immune responses, adaptation mechanisms, expression patterns, and interference methods. Type I systems utilize a complex arrangement of Cas9 proteins featuring both helicase and DNase capabilities, while Type III systems employ specialized repeat-associated mysterious proteins within the broader Cas9 family [14, 15].

These systems are further categorized into two classes based on their effector units. Class 1 encompasses Types I, III, and IV, characterized by multi-subunit effector complexes. Class 2, comprising Types II, V, and VI, features single-subunit effectors [14, 15]. Type II, which employs a single Cas9 protein for nuclease activity, has garnered particular attention in genome engineering applications [14, 16].

Thus, the objective of this chapter is to introduce CRISPR-Cas9 technology and describe current applications and future perspectives of the system with its mechanism of action on lung cancer therapy.

1.2 Molecular Basis of Lung Cancer Development

Lung cancer's molecular pathogenesis presents a complex and diverse landscape. The disease emerges through various genetic and epigenetic alterations, including point mutations, amplifications, insertions, deletions, and chromosomal translocations. These changes typically result in the enhancement of growth-promoting pathways while simultaneously suppressing tumor-inhibiting mechanisms [17]. Research has shown that non-small cell lung cancer (NSCLC) subtypes, specifically adenocarcinomas and squamous cell carcinomas, exhibit distinct molecular profiles despite their relative infrequency [18, 19].

The development of lung cancer can be understood as a gradual accumulation of genetic and epigenetic modifications within cellular nuclei over extended periods [20]. Cancer progression begins when cells escape normal regulatory controls governing division and positioning. While these cells maintain similar cycle patterns to healthy cells, they become unresponsive to regulatory signals and intercellular communication.

Neoplastic transformation is driven by a constellation of molecular and cellular alterations, including disrupted regulation of the cell cycle, genetic changes in proto-oncogenes and tumor suppressor genes, and impaired DNA repair mechanisms. These are compounded by increased production of growth factors and angiogenic signals, mutations in apoptotic pathways that confer resistance to programmed cell death, upregulated telomerase activity that enables replicative immortality, and an enhanced ability of cells to invade surrounding tissues and metastasize. Genomic instability, occurring early in carcinogenesis, plays a crucial role in disease progression. This instability results from the progressive accumulation of genetic abnormalities, leading to compromised DNA structural integrity and increased susceptibility to additional mutations [21, 22].

Cell cycle regulation abnormalities are fundamentally linked to mutations in both proto-oncogenes and tumor suppressor genes. Cancer development essentially involves either the loss of proliferation control or enhanced cell division, rendering cells unresponsive to growth-inhibiting signals. In lung cancer cells, the most frequently mutated tumor suppressor genes include TP53, RB, and p16 [23]. Similarly, the MYC, RAS, and HER gene families represent the most commonly altered proto-oncogenes, with ALK gene rearrangements also playing a significant role in lung cancer development [24].

Growth factors comprise a diverse group of peptide molecules produced by various cell types, influencing cellular proliferation, differentiation, metastatic potential, and programmed cell death. These factors interact with cell surface receptors, facilitating signal transmission from the external environment to the cell interior. In NSCLC, the epidermal growth factor (EGF) and its receptor (EGFR) are particularly crucial, with their dysfunction representing a key element in lung cancer pathogenesis [25].

Blood vessel formation plays a vital role in both healthy and diseased tissues. While normal angiogenesis is self-limiting, pathological blood vessel formation is characterized by prolonged endothelial cell division and extended cell survival. Vascular endothelial growth factor (VEGF) stands as one of the most potent pro-angiogenic factors. In cancerous growths, continuous VEGF pathway activation and the dominance of pro-angiogenic over anti-angiogenic factors facilitate tumor expansion. Notably, tumors exceeding 3 mm in diameter require their own blood supply network to sustain growth [26].

The development of a tumor's own blood supply represents a critical milestone in cancer progression. VEGF mRNA is detected in most cancer cells, including those in lung cancer. Notably, endothelial cells exhibit higher VEGFR expression compared to VEGF itself, suggesting a paracrine mechanism where VEGF secreted by cancer cells activates receptors on endothelial cells. Research has shown that VEGF concentrates within 0.5 mm of tumor boundaries [26]. The resulting tumor vasculature is characterized by irregular arrangement, inconsistent diameter, and structural fragility, potentially leading to hemoptysis — a clinical symptom that should alert physicians to possible malignancy.

In lung cancer pathogenesis, diminished cellular apoptotic response to environmental signals plays a crucial role. Apoptosis, or programmed cell death, is fundamental to maintaining bodily homeostasis.

Lung cancer development requires the accumulation of multiple genetic alterations. Recent advances in molecular biology have enabled deeper understanding of cancer-related genomic changes. The p53 gene mutations play a central role in carcinogenesis, and when combined with alterations in other genes (Rb, MYC, RAS, EGFR), significantly increase the likelihood of neoplastic transformation.

In clinical settings, identifying specific genetic abnormalities serves as molecular predictive factors, enabling more targeted and effective cancer treatments with improved prognosis. While comprehensive predictive testing using all known markers is not yet standard practice, certain markers have become crucial in lung cancer diagnostics and treatment protocols. These include EGFR mutation profiling for EGFR tyrosine kinase inhibitor targeted therapy qualification and ALK gene rearrangement testing for ALK inhibitor therapy.

The scientific community anticipates that ongoing advances in molecular diagnostics may soon enable early, non-invasive lung cancer detection, potentially improving treatment outcomes through earlier intervention.

1.3 Mechanism of CRISPR/Cas9 and its Application in Lung Cancer

Genome editing using CRISPR-Cas9 can be implemented through several distinct approaches. The primary and most straightforward method utilizes a plasmid-based system that encodes both the Cas9 protein and sgRNA within a single vector, eliminating the need for multiple component transfections. In this approach, the vector expresses both elements, which then form the sgRNA-Cas9 complex inside cells to modify targeted genomic sequences [9, 12, 15]. Alternative methods include the combination of Cas9 mRNA with sgRNA, where the complex forms after cellular translation of Cas9 mRNA to protein, or the direct cellular delivery of pre-assembled sgRNA-Cas9 complexes [15].

The system operates through two primary components working in concert [16]. The first component, sgRNA, comprises crRNA (CRISPR RNA), which identifies and targets specific DNA sequences for modification, and tracrRNA (trans-activating CRISPR RNA), which recruits the second component — the Cas9 endonuclease protein. This protein creates site-specific double-strand DNA breaks (DSB) [12]. The bacterial type II CRISPR-Cas9 system has become preferred for RNA-guided nuclease engineering due to its efficiency and simplicity [15], though it requires proto-spacer adjacent motif sequences.

The DNA cleavage process involves two distinct Cas9 domains: the HNH domain (named for its characteristic histidine and asparagine residues) cuts the complementary strand, while the RuvC-like domain (named after an *E. coli* DNA repair protein) cleaves the non-complementary strand [14]. Following cleavage, cellular DNA repair mechanisms introduce various genetic modifications, including substitutions, deletions, and insertions, through either non-homologous end joining (NHEJ) or homologous-dependent repair (HDR) pathways [12, 13, 15].

Research confirms that the sgRNA-Cas9 complex functions by scanning and binding to specific genomic sequences through complementary base-pairing. After identifying the protospacer adjacent motif sequence near the target, it precisely cuts the double-stranded DNA. This break triggers either NHEJ or HDR repair pathways. In cases where no homologous repair template is available, NHEJ creates random insertions or deletions (indels), disrupting the target sequence through its error-prone repair mechanism [27, 28].

Based on GLOBOCAN 2020 estimates, lung cancer accounted for approximately 2.2 million newly diagnosed cases worldwide in 2020, corresponding to an age-standardized incidence rate of 22.4 per 100,000 population. In the same year, the disease was responsible for nearly 1.8 million deaths globally, with an age-standardized mortality rate of 18.0 per 100,000 [68]. While initial treatments relied on surgery and radiation, therapy later evolved to include selective tyrosine kinase inhibitors such as gefitinib and erlotinib, which target EGFR's tyrosine kinase activity. However, these treatments faced challenges including technical limitations and non-specific toxicity [29, 30]. The EGFR membrane glycoprotein consists of extracellular ligand-binding, transmembrane, and intracellular tyrosine kinase domains. Ligand activation triggers intracellular kinase activity, promoting cell proliferation, blood vessel formation, invasion, metastasis, reduced cell death, and enhanced glycolysis. Unfortunately, drug resistance has emerged as a significant challenge to these treatments [30, 31].

CRISPR-Cas9 represents a revolutionary biotechnology advancement in lung cancer treatment [2]. The system operates through two mechanisms. The primary approach involves designing sgRNA targeting mutated EGFR sequences, followed by Cas9 protein activity. Researchers developed CRISPR systems with sequences complementary to mutated EGFR for patient treatment. When these complementary sequences bind to mutated EGFR, the Cas9 endonuclease creates DNA breaks (either single- or double-stranded, depending on the enzyme variant), which are then addressed by cellular DNA repair mechanisms [30].

Restricting receptor mutation prevents ligand activator binding, thereby inhibiting cell proliferation, new blood vessel formation, and cancer spread. CRISPR-Cas9-mediated EGFR inhibition enhances major histocompatibility complex class I expression, leading to improved tumor cell recognition and destruction by cytotoxic lymphocytes [29]. However, off-target effects present significant challenges, potentially causing genomic instability, gene dysfunction, and epigenetic modifications. These effects, particularly crucial in therapeutic applications, can be categorized into off-target binding and cleavage. While Cas9 can bind to partially complementary sequences without cleaving them [4], several strategies can minimize these effects, including using *in vitro* assembled sgRNA with sustained Cas9 association or employing modified Cas9 variants that create single-strand nicks [27].

The second major therapeutic approach involves modifying immune cells, particularly lymphocytes. In Chinese clinical trials, researchers extracted T cells from patients' blood and used CRISPR-Cas9 to eliminate the PD-1 protein-encoding gene. These modified cells were then cultivated in laboratory conditions before reintroduction into patients [2]. The process involves treating extracted lymphocytes with CRISPR-Cas9 systems containing sgRNA matching the PD-1 protein sequence. Following DNA cleavage and cellular repair, PD-1 gene expression is blocked, preventing cancerous cells from interacting with immune lymphocyte receptors [2].

This reduced interaction between cancer ligands and receptors enables T cell receptors to better identify and target problematic cells. Before reintroduction, modified lymphocytes undergo screening for viability and proliferation capacity to exclude potential mutations [2]. Additionally, PD-1 protein elimination on immune cells facilitates caspase activation, promoting programmed cell death in cancer cells [32].

Research demonstrates that T cells lacking PD-1 exhibit enhanced antitumor cytotoxic activity. However, this approach faces challenges, particularly the heightened activity of modified T cells, along with concerns regarding safe and effective delivery methods and potential side effects.

A phase I clinical trial evaluated the safety of CRISPR-Cas9-mediated PD-1 gene knockout therapy in advanced NSCLC patients showing positive PD-1 expression. The trial included nine enrolled patients, with eight receiving PD-1-deficient T cell treatment (**Table 1.1**). Despite initial concerns, patients receiving the modified T cell therapy showed promising tolerance to the treatment. Researchers recommended expanding the studies to determine optimal dosing protocols and better understand the immune response patterns.

1.4 Targeting Oncogenes with CRISPR/Cas9 in Lung Cancer

Oncogenes disrupt normal cellular regulation, leading to malignant transformation and uncontrolled growth in eukaryotic cells. The concept of oncogene addiction, where cancer cells depend on single oncogenes for survival, provides the theoretical foundation for CRISPR/Cas9 applications in cancer treatment [33]. The technology's precise DNA sequence recognition capabilities have enabled specific targeting of overexpressed or hyperactivated genes [34].

Recent lung cancer research has focused on CRISPR/Cas9 editing of several oncogenes, including EGFR, FAK, NESTIN, RSF1, CTNND2, and IGF1R [35–42]. These genes, through mutation or overexpression, promote lung cancer development and enhance metastatic potential.

Recent experimental studies have elucidated key genetic targets influencing lung cancer progression and therapeutic response. Knockout of the EGFR mutant allele markedly inhibited

Table 1.1 CRISPR-Cas9 therapeutic applications.

CRISPR/Cas Method	Components	Mechanism(s) of Action	Target	Reference
Plasmid-based system	Cas9 protein + sgRNA encoded on same vector	Forms sgRNA-Cas9 complex within cells to edit genomic sequences	EGFR mutations	[15]
Cas9 mRNA + sgRNA	Cas9 mRNA + synthetic sgRNA	Cas9 mRNA translated to protein, forms complex with sgRNA	Various genomic targets	[15]
Pre-assembled complex	*In vitro* assembled sgRNA-Cas9 complex	Direct delivery of functional complex	Various genomic targets	[15]
EGFR targeting	Custom sgRNA + Cas9 protein	Targets mutated EGFR sequences, creates DSBs	EGFR oncogene	[30]
PD-1 knockout in T-cells	sgRNA targeting PD-1 + Cas9	Knocks out PD-1 gene in patient T-cells	PD-1 protein on lymphocytes	[32]
DNA repair mechanisms	NHEJ pathway	Error-prone repair creating indels	DSB sites	[15]
DNA repair mechanisms	HDR pathway	Homology-directed precise repair	DSB sites	[12]
Off-target reduction	Modified Cas9 variants	Single-strand nicking instead of DSBs	Non-specific sites	[27]

proliferation across multiple NSCLC cell lines (H1975, A549, H1650) and led to substantial tumor volume reduction in xenograft models (81.5% and 78.3% compared to controls) [37]. Disruption of the FAK gene in KRAS-mutant cells heightened DNA damage and sensitized tumors to radiation [41]. Silencing NESTIN in A549 and H1299 cells promoted apoptosis and suppressed proliferation and invasion by impeding epithelial-to-mesenchymal transition [40]. RSF1 deletion in H460 and H1299 cells triggered G1-phase arrest, enhanced apoptotic activity, and reduced cellular motility [36]. CTNND2 knockout depleted δ-catenin, thereby diminishing tumorigenic and metastatic potential via Wnt pathway inhibition [43]. Furthermore, IGF1R deletion in HCC827 cells modulated mesenchymal markers and contributed to erlotinib resistance through MET amplification [38]. These findings suggest CRISPR/Cas9-mediated oncogene editing shows promise as a potential lung cancer treatment strategy.

1.5 Restoring Tumor Suppressor Functions

Inactivation of tumor suppressor genes plays a pivotal role in cancer initiation and progression [44, 45]. These genes typically encode proteins that regulate cell proliferation, promote differentiation, restrict cellular migration, and suppress tumorigenesis [46]. Loss of function via mutation, deletion, or epigenetic silencing can lead to oncogene activation and malignant transformation. Numerous cancers exhibit reduced expression or mutational inactivation of tumor-suppressor genes [47], positioning them as strategic targets for CRISPR/Cas9-based therapeutic interventions.

CRISPR/Cas9 technology holds promise for restoring tumor-suppressor gene function and curbing cancer development. In lung cancer models, several key findings underscore this potential. Keap1 knockout in Kras-driven lung adenocarcinoma mice led to Nrf2 hyperactivation and accelerated tumor growth [48]. Deletion of mitofusin 2 in A549 cells enhanced cell survival, proliferation, colony formation, invasion, and metastatic capacity through upregulation of the mTORC2/Akt signaling axis [47]. Similarly, knockout of the tumor-suppressor miR-1304 increased heme oxygenase-1 expression, promoting cell viability and growth [49].

1.6 CRISPR/Cas9 in Overcoming Chemoresistance in Lung Cancer

Chemotherapy remains a cornerstone of systemic cancer treatment, employed either as a standalone modality or in combination with surgery and radiotherapy to suppress tumor growth, prevent metastasis, and induce cancer cell death. Despite its widespread use, the emergence of drug resistance poses a significant challenge, often resulting in suboptimal therapeutic outcomes and disease progression. Targeting drug resistance pathways through gene editing offers a promising strategy to enhance tumor cell responsiveness to chemotherapeutic agents [7].

Recent CRISPR/Cas9-based investigations have focused on modulating genes that influence sensitivity to key lung cancer chemotherapeutics, including cisplatin, carboplatin, and paclitaxel. Notably, RSF1 gene knockout combined with paclitaxel treatment in H460 and H1299 cells induced G1-phase cell-cycle arrest, increased apoptosis, and suppressed migration and proliferation. *In vivo*, RSF1 deletion significantly improved paclitaxel efficacy, reducing tumor weight ($P < 0.01$) and volume ($P < 0.05$) in H460 xenografts [36].

Additional findings reinforce the therapeutic potential of gene editing. ERCC1 knockout heightened cisplatin sensitivity in lung cancer cell lines [50]. NRF2 deletion in A549 cells markedly increased responsiveness to cisplatin (tumor volume: 130 mm^3 vs. 660 mm^3) and carboplatin (200 mm^3 vs. 660 mm^3) [51]. Furthermore, Aurora B knockout restored TP53 expression and enhanced sensitivity to both cisplatin and paclitaxel in NSCLC models [52].

1.7 CRISPR/Cas9 in Association with Other Therapeutic or Diagnostic Aspects of Lung Cancer

1.7.1. *CRISPR/Cas9 and Immunotherapy*

CRISPR/Cas9 technology has revolutionized the genetic modification of T cells in cancer immunotherapy, particularly through CAR-T cell therapy [53]. This innovative approach involves extracting patients' T cells, genetically altering them to target cancer cells, and enhancing the antitumor characteristics within the tumor microenvironment.

A significant milestone occurred in June 2016 when the USA's National Institutes of Health sanctioned the first CRISPR/Cas9 CAR-T cell therapy clinical trial. This groundbreaking study involved genetically engineered T cells being reintroduced into cancer patients to specifically eliminate tumor cells [54]. Later that year, Chinese researchers achieved another breakthrough by conducting the first human CRISPR/Cas9 trial, where they disabled the PD1 (PDCD1) gene in T cells [55].

The PD-1 protein typically inhibits immune responses, a mechanism that cancer cells exploit for unrestricted growth and metastasis. The modified T cells, after laboratory expansion, were infused back into patients' bloodstreams to restore immune system balance and combat cancer. Research has demonstrated that cancer cells can evade immune detection through PD-1/PD-L1 interactions. Studies in mice showed that CRISPR/Cas9-mediated disruption of the PD-L1 3′-UTR allowed EG7-OVA cancer cells to escape immune surveillance by increasing PD-L1 expression. This finding suggests that PD-L1 3′-UTR disruption could serve as a biomarker for identifying cancers that actively evade immune responses through PD-L1 overexpression [56].

While CRISPR/Cas9-based immunomodulation has shown promise in cancer treatment research, including lung cancer, clinical studies specifically focusing on lung cancer immunotherapy using this gene editing technology remain scarce, despite several clinical trials being conducted.

1.7.2. *CRISPR/Cas9 in miRNA Detection*

MicroRNAs (miRNAs) play crucial roles in disease processes and show promise as cancer biomarkers. However, current miRNA detection methods face challenges due to their intricate nature, expensive procedures, and limited sensitivity, necessitating improved detection techniques.

Researchers have developed an innovative detection platform that combines three key technologies: isothermal amplification based on rolling circle amplification, CRISPR/Cas9, and split horseradish peroxidase techniques [57]. This integrated approach enables highly sensitive miRNA detection with single-nucleotide precision. The system has demonstrated particular success in detecting specific miRNAs, such as let-7a, in clinical serum samples, effectively distinguishing NSCLC patients from healthy individuals. The study revealed a statistically significant reduction in let-7a levels among NSCLC patients compared to healthy controls ($P = 0.0004$) [57]. This groundbreaking application of CRISPR/Cas9 technology for miRNA detection represents a promising advancement in lung cancer screening, diagnosis, and prognosis. The method's ability to detect early-stage cancer markers could potentially improve the timing and effectiveness of lung cancer treatment interventions.

1.7.3. *CRISPR/Cas9 Barcoding*

Tumor cells' inherent genetic diversity drives their evolution and environmental adaptability. A novel approach combining CRISPR/Cas9 technology with specific DNA barcodes, a system traditionally used for species identification through standardized DNA segments, enables researchers to monitor and analyze specific cancer cell populations carrying mutations of interest [58]. This innovative methodology has proven valuable in studying resistance mechanisms to EGFR inhibitors in lung cancer cells and assessing the effectiveness of combination therapies [59]. The CRISPR barcoding technique facilitates straightforward comparisons of different mutations' effects within heterogeneous cell populations.

This rapid and adaptable approach enables researchers to examine various genomic modifications across multiple functional assays. It successfully replicates the interactions between genetically distinct cancer cells, both with and without therapeutic intervention, creating a more accurate model of treatment response dynamics. The technique's capability to simultaneously correct mutations in oncogenic driver genes while tracking thousands of gene markers in cancer cells represents a significant advancement [59].

The implementation of CRISPR barcoding enhances functional analysis of specific mutations, marking a promising development in lung cancer treatment research. This approach is expected to significantly contribute to advancing therapeutic strategies in lung cancer.

1.7.4. *Allele Frequency and Mutation Rate Detection*

Researchers have developed an innovative small-allele enrichment technique utilizing deactivated Cas9 (dCas9), which capitalizes on the CRISPR/Cas9 system's precise single-base pair targeting and versatility. This method has proven particularly effective in detecting the three most prevalent EGFR mutations in NSCLC: exon 19 deletion, T790M, and L858R [60].

The dCas9 technique demonstrates superior performance compared to traditional qPCR methods in determining both allele frequency and mutation rate. Notably, in an analysis of cell-free DNA from NSCLC patients, the dCas9 method detected over 60% more mutations than qPCR [60].

This application of CRISPR/Cas9 technology represents a significant advancement in genomic editing, substantially improving the diagnostic capabilities of cell-free DNA analysis. The enhanced detection efficiency offered by this method has important implications for targeted lung cancer therapy, potentially leading to more accurate and effective treatment strategies.

Collectively in **Figure 1.1**, the relationship between CRISPR/Cas9 technology and other common diagnostic and therapeutic aspects of lung cancer are summarily illustrated.

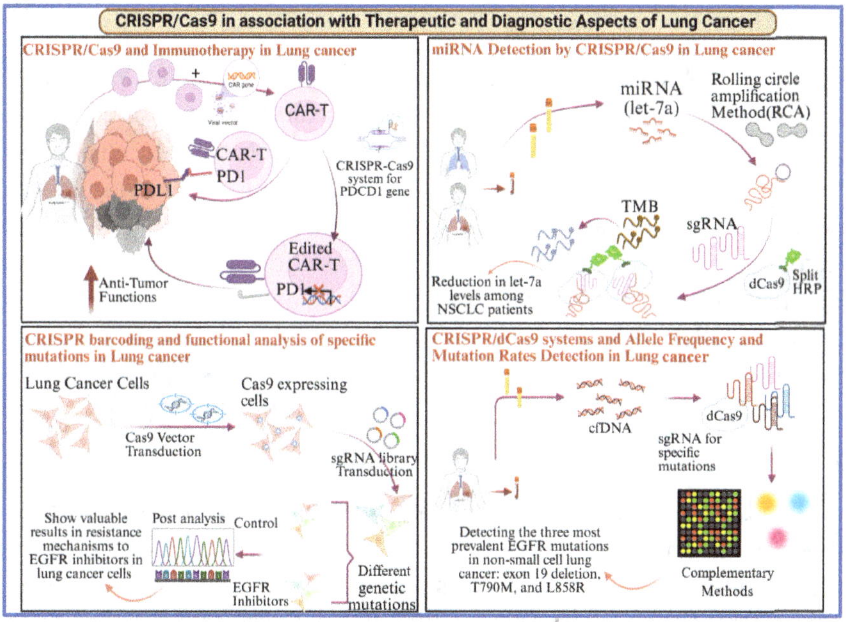

Figure 1.1 Applications of CRISPR/Cas9 systems in the therapeutic and diagnostic landscape of lung cancer. The diverse roles of CRISPR/Cas9 technologies in lung cancer intervention, encompassing immunotherapy, biomarker detection, functional genetic profiling, and mutation analysis are illustrated here. **Top left:** CRISPR/Cas9-mediated editing of T-cell PDCD1 (encoding PD-1) enhances CAR-T cell therapy by disrupting PD-1 expression, thereby improving anti-tumor immune responses in the lung tumor microenvironment. **Top right**: detection of miRNAs, such as let-7a, in lung cancer is achieved via CRISPR/Cas9-based approaches incorporating rolling circle amplification and dCas9-sgRNA complexes, enabling precise and sensitive measurement of circulating biomarkers for NSCLC. **Bottom left**: CRISPR barcode and sgRNA libraries allow high-throughput functional analysis of specific genetic mutations in lung cancer cells, aiding in elucidation of resistance mechanisms to EGFR inhibitors and informing targeted therapy design. **Bottom right**: CRISPR/dCas9 systems facilitate detection of allele frequency and mutation rates through the analysis of circulating free DNA (cfDNA), enabling identification of prevalent EGFR mutations (exon 19 deletion, T790M, L858R) in NSCLC. Complementary high-throughput methods enhance mutation mapping and precision diagnostics.

1.8 Future Perspectives

CRISPR-Cas9 technology marks a paradigm shift in cancer biology [5], distinguished by its precision, adaptability, and operational simplicity [61, 62]. By enabling targeted genomic modifications in cancer cells—a feat previously limited by technical constraints, this system opens new avenues for therapeutic intervention [63–65]. Its exceptional versatility and efficiency position CRISPR-Cas9 as a potentially transformative platform for next-generation cancer treatments [66, 67], with the capacity to redefine molecular oncology [63].

1.9 Conclusion

CRISPR/Cas9 has transformed lung cancer research from descriptive genetics to actionable genome engineering, enabling precise manipulation of disease drivers and systematic discovery of vulnerabilities that underlie treatment failure. Evidence across cellular and animal models shows that CRISPR-enabled interrogation of EGFR-, KRAS-, and ALK-centric networks can elucidate and reverse resistance phenotypes, laying the groundwork for combination strategies and allele-selective interventions. Realizing clinical impact will depend on continued gains in editing fidelity, comprehensive off-target surveillance, and safe, tumor-directed delivery vehicles compatible with pulmonary biology. As high-precision editors (including base and prime editors) and non-viral delivery platforms mature, CRISPR/Cas9 is poised to complement targeted therapy and immunotherapy, advancing a more personalized, mechanism-driven era of lung cancer treatment.

References

1. Yin H, Song CQ, Dorkin JR, Zhu LJ, Li Y, Wu Q, et al. Therapeutic genome editing by combined viral and non-viral delivery of CRISPR system components in vivo. Nat Biotechnol. 2016;34(3):328–33.
2. Castillo A. Gene editing using CRISPR-Cas9 for the treatment of lung cancer. Colomb Med (Cali). 2016;47(4):178–80.

3. Platt RJ, Chen S, Zhou Y, Yim MJ, Swiech L, Kempton HR, et al. CRISPR-Cas9 knockin mice for genome editing and cancer modeling. Cell. 2014;159(2):440–55.
4. Wen WS, Yuan ZM, Ma SJ, Xu J, Yuan DT. CRISPR-Cas9 systems: versatile cancer modelling platforms and promising therapeutic strategies. Int J Cancer. 2016;138(6):1328–36.
5. Bhattacharjee R, Das Purkayastha K, Adapa D, Choudhury A. CRISPR/Cas9 genome editing system in the diagnosis and treatment of cancer. Journal of RNAi & Gene Silencing. 2017;13(1):585–91.
6. Gwiazda KS, Grier AE, Sahni J, Burleigh SM, Martin U, Yang JG, et al. High Efficiency CRISPR/Cas9-mediated Gene Editing in Primary Human T-cells Using Mutant Adenoviral E4orf6/E1b55k "Helper" Proteins. Mol Ther. 2016;24(9):1570–80.
7. Chen Y, Zhang Y. Application of the CRISPR/Cas9 System to Drug Resistance in Breast Cancer. Adv Sci (Weinh). 2018;5(6):1700964.
8. Wang T, Wei JJ, Sabatini DM, Lander ES. Genetic screens in human cells using the CRISPR-Cas9 system. Science. 2014;343(6166):80–4.
9. Ran FA, Cong L, Yan WX, Scott DA, Gootenberg JS, Kriz AJ, et al. In vivo genome editing using Staphylococcus aureus Cas9. Nature. 2015;520(7546):186–91.
10. Gori JL, Hsu PD, Maeder ML, Shen S, Welstead GG, Bumcrot D. Delivery and Specificity of CRISPR-Cas9 Genome Editing Technologies for Human Gene Therapy. Hum Gene Ther. 2015;26(7):443–51.
11. Shinmyo Y, Tanaka S, Tsunoda S, Hosomichi K, Tajima A, Kawasaki H. CRISPR/Cas9-mediated gene knockout in the mouse brain using in utero electroporation. Sci Rep. 2016;6:20611.
12. Ratan ZA, Son YJ, Haidere MF, Uddin BMM, Yusuf MA, Zaman SB, et al. CRISPR-Cas9: a promising genetic engineering approach in cancer research. Ther Adv Med Oncol. 2018;10:1758834018755089.
13. Jamal M, Ullah A, Ahsan M, Tyagi R, Habib Z, Khan FA, Rehman K. Treating Genetic Disorders Using State-Of-The-Art Technology. Curr Issues Mol Biol. 2018;26:33–46.
14. Kim EJ, Kang KH, Ju JH. CRISPR-Cas9: a promising tool for gene editing on induced pluripotent stem cells. Korean J Intern Med. 2017;32(1):42–61.
15. Liu C, Zhang L, Liu H, Cheng K. Delivery strategies of the CRISPR-Cas9 gene-editing system for therapeutic applications. J Control Release. 2017;266:17–26.

16. Sánchez-Rivera FJ, Jacks T. Applications of the CRISPR-Cas9 system in cancer biology. Nat Rev Cancer. 2015;15(7):387–95.
17. Cooper WA, Lam DC, O'Toole SA, Minna JD. Molecular biology of lung cancer. J Thorac Dis. 2013;5 Suppl 5(Suppl 5):S479–90.
18. Boolell V, Alamgeer M, Watkins DN, Ganju V. The Evolution of Therapies in Non-Small Cell Lung Cancer. Cancers (Basel). 2015;7(3):1815–46.
19. Roh MS. Molecular pathology of lung cancer: current status and future directions. Tuberc Respir Dis (Seoul). 2014;77(2):49–54.
20. Massion PP, Carbone DP. The molecular basis of lung cancer: molecular abnormalities and therapeutic implications. Respir Res. 2003;4(1):12.
21. Dakal TC, Dhabhai B, Pant A, Moar K, Chaudhary K, Yadav V, et al. Oncogenes and tumor suppressor genes: functions and roles in cancers. MedComm (2020). 2024;5(6):e582.
22. Ferguson LR, Chen H, Collins AR, Connell M, Damia G, Dasgupta S, et al. Genomic instability in human cancer: Molecular insights and opportunities for therapeutic attack and prevention through diet and nutrition. Semin Cancer Biol. 2015;35 Suppl(Suppl):S5-S24.
23. Chen T, Ashwood LM, Kondrashova O, Strasser A, Kelly G, Sutherland KD. Breathing new insights into the role of mutant p53 in lung cancer. Oncogene. 2025;44(3):115–29.
24. Kontomanolis EN, Koutras A, Syllaios A, Schizas D, Mastoraki A, Garmpis N, et al. Role of Oncogenes and Tumor-suppressor Genes in Carcinogenesis: A Review. Anticancer Res. 2020;40(11):6009–15.
25. Takahashi T, Sakai K, Kenmotsu H, Yoh K, Daga H, Ohira T, et al. Predictive value of EGFR mutation in non-small-cell lung cancer patients treated with platinum doublet postoperative chemotherapy. Cancer Sci. 2022;113(1):287–96.
26. Apte RS, Chen DS, Ferrara N. VEGF in Signaling and Disease: Beyond Discovery and Development. Cell. 2019;176(6):1248–64.
27. Martinez-Lage M, Puig-Serra P, Menendez P, Torres-Ruiz R, Rodriguez-Perales S. CRISPR/Cas9 for Cancer Therapy: Hopes and Challenges. Biomedicines. 2018;6(4):105.
28. Pandey VK, Tripathi A, Bhushan R, Ali A, Dubey PK, Therapy G. Application of CRISPR/Cas9 genome editing in genetic disorders: a systematic review up to date. J Genet Syndr Gene Ther. 2017; 8(2):1–10.

29. Lizotte PH, Hong RL, Luster TA, Cavanaugh ME, Taus LJ, Wang S, et al. A High-Throughput Immune-Oncology Screen Identifies EGFR Inhibitors as Potent Enhancers of Antigen-Specific Cytotoxic T-lymphocyte Tumor Cell Killing. Cancer Immunol Res. 2018;6(12):1511–23.
30. Tang H, Shrager JB. CRISPR/Cas-mediated genome editing to treat EGFR-mutant lung cancer: a personalized molecular surgical therapy. EMBO Mol Med. 2016;8(2):83–5.
31. Jiang C, Lin X, Zhao Z. Applications of CRISPR/Cas9 Technology in the Treatment of Lung Cancer. Trends Mol Med. 2019;25(11):1039–49.
32. Zhao Z, Shi L, Zhang W, Han J, Zhang S, Fu Z, Cai J. CRISPR knock out of programmed cell death protein 1 enhances anti-tumor activity of cytotoxic T lymphocytes. Oncotarget. 2018;9(4):5208–15.
33. White MK, Khalili K. CRISPR/Cas9 and cancer targets: future possibilities and present challenges. Oncotarget. 2016;7(11):12305–17.
34. Gilbert LA, Larson MH, Morsut L, Liu Z, Brar GA, Torres SE, et al. CRISPR-mediated modular RNA-guided regulation of transcription in eukaryotes. Cell. 2013;154(2):442–51.
35. Bu X, Kato J, Hong JA, Merino MJ, Schrump DS, Lund FE, Moss J. CD38 knockout suppresses tumorigenesis in mice and clonogenic growth of human lung cancer cells. Carcinogenesis. 2018;39(2):242–51.
36. Chen X, Sun X, Guan J, Gai J, Xing J, Fu L, et al. Rsf-1 Influences the Sensitivity of Non-Small Cell Lung Cancer to Paclitaxel by Regulating NF-κB Pathway and Its Downstream Proteins. Cell Physiol Biochem. 2017;44(6):2322–36.
37. Cheung AH, Chow C, Zhang J, Zhou Y, Huang T, Ng KC, et al. Specific targeting of point mutations in EGFR L858R-positive lung cancer by CRISPR/Cas9. Lab Invest. 2018;98(7):968–76.
38. Hussmann D, Madsen AT, Jakobsen KR, Luo Y, Sorensen BS, Nielsen AL. IGF1R depletion facilitates MET-amplification as mechanism of acquired resistance to erlotinib in HCC827 NSCLC cells. Oncotarget. 2017;8(20):33300–15.
39. Koo T, Yoon AR, Cho HY, Bae S, Yun CO, Kim JS. Selective disruption of an oncogenic mutant allele by CRISPR/Cas9 induces efficient tumor regression. Nucleic Acids Res. 2017;45(13):7897–908.
40. Liu F, Zhang Y, Lu M, Wang C, Li Q, Gao Y, et al. Nestin servers as a promising prognostic biomarker in non-small cell lung cancer. Am J Transl Res. 2017;9(3):1392–401.

41. Tang KJ, Constanzo JD, Venkateswaran N, Melegari M, Ilcheva M, Morales JC, et al. Focal Adhesion Kinase Regulates the DNA Damage Response and Its Inhibition Radiosensitizes Mutant KRAS Lung Cancer. Clin Cancer Res. 2016;22(23):5851–63.
42. Yi J, Wei X, Li X, Wan L, Dong J, Wang R. A genome-wide comprehensive analysis of alterations in driver genes in non-small-cell lung cancer. Anticancer Drugs. 2018;29(1):10–8.
43. Huang F, Chen J, Wang Z, Lan R, Fu L, Zhang L. δ-Catenin promotes tumorigenesis and metastasis of lung adenocarcinoma. Oncol Rep. 2018;39(2):809–17.
44. Chen ML, Chang JH, Yeh KT, Chang YS, Chang JG. Epigenetic changes in tumor suppressor genes, P15, P16, APC-3 and E-cadherin in body fluid. Kaohsiung J Med Sci. 2007;23(10):498–503.
45. Solomon H, Brosh R, Buganim Y, Rotter V. Inactivation of the p53 tumor suppressor gene and activation of the Ras oncogene: cooperative events in tumorigenesis. Discov Med. 2010;9(48):448–54.
46. Sun H, Huang D, Liu G, Jian F, Zhu J, Zhang L. SIRT4 acts as a tumor suppressor in gastric cancer by inhibiting cell proliferation, migration, and invasion. Onco Targets Ther. 2018;11:3959–68.
47. Xu K, Chen G, Li X, Wu X, Chang Z, Xu J, et al. MFN2 suppresses cancer progression through inhibition of mTORC2/Akt signaling. Sci Rep. 2017;7:41718.
48. Romero R, Sayin VI, Davidson SM, Bauer MR, Singh SX, LeBoeuf SE, et al. Keap1 loss promotes Kras-driven lung cancer and results in dependence on glutaminolysis. Nat Med. 2017;23(11):1362–8.
49. Li CG, Pu MF, Li CZ, Gao M, Liu MX, Yu CZ, et al. MicroRNA-1304 suppresses human non-small cell lung cancer cell growth in vitro by targeting heme oxygenase-1. Acta Pharmacol Sin. 2017;38(1):110–9.
50. Heyza JR, Lei W, Watza D, Zhang H, Chen W, Back JB, et al. Identification and Characterization of Synthetic Viability with ERCC1 Deficiency in Response to Interstrand Crosslinks in Lung Cancer. Clin Cancer Res. 2019;25(8):2523–36.
51. Bialk P, Wang Y, Banas K, Kmiec EB. Functional Gene Knockout of NRF2 Increases Chemosensitivity of Human Lung Cancer A549 Cells In Vitro and in a Xenograft Mouse Model. Mol Ther Oncolytics. 2018;11:75–89.
52. Yu J, Zhou J, Xu F, Bai W, Zhang W. High expression of Aurora-B is correlated with poor prognosis and drug resistance in non-small cell lung cancer. Int J Biol Markers. 2018;33(2):215–21.
53. Wu HY, Cao CY. The application of CRISPR-Cas9 genome editing tool in cancer immunotherapy. Brief Funct Genomics. 2019;18(2):129–32.

54. Zhan T, Rindtorff N, Betge J, Ebert MP, Boutros M. CRISPR/Cas9 for cancer research and therapy. Semin Cancer Biol. 2019;55:106–19.
55. Cyranoski D. Chinese scientists to pioneer first human CRISPR trial. Nature. 2016;535(7613):476–7.
56. Kataoka K, Shiraishi Y, Takeda Y, Sakata S, Matsumoto M, Nagano S, et al. Aberrant PD-L1 expression through 3′-UTR disruption in multiple cancers. Nature. 2016;534(7607):402–6.
57. Qiu XY, Zhu LY, Zhu CS, Ma JX, Hou T, Wu XM, et al. Highly Effective and Low-Cost MicroRNA Detection with CRISPR-Cas9. ACS Synth Biol. 2018;7(3):807–13.
58. Liu F, Zhang X, Yang Y. Simulation of CRISPR-Cas9 editing on evolving barcode and accuracy of lineage tracing. Sci Rep. 2024;14(1):19213.
59. Guernet A, Mungamuri SK, Cartier D, Sachidanandam R, Jayaprakash A, Adriouch S, et al. CRISPR-Barcoding for Intratumor Genetic Heterogeneity Modeling and Functional Analysis of Oncogenic Driver Mutations. Mol Cell. 2016;63(3):526–38.
60. Aalipour A, Dudley JC, Park SM, Murty S, Chabon JJ, Boyle EA, et al. Deactivated CRISPR Associated Protein 9 for Minor-Allele Enrichment in Cell-Free DNA. Clin Chem. 2018;64(2):307–16.
61. Lu Y, Xue J, Deng T, Zhou X, Yu K, Deng L, et al. Safety and feasibility of CRISPR-edited T cells in patients with refractory non-small-cell lung cancer. Nat Med. 2020;26(5):732–40.
62. Zhang B. CRISPR/Cas gene therapy. J Cell Physiol. 2021;236(4):2459–81.
63. Li H, Yang Y, Hong W, Huang M, Wu M, Zhao X. Applications of genome editing technology in the targeted therapy of human diseases: mechanisms, advances and prospects. Signal Transduct Target Ther. 2020;5(1):1.
64. Ma CC, Wang ZL, Xu T, He ZY, Wei YQ. The approved gene therapy drugs worldwide: from 1998 to 2019. Biotechnol Adv. 2020;40:107502.
65. Xu M, Weng Q, Ji J. Applications and advances of CRISPR/Cas9 in animal cancer model. Brief Funct Genomics. 2020;19(3):235–41.
66. Hanna RE, Doench JG. Design and analysis of CRISPR-Cas experiments. Nat Biotechnol. 2020;38(7):813–23.
67. Hong W, Huang M, Wei Y, Wei X. A new and promising application of gene editing: CRISPR-controlled smart materials for tissue engineering, bioelectronics, and diagnostics. Sci China Life Sci. 2019;62(11):1547–9.
68. Li C, Lei S, Ding L, Xu Y, Wu X, Wang H, Zhang Z, Gao T, Zhang Y, Li L. Global burden and trends of lung cancer incidence and mortality. Chin Med J (Engl). 2023;136(13):1583–90.

https://doi.org/10.1142/9789819826759_0002

CHAPTER 2

CRISPR/Cas9 in the Treatment of Breast Cancer

Mehrdad Hashemi[1,2], *Alireza Khosravinejad*[1,3], *Mina Alimohammadi*[4], *Behdokht Jamali*[5], *Reza Mohajer Shirazi*[1,3], *Kimia Sadat Esfahani*[1,3], *Ali Shirazi*[1,3], *Rojin Ghannad Zadeh*[1,6], *Faranak Jamshidian*[1,7], *Neda Zali*[3], *Najma Farahani*[1,*], *Afshin Taheriazam*[1,8,*], *Payman Rahimzadeh*[9,*], *Maliheh Entezari*[1,2,*]

[1]Farhikhtegan Medical Convergent Sciences Research Center, Farhikhtegan Hospital, Faculty of Medicine, TeMs. C., Islamic Azad University, Tehran, Iran

[2]Department of Genetics, Faculty of Advanced Sciences and Technology, TeMs. C, Islamic Azad University, Tehran, Iran

[3]Basic and Molecular Epidemiology of Gastrointestinal Disorders Research Center, Research Institute for Gastroenterology and Liver Diseases, Shahid Beheshti University of Medical Sciences, Tehran, Iran

[4]Department of Immunology, School of Medicine, Shahid Beheshti University of Medical Sciences, Tehran, Iran

[5]Department of Microbiology and Genetics, Kherad Institute of Higher Education, Bushehr, Iran

* **Corresponding authors:** Najmafarahani@gmail.com (N.F.); a.taheriazam@iautmu.ac.ir (A.T.); P.rahimzadeh76@gmail.com (P.R.); mentezari@iautmu.ac.ir (M.E.)

[6]Department of Art & Sciences, Faculty of Biology,
University of North Florida, Jacksonville, Florida, USA
[7]Department of Biology, ET.C., Islamic Azad University,
Tehran, Iran
[8]Department of Orthopedics, Faculty of Medicine,
TeMs. C, Islamic Azad University, Tehran, Iran
[9]Surgical Research Society (SRS), Students' Scientific Research
Center, Tehran University of Medical Sciences, Tehran, Iran

Abstract

Breast cancer remains the most frequently diagnosed malignancy in women and a leading cause of cancer mortality, driven by profound inter- and intratumoral heterogeneity arising from germline predisposition, somatic mutations, and epigenetic dysregulation. CRISPR/Cas9, an RNA-guided nuclease platform, offers precise insertion, correction, and deletion of disease-relevant loci, enabling direct interrogation and therapeutic rewriting of oncogenic pathways across breast cancer subtypes, including triple-negative disease. Applications span functional genomics (loss- and gain-of-function mapping, synthetic lethality discovery), epigenome engineering with catalytically inactive Cas9 fusions, and immuno-oncology modulation, alongside emerging non-viral and targeted delivery systems that improve translational feasibility. Early preclinical studies demonstrate reversal of resistance phenotypes, reactivation of tumor suppressors, and attenuation of metastatic traits, while highlighting practical constraints — off-target activity, p53-coupled DNA damage responses, heterogeneity of editing across tumor ecosystems, and delivery, ethical, and regulatory hurdles. This chapter synthesizes the state of CRISPR/Cas9 for breast cancer therapy, outlines design principles for high-fidelity editing and rational combinations, and charts a roadmap toward clinically scalable, personalized genome and epigenome interventions.

Keywords: breast neoplasms; CRISPR/Cas9; p53; HER2; triple-negative breast cancer; gene editing

2.1 Introduction

Breast cancer stands as the predominant cause of cancer-related mortality and ranks second in overall death rates among women [1]. While primarily affecting females, accounting for approximately 28% of new cancer cases, breast cancer has also been documented in males, albeit rarely [2].

The disease is characterized by significant heterogeneity and irregular signaling pathways that contribute to its initiation and progression [3]. Clinical diversity stems from both hereditary (10%) and somatic (90%) alterations [4]. Despite advances in medicine, accurately predicting the prognosis of metastatic breast cancer remains challenging at both histopathological and molecular levels [4].

The metastatic process in breast cancer is driven by irregular gene expression patterns that activate various downstream signaling cascades [5]. While germline mutations commonly occur across genes with varying penetrance sensitivity [6], somatic variations develop throughout life, encompassing both genomic mutations and epigenetic dysregulation. These genetic and epigenetic modifications orchestrate cancer cell metabolic requirements, including altered lipid metabolism, which promotes cell proliferation and tumor development [7].

CRISPR/Cas9 has emerged as a promising therapeutic tool with diverse applications in cancer research [8]. The system's Cas9 nuclease enables precise genetic modifications, including insertion, correction, or removal of defective genes. Although certain limitations exist in its application across various cancer types, ongoing research continues to address these challenges. This discussion explores various CRISPR/Cas9-based therapeutic strategies for breast cancer treatment.

2.2 Genetic and Molecular Landscape of Breast Cancer

Understanding breast cancer's pathophysiology and molecular subtypes is essential for comprehending its development, progression, and treatment response. This knowledge is fundamental for developing targeted therapies and personalized treatment approaches to improve patient outcomes.

Extensive research has uncovered the intricate molecular features and progression dynamics of breast cancer. The disease's development is primarily explained by two models: clonal evolution and the cancer stem cell hypothesis, with the added complexity that tumor stem cells themselves may undergo clonal evolution [9]. The progression from normal glandular tissue to malignant cancer is marked by a variety of morphological transformations and genetic modifications. The identification of the BRCA1 and BRCA2 genes, as well as PI3CA and TP53 pathogenic variants, which produce proteins essential for DNA repair through homologous recombination, has significantly deepened our understanding of both hereditary and sporadic breast cancer cases. Genetic mutations form the foundation of carcinogenesis. When cells carrying heterozygous BRCA1/2 mutations experience significant external damage, they may transform into malignant cells, leading to genomic instability and cellular dysfunction. This genetic instability can trigger additional genetic alterations, including non-inherited somatic mutations in PIK3CA and TP53 [10, 11]. Key mechanisms driving the disease include genetic mutations, hormonal imbalances, and interactions with the immune system.

Chromosomal instability is recognized as a hallmark of cancer [12], contributing to somatic copy number changes and fostering genetic diversity among tumor subclones as the disease advances [13]. As tumors evolve, cancer cells utilize a range of strategies to escape immune detection and adapt to environmental challenges, such as losing DNA segments, repressing gene transcription, silencing genes through epigenetic mechanisms, and undergoing whole-genome duplication [13]. These intricate genomic alterations allow cells to accumulate irreversible, harmful mutations that help them survive the selective pressures of human germline evolution, ultimately increasing their fitness, reducing cell death, and promoting malignancy [14]. Hormonal influences are also pivotal in the onset of sporadic breast cancer, including factors like hormone replacement therapy during menopause, high dietary estrogen intake, and overall endocrine disruption. Estrogen's interaction with nuclear estrogen receptors, encoded by the ESR1 gene, is particularly important in initiating breast cancer. Imbalances between estrogen and progesterone can drive cell proliferation and lead to DNA damage. Elevated estrogen levels further stimulate the growth of malignant cells and the expansion of supportive stromal tissue, aiding tumor progression [15]. When activated by their ligands, estrogen receptors regulate gene expression by binding to estrogen response elements in gene promoters [16]. Additionally, estrogen receptors can directly interact with proteins in growth signaling pathways, boosting the transcription of genes involved in cell division and survival [17]. Breast cancer arises within a complex tumor microenvironment composed of various cell types and extracellular matrix components. While cancer-associated fibroblasts are the most abundant, the microenvironment also includes lymphocytes, macrophages, etc., that modulate immune responses; for instance, breast cancer-associated macrophages promote tumorigenesis by suppressing succinate dehydrogenase in tumor cells [18]. In early tumor development, the immune microenvironment — through cytokines released by activated CD8+ and CD4+ T cells — can suppress tumor growth. However, as tumors become more aggressive, they begin to express immune checkpoint molecules such as CTLA-4 and PD-L1, which dampen immune activity. Cancer cells also shape the microenvironment by influencing cancer-associated fibroblasts and cytokine production, thereby promoting tumor advancement [19]. Breast cancer uses a variety of immune evasion tactics that impact disease progression and resistance to immunotherapy. As the disease evolves, it becomes more genomically complex and heterogeneous, creating selective pressures and leading to diverse responses to treatment [20]. For example, breast cancer cells can imitate anti-inflammatory processes found in the central nervous system to avoid immune destruction, relying on immunological synapse mechanisms [21]. Triple-negative breast cancer (TNBC), which typically has lower clonal diversity and fewer neoantigens, escapes immune detection through the Lgals2-CSF1-CSF1R pathway [22]. The interplay between breast cancer cells and the host's immune system results in multiple, simultaneous immune escape strategies within individual patients. This highlights the need for combination immunotherapy approaches and the development of reliable biomarkers to guide treatment.

2.3 Targeting Oncogenes in Breast Cancer with CRISPR/Cas9

CRISPR/Cas9 has rapidly become a cornerstone in both basic and translational cancer research, owing to its precision, flexibility, and broad applicability. This genome-editing platform enables targeted manipulation of oncogenes and tumor suppressor genes, thereby inhibiting cancer progression through diverse mechanisms such as gene knockout, transcriptional repression, sequence editing, and epigenetic modulation.

The editing process is primarily mediated through two distinct DNA repair pathways. Non-homologous end-joining, the more prevalent mechanism across cell types, introduces random insertions or deletions at double-strand break sites. While efficient, it is inherently error-prone and often leads to frameshift mutations that produce truncated or non-functional proteins. In contrast, homology-directed repair offers a high-fidelity alternative by utilizing a homologous donor DNA template to precisely correct genetic lesions [23].

CRISPR/Cas9 has shown particular efficacy in silencing both cellular and viral oncogenes across multiple cancer models, with especially promising outcomes in breast cancer research. These findings underscore the system's potential as a transformative tool for dissecting cancer biology and developing targeted therapeutic strategies.

2.3.1 *MYC*

Targeting MYC, a key oncogene elevated by 30–50% in high-grade breast cancers [24], remains a major therapeutic challenge due to its elusive pharmacological profile. Schuijers et al. demonstrated that CRISPR/Cas9-mediated reduction of MYC expression effectively suppressed cancer cell proliferation [24]. CRISPR/Cas9 has further enabled the disruption of MYC enhancer-docking sites and modification of its regulatory elements, thereby impeding transcription factor binding and reducing MYC protein levels. Beyond conventional gene knockout, the CRISPR/Cas system encompasses two additional modalities: CRISPR interference (CRISPRi) for transcriptional repression and CRISPR activation (CRISPRa) for gene upregulation. These approaches offer promising applications in breast cancer therapy, with CRISPRi targeting oncogenes and CRISPRa reactivating silenced tumor suppressor genes. CRISPRa strategies often employ dCas9 chimeras fused to transcriptional activators or epigenetic modifiers such as demethylases.

2.3.2 *CXCR7 and CXCR4*

Yang and colleagues used CRISPR/Cas9 technology to generate both single and double knockouts of the CXCR7 and CXCR4 genes in MDA-MB-231 breast cancer cells [25]. Clinical investigations have shown that high levels of CXCL12 and its receptors, CXCR4 and CXCR7, are linked to greater metastatic behavior and poorer outcomes in patients with TNBC [26]. These receptors contribute to enhanced cell movement, invasiveness, new blood vessel formation, and tumor growth. The study by Yang et al. found that knocking out both CXCR4 and CXCR7 together led to a marked reduction in TNBC progression, highlighting their combined effect in promoting the disease [25]. The CRISPR/Cas9 system is also effective for targeting regions outside of protein-coding genes, such as non-coding RNAs. Hannafon et al. demonstrated this capability by creating MCF-7 cell lines with CRISPR/Cas9-mediated knockouts of miR-23b and miR-27b. Their findings indicated that, although both miRNAs generally act as oncogenes, miR-27b can also exhibit tumor-suppressive activity under certain conditions [27].

2.3.3 *MASTL*

In recent years, MASTL kinase, a Great Wall in breast cancer, has emerged as a crucial regulator of protein phosphatase 2A (PP2A) during mitotic division. Research has identified altered expression patterns and somatic mutations of PP2A subunit B55 across various cancers, including breast cancer [28]. MASTL functions by phosphorylating two proteins — endosulfine and ARPP19 — which subsequently inhibit PP2A-B55 complexes. Studies have also shown that CDK substrate phosphorylation influences PP2A-B55 complexes [29]. The inhibition of MASTL and subsequent PP2A reactivation are essential for maintaining normal cell growth through proper mitotic exit.

Research by Alvares-Fernández et al. demonstrated that using CRISPR/Cas9 to inhibit MASTL kinase activity effectively reduced cell proliferation in human cell lines. This finding is particularly significant as MASTL shows higher expression in cancer cells compared to normal cells *in vivo* [28]. Consequently, CRISPR/Cas9-mediated MASTL inhibition represents a promising therapeutic strategy for breast cancer treatment.

2.3.4 *FASN*

The FASN gene, which codes for fatty acid synthase, is essential for *de novo* fatty acid synthesis and phospholipid production, and has been identified as an oncogene [7]. Studies have demonstrated a positive association between FASN protein expression and the progression of various cancers, including stomach, lung, breast, prostate, colon, and ovarian carcinomas. Cancer cells require increased FASN activity to meet their phospholipid demands for cell division, making it a promising therapeutic target [30].

Research investigating CRISPR/Cas9-generated FASN mutants in the MCF-7 breast cancer cell line has yielded significant results. The studies revealed that FASN mutations inhibit MCF-7 cell progression, suggesting these mutations play a distinct and non-redundant role in breast cancer development [31]. These findings further support FASN as a potential therapeutic target in breast cancer treatment.

2.3.5 *HER2*

The CRISPR system has been utilized to analyze HER2, an oncoprotein that shows promise as a therapeutic target in cancer treatment [32]. The significance of HER2 in breast cancer is particularly noteworthy, as approximately 20% of breast cancer patients exhibit HER2 gene amplification, leading to more aggressive disease progression compared to other cancer types [32]. Research has shown that mutations in exon12 of HER2 exhibit dominant-negative characteristics and potentially inhibit the HER2-MAPK/ERK signaling cascade, with this inhibitory effect being enhanced when combined with poly-ADP ribose polymerase (PARP) inhibitor treatment [32]. Studies have revealed that modifying a single copy of HER2 through CRISPR/Cas9 techniques does not significantly impact total HER2 protein levels, suggesting partial HER2 genetic alterations [32].

2.3.6 *FOXA1*

The pioneer transcription factor, fork-head box protein A (FOXA1), plays a crucial role in both organogenesis and the progression of various cancers, including breast cancer [33]. While FOXA1 exhibits its binding capability to approximately 90% of genes in the human cancer genome, only 17% of these FOXA1 interactions actively participate in gene transcriptional regulation, with this functional subset displaying cancer cell-type specificity [33]. Research has demonstrated that FOXA1 establishes distinct genomic signatures and modulates gene expression differently across various human cancer cell lines [34]. These variations in regulation may be attributed to diverse epigenetic mechanisms, particularly histone modifications. Through CRISPR/Cas9 technology, researchers have explored cell-specific FOXA1 regulation, revealing distinctive FOXA1 binding patterns, genetic variants, and potential epigenetic regulatory mechanisms [34]. Furthermore, CRISPR-based modification of FOXA1 binding sites has enabled manipulation of cell-specific gene transcription, resulting in decreased breast cancer progression [34]. In TNBC, ubiquitous transcriptional processes and specific cyclin-dependent kinases play regulatory roles, which have been investigated using CRISPR/Cas genome editing [35]. Studies have shown that targeting CDK7 can effectively induce cancer cell death through apoptosis [36].

2.3.7 *CDK7*

Cyclin-dependent kinase 7 (CDK7) acts as the catalytic subunit of CDK-activating kinase, playing a key role in phosphorylating T loops and activating several cyclin-dependent kinases, such as CDK1, CDK2, CDK4, and CDK6 [37]. Research has shown that CDK7 is vital for both the initiation and progression of TNBC. When the CDK7 gene was knocked out in TNBC cells using CRISPR/Cas9, there was a notable reduction in cell growth and tumor formation. Comparisons with CRISPR/Cas9-mediated knockouts of other transcription-related CDKs (including CDK8, CDK9, CDK12, CDK13, and CDK19) revealed that CDK7 is especially important for the survival and proliferation of TNBC cells. Further CRISPR/Cas9 studies targeting major TNBC driver genes — such as EGFR, FOSL1, FOXC1, MYC, and SOX9 — demonstrated that CDK7 regulates these critical genes involved in cell proliferation [36]. Altogether, these findings indicate that targeting CDK7 with CRISPR/Cas9 could be a promising strategy for controlling cancer cell growth.

2.3.8 *UBR5*

The nuclear phosphoprotein UBR5, which shows elevated expression in TNBC samples, functions as a critical regulator in developing endocrine therapy resistance through two mechanisms: enhancing unfolded protein levels and decreasing ERα degradation, with ERα being crucial for TNBC development and progression [38]. Studies have demonstrated that when UBR5 (E3-Ubiquitin Ligase) is eliminated using CRISPR/Cas9 technology, it disrupts both tumor growth and metastatic processes in TNBC murine mammary models studied *in vivo* [39]. These findings have led researchers to identify UBR5 as a key driver in breast cancer progression, influencing both tumor development and metastatic spread.

The most substantial oncogenic targets being manipulated by CRISPR/Cas9 system are summarized in **Table 2.1**.

2.4 Restoring Tumor Suppressor Functions

FOXP3, located on the X chromosome, acts as a tumor suppressor gene, and studies have shown that mice carrying heterozygous FOXP3 mutations develop breast cancer [41]. Given that breast cancer is characterized by decreased FOXP3 expression, researchers have utilized CRISPRi/a technology to reactivate endogenous FOXP3, enhancing its expression and subsequently reducing breast cancer growth [42]. Research has demonstrated the possibility of generating breast organoids from normal breast epithelial cells, which can undergo genetic modification via CRISPR/Cas9 to induce tumor formation. Specifically, when CRISPR/Cas9 was employed to modify four tumor suppressor genes (P53, PTEN, RB1, and NF1) in breast organoids, it resulted in the development of ER-α luminal breast cancer [43]. This finding suggests that the deactivation of these particular tumor suppressor genes serves as a crucial mechanism for breast cancer development under *in vivo* conditions. These insights indicate that CRISPRi/a-mediated activation of these tumor suppressor genes could enhance our understanding of their regulatory pathways, potentially leading to improved therapeutic strategies for breast cancer management.

2.5 CRISPR/Cas9 and Breast Cancer Immunotherapy

Impaired immune function is a key factor in tumor formation, as cancer cells utilize multiple strategies to avoid immune detection

Table 2.1 CRISPR-Cas9 applications in breast cancer research.

Target Gene or Region	CRISPR-based Approach	Mechanism(s) of Action	Reference
PTEN/BRCA1	CRISPRa with dCas9-TET chimera	Demethylation of promoter regions, gene activation	[40]
CXCR4 & CXCR7	CRISPR/Cas9 knockout	Co-knockout suppresses cell motility, invasion, angiogenesis	[25]
FASN	CRISPR/Cas9 mutation	Inhibits fatty acid synthesis, reduces cancer cell progression	[31]
HER2	CRISPR/Cas9 editing	Creates dominant-negative mutants, suppresses HER2-MAPK/ERK pathway	[32]
FOXA1	CRISPR/Cas9 editing of binding sites	Manipulates cell-specific gene transcription, reduces cancer progression	[33]
CDK7	CRISPR/Cas9 knockout	Inactivation impedes cell growth and tumor formation in TNBC	[37]
UBR5	CRISPR/Cas9 knockout	Deregulates tumor growth and metastasis, reduces endocrine therapy resistance	[39]
miR-23b/ miR-27b	CRISPR/Cas9 miRNA knockout	Modulates oncogenic/tumor suppressor activities	[27]
MASTL	CRISPR/Cas9 inhibition	Reduces cell proliferation by reactivating PP2A complexes	[28]

and foster an environment that suppresses immune activity. Genetic editing using CRISPR/Cas systems has shown promise in tackling issues related to immune dysfunction [44]. In the context of breast cancer, CRISPR/Cas9 has been applied to boost anti-tumor immune responses through various approaches (**Figure 2.1**). Treatments based on T-lymphocytes have attracted considerable interest because these cells can differentiate between self and foreign antigens due to their diverse T cell repertoire. Conventional immunotherapy methods involve modifying a patient's T cells to express specific T cell receptors (TCRs) or chimeric antigen

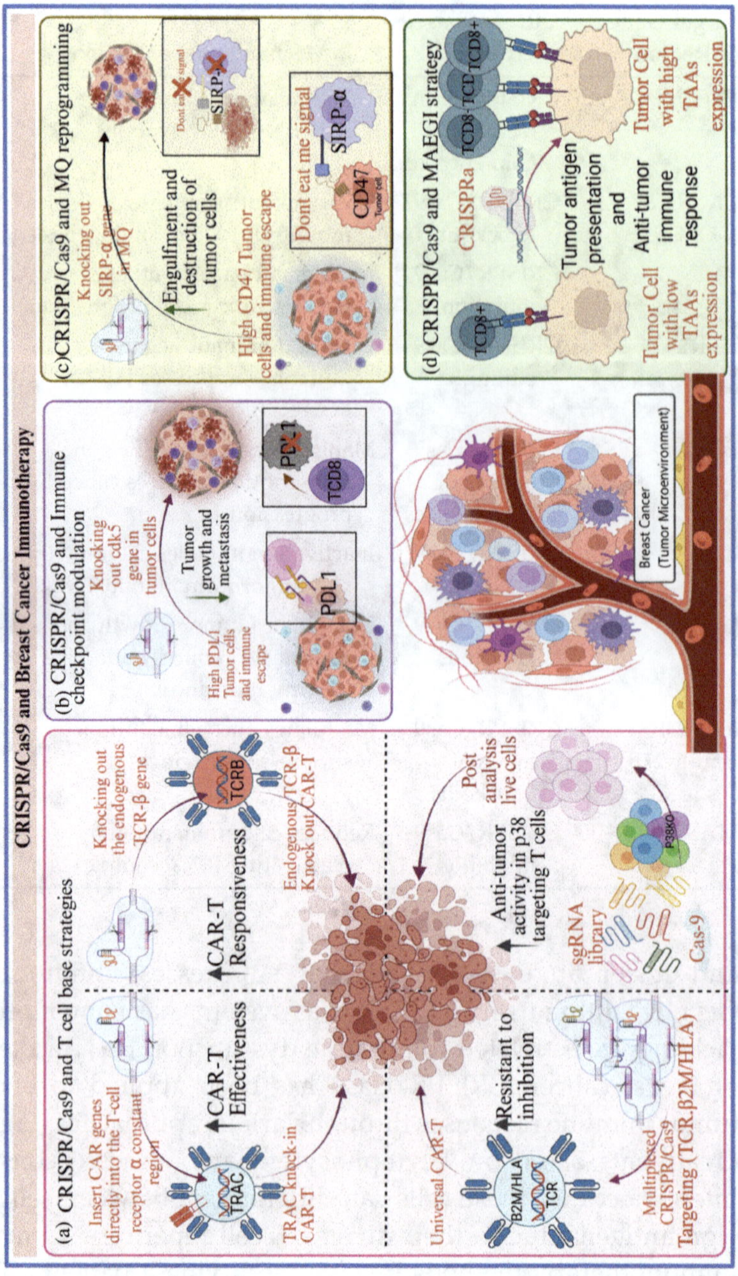
CRISPR/Cas9 and Breast Cancer Immunotherapy
(a) CRISPR/Cas9 and T cell base strategies
Insert CAR genes directly into the T-cell receptor α constant region
TRAC
TRAC knock-in CAR-T
CAR-T Effectiveness
Knocking out the endogenous TCR-β gene
TCRB
CAR-T Responsiveness
Endogenous TCR-β Knock out CAR-T
Universal CAR-T
B2M/HLA
TCR
Resistant to inhibition
Multiplexed CRISPR/Cas9 Targeting (TCR.β2M/HLA)
Anti-tumor activity in p38 targeting T cells
Post analysis live cells
sgRNA library
Cas-9
P38KO
(b) CRISPR/Cas9 and Immune checkpoint modulation
Knocking out cdk5 gene in tumor cells
Tumor growth and metastasis
High PDL1 Tumor cells and immune escape
PDL1
TCD8
Breast Cancer (Tumor Microenvironment)
(c) CRISPR/Cas9 and MQ reprogramming
Knocking out SIRP-α gene in MQ
Engulfment and destruction of tumor cells
High CD47 Tumor cells and immune escape
Dont eat me signal
SIRP-α
CD47
(d) CRISPR/Cas9 and MAEGI strategy
TCD8+
CRISPRa
Tumor antigen presentation and Anti-tumor immune response
Tumor Cell with low TAAs expression
Tumor Cell with high TAAs expression

Figure 2.1 CRISPR/Cas9 applications in the immunotherapy and microenvironment modulation of breast cancer. The multifaceted roles of CRISPR/Cas9-mediated genome editing in advancing breast cancer immunotherapy are summarized here. **(a) CRISPR/Cas9 and T cell-based strategies:** Engineered CAR-T cell effectiveness and responsiveness are enhanced by inserting CAR genes into the TRAC locus and eliminating endogenous TCR-β genes. The multiplexed targeting of TCR, B2M, and HLA loci generates universal CAR-T cells that are resistant to inhibition within the tumor microenvironment. High-throughput CRISPR/Cas9 screens in T cells (e.g., targeting p38) enable identification of key regulators of anti-tumor activity, with live cell analysis post-editing. **(b) CRISPR/Cas9 and immune checkpoint modulation:** CRISPR/Cas9 knockout of genes mediating immune checkpoint pathways, such as PD-L1 or cdk5 in tumor cells, reduces tumor growth, impedes immune escape, and suppresses metastasis by enhancing T cell-mediated cytotoxicity. **(c) CRISPR/Cas9 and macrophage reprogramming:** Targeted disruption of the SIRP-α gene in macrophages abolishes the "don't eat me" signal conveyed by CD47-overexpressing tumor cells, thereby facilitating macrophage-mediated phagocytosis and destruction of breast cancer cells. **(d) CRISPR/Cas9 and MAEGI strategy:** CRISPRa platforms increase TAA expression, promoting more effective antigen presentation and potentiating TCD8+ cytotoxic T lymphocyte responses against tumor cells, whether baseline TAA expression is high or low. Collectively, these CRISPR/Cas9-driven strategies provide powerful avenues for modifying immune cell function, overcoming immunosuppression, and enhancing tumor antigenicity, underpinning the next generation of precision immunotherapies for breast cancer.

receptors (CARs) that can recognize tumor-associated antigens (TAA) [45]. However, this process is often lengthy and relies heavily on the unique characteristics of the patient's T cells [44]. The advent of CRISPR/Cas9 has made it possible to insert CAR genes directly into the TCR α constant region, effectively substituting the native TCR with a CAR. Research using mouse models of acute myeloid leukemia has demonstrated that this targeted CAR expression increases T cell effectiveness while minimizing terminal differentiation and lymph node depletion [46], indicating potential benefits for breast cancer therapy. Additionally, CRISPR/Cas9 has been used to refine T lymphocytes engineered to express cancer antigen-specific TCRs. By knocking out the endogenous TCR-β gene in recipient cells, CRISPR-edited T cells have shown a thousand-fold increase in responsiveness to cancer antigens compared to traditional TCR-transduced T cells. Likewise, CRISPR/Cas9 modifications have enabled the creation of universal CAR-T cells that are resistant to inhibition [47].

CRISPR/Cas9-based genetic screen conducted on primary T cells identified 25 kinases involved in TCR signaling that were disrupted [48]. Among these, p38 kinase was found to be a key player in regulating cell proliferation, differentiation, and responses to cellular stress. Higher levels of p38α were linked to increased cell expansion, decreased oxidative and genomic stress, and less terminal differentiation. These results indicate that targeting p38 with inhibitors could potentially boost the anti-tumor activity of T cells, offering a promising direction for cancer therapy [48]. Recent advances have also focused on targeting PD-L1 on tumor cells using monoclonal antibodies as a therapeutic strategy. Tumor cells often show increased PD-L1 expression which, when interacting with the PD-1 receptor on immune cells, helps tumors evade immune attack and fosters an immunosuppressive environment. Although clinical trials using monoclonal antibodies to block the PD-L1/PD-1 interaction have had limited success, they have paved the way for new cancer treatment strategies. Research by Deng et al. demonstrated that knocking out the Cdk5 gene in tumor cells using CRISPR-Cas9 reduced PD-L1 expression, which in turn suppressed tumor growth in a mouse melanoma model and decreased lung metastasis in TNBC [49]. This intervention also strengthened T cell-mediated immune responses in the tumor microenvironment, as shown by an increase in CD8+ T cells and a reduction in regulatory T cells, suggesting a promising alternative to traditional immune checkpoint blockade therapies. Macrophages play multiple roles in cancer progression. The interaction between signal-regulatory protein alpha (SIRP-α) on macrophages and CD47 on cancer cells generates a "do not eat me" signal, allowing cancer cells to avoid being destroyed by the immune system [50]. Elevated CD47 levels have been detected in several cancers, such as ovarian carcinoma, mouse myeloid leukemia, and leukemic stem cells [51]. Therefore, using CRISPR/Cas9 to create macrophages that lack SIRP-α could be a novel approach for breast cancer therapy. These engineered macrophages would be unable to receive the inhibitory signal from cancer cells, thereby promoting the engulfment and destruction of tumor cells [50]. A novel strategy called multiplexed activation of endogenous genes as immunotherapy (MAEGI) has been developed to overcome the limitations of conventional immunotherapies. This method uses CRISPRa to simultaneously activate several endogenous genes, leading to improved tumor antigen presentation and a much stronger anti-tumor immune response [52]. When used as a cell-based vaccine, MAEGI has shown the potential to enhance both preventive and therapeutic vaccine efficacy. Additionally, this approach can remodel the tumor microenvironment and improve T cell infiltration. Given these benefits, MAEGI may offer a more flexible and effective way to generate robust immune responses against breast cancer compared to current treatment options [52].

2.6 CRISPR/Cas9 against Triple-negative Breast Cancer Drug Resistance

Drug resistance is estimated to contribute to nearly 90% of cancer-related fatalities, representing a significant obstacle in effective cancer treatment [53]. Studies have revealed that numerous genes involved in mechanisms such as drug efflux, DNA repair, programmed cell death (apoptosis), and various cellular signaling pathways are associated with the development of resistance to cancer therapies [54]. Among these, several have been targeted using the CRISPR/Cas9 system, demonstrating promising outcomes in terms of lowering drug resistance and improving the effectiveness of anticancer therapies [55]. Moreover, high-throughput screening libraries utilizing CRISPR/Cas9 gene knockout techniques have been employed to pinpoint and validate potential targets for modifying genes related to drug resistance [56]. To understand the genetic basis of paclitaxel resistance, researchers have combined RNA sequencing with genome-wide single-guide RNA library screening, which led to the identification of eight candidate genes — including histone deacetylase 9 — that are linked to drug resistance in patients experiencing relapse of TNBC [53]. In another investigation, elevated expression of dual serine/threonine and tyrosine protein kinase (DSTYK) was detected in surviving TNBC patients undergoing anticancer drug treatment. Notably, knocking down DSTYK using CRISPR/Cas9 significantly increased apoptosis in drug-resistant cancer cells in both *in vitro* models (SUM102PT and MDA-MB-468 cell lines) and in *in vivo* TNBC models [57].

TNBCs often display abnormal activation of the MAPK signaling pathway, yet treatments targeting MEK have shown limited clinical success. Through CRISPR/Cas9-based genomic library screening, researchers discovered that suppressing PSMG2 (proteome assembly chaperone 2) increases the sensitivity of BT549 and MB468 TNBC cells to the MEK inhibitor AZD6244. When PSMG2 is knocked down using CRISPR/Cas9, it disrupts normal proteasome activity, resulting in the degradation of autophagy-regulated PDPK1. This process further enhances the combined tumor-killing effects of AZD6244 (a MEK inhibitor) and MG132 (a proteasome inhibitor) in mouse models of TNBC. As a result, using both proteasome and MAP kinase (MEK) inhibitors together has been shown to more effectively suppress tumor cell growth [58]. Additionally, CRISPR/Cas9 has been employed to identify genes whose loss of function leads to drug resistance in TNBC [59]. Ge and colleagues investigated how TNBC cells develop resistance to JQ1, a BET bromodomain inhibitor. Their CRISPR/Cas9 experiments revealed that deleting the rb1 gene caused TNBC cells to become resistant to JQ1, highlighting the crucial role of rb1 in mediating the response to this drug. They also found that paclitaxel, which inhibits CDK4/6 kinase and microtubules, when used in combination with BET bromodomain inhibitors like JQ1, may offer a promising strategy to overcome drug resistance in TNBC [60].

Recent research has revealed that the transcriptional profiles of lncRNAs contribute to resistance against neoadjuvant therapies in TNBC. Specifically, elevated levels of five distinct MALAT1 lncRNA transcripts have been observed in TNBC cases. Moreover, removing MALAT1 using CRISPR/Cas9 technology made BT-549 TNBC cells more responsive to paclitaxel and doxorubicin, suggesting that MALAT1 plays a significant role in mediating drug resistance in TNBC [61]. BRCA1 mutations are highly variable, making them difficult to target directly. Since PARP1 acts as a synthetic lethal partner to BRCA1, inhibiting PARP1 could potentially increase the effectiveness of chemotherapy in TNBC. CRISPR/Cas9-mediated deletion of PARP1 has been shown to boost the sensitivity of mBRCA1 mutant TNBC cells to drugs like doxorubicin, gemcitabine, and docetaxel, indicating PARP1's involvement in drug resistance [55]. It is also well established that mutations in the tumor suppressor genes BRCA1 or BRCA2 raise the risk of developing breast cancer, and patients with these mutations are typically treated with PARP inhibitors. Additionally, CRISPR/Cas9 knockdown of the nucleotide salvage factor DNPH1 has been found to increase the vulnerability of BRCA-deficient cells to PARP inhibitors by eliminating the toxic nucleotide 5-hydroxymethyl-deoxyuridine monophosphate [62]. Therefore, combining CRISPR/Cas9 with PARP1 inhibitors could represent a promising therapeutic strategy for TNBC [63].

The P-glycoprotein (P-gp) gene, which is associated with multidrug resistance, is upregulated in about 41% of TNBC cases [64]. P-gp-driven drug efflux is recognized as a major factor in breast cancer drug resistance. The use of P-gp inhibitors has been shown to increase the effectiveness of anticancer drugs in breast cancer [65]. Thus, targeting P-gp through CRISPR/Cas9-mediated deletion or silencing, in combination with P-gp inhibitors could be a valuable approach to overcoming drug resistance in TNBC. The ATP-binding cassette transporter G2 (ABCG2) is another gene known to promote drug resistance in TNBC [66]. Although there are currently no studies directly linking CRISPR/Cas9 to the silencing of ABCG2, it has been reported that loss of the tumor suppressor gene PTEN can lead to increased ABCG2 expression [66, 67]. Therefore, using CRISPR/Cas9 to delete ABCG2, possibly in combination with ABCG2 inhibitors, may offer a promising therapeutic strategy to address drug resistance in TNBC.

2.7 Challenges, Safety, and Ethical Considerations

Drug resistance represents a major challenge in breast cancer treatment [68]. While CRISPR/Cas9 technology offers potential solutions through targeting drug resistance-related genes, Cas9's off-target activity remains a significant limitation. Despite various approaches to address this issue, the mechanisms underlying guide RNA (gRNA) specificity remain incompletely understood [69, 70].

Several methods have been developed to detect CRISPR/Cas9-edited alleles, including the "pop-in/pop-out" technique developed by Kühn and Chu, which has simplified edited allele isolation [71].

A major clinical limitation of CRISPR/Cas9 implementation is the presence of Cas9-specific T-cells, which can restrict nuclease activity and overall editing efficiency. Additionally, the immune system may recognize and eliminate edited cells. Multiple studies have highlighted these immunological concerns in clinical applications [72–74]. Further research is needed to understand Cas9-specific T-cell function during treatment and potentially develop immune-evasive Cas9 variants or incorporate immune-compromising agents within Cas9-containing cassettes.

Delivery systems for hard-to-transfect cells/tissues present another challenge. Non-viral delivery methods, including nanoparticles, electroporation, and direct injection, typically require large plasmid quantities and specialized equipment. While viral and bacteriophage-derived vectors offer simpler delivery options, they require extensive preclinical safety studies to assess genotoxicity and cellular toxicity [75], along with comprehensive pharmacokinetic and pharmacodynamic characterization.

Recent innovations in delivery systems include encapsulating CRISPR components in lipopolymers with cancer-specific aptamers, showing improved efficiency compared to traditional delivery methods [76]. Wang et al. [77] developed a delivery system using PEGylated nanoparticles based on α-helical polypeptide PPABLG, which achieved efficient cellular internalization and endosomal escape through the polypeptide's membrane-penetrating properties.

A significant challenge in CRISPR/Cas9 therapeutic applications is the potential for off-target effects, where Cas9 may cut DNA at unintended locations. Precise gRNA design, particularly regarding the 5′ end sequence composition, is crucial for minimizing these off-target effects. Over the past decade, various algorithms have been developed to optimize on-target specificity while reducing off-target activity. Additionally, Cas9 activity levels significantly influence off-target effects [78], with higher activity levels potentially increasing non-specific DNA cleavage.

Several strategies have been developed to optimize Cas9 activity. One approach involves placing the Cas9-encoding gene under the control of a tetracycline-responsive element promoter, allowing conditional Cas9 expression in response to tetracycline/doxycycline. Similar control can be achieved by placing gRNA under the same promoter, helping to minimize off-target cleavage [79–81].

Another effective strategy involves creating a 4-hydroxytamoxifen-dependent Cas9 variant by fusing the estrogen receptor's hormone-binding domain to Cas9. This modification ensures Cas9 is only released into the cytoplasm in the presence of 4-hydroxytamoxifen, providing better control over Cas9 activity [82].

Alternative strategies have utilized the self-removing characteristics of protein segments known as "inteins," which are capable of excising themselves and reconnecting the remaining protein fragments via a peptide bond. This mechanism enables the Cas9 nuclease to become functional only when 4-hydroxytamoxifen is present [83]. Notably, these two methods for regulating Cas9 expression could soon be harnessed to develop vectors for therapeutic applications. Additionally, for Cas9 to identify its target site, it must recognize a particular short sequence called the protospacer adjacent motif. To address this limitation, scientists have engineered Cas9 variants with modified protospacer adjacent motif recognition abilities [84]. In another approach, a split version of Cas9 was combined with a protein domain that is expressed at low levels. This configuration allows Cas9 to be activated by blue light, giving researchers precise control over Cas9 activity both in laboratory and living systems [85]. The accuracy of Cas9 targeting is generally influenced by several elements, such as the design of the gRNA, the structure of the Cas9 enzyme, the proportion of gRNA to Cas9, and the uniqueness of the target DNA sequence. To minimize unintended (off-target) effects, several strategies have been proposed. These include shortening the gRNA to 20 nucleotides, which can boost specificity by up to 5,000 times [84]. Another method involves mutating the active site of Cas9 so that it requires two enzyme units to create a double-strand break [86]. Additionally, fusing a catalytically inactive Cas9 (dCas9) with the FokI nuclease has been suggested to enhance specificity [87]. Modifying the electric charge of Cas9's HNH and RuvC domains has also been shown to reduce off-target activity [80]. Delivering Cas9 as a protein, rather than as DNA encoding Cas9 in a plasmid, may further improve on-target effects and decrease off-target mutations [88]. For CRISPR/Cas9 to be used in medical treatments, especially for cancers like breast cancer, it is essential to develop reliable methods for controlling Cas9 activity. The simpler and more effective these methods are, the more likely they are to be adopted for therapeutic use.

2.8 Future Perspectives

CRISPR represents a groundbreaking advancement in gene editing, transforming the field of biology through its unprecedented accuracy and simplicity in altering the genomes of virtually any organism. This technology has swiftly moved from theory to practice; for instance, researchers have developed gene-edited monkey models and have also used the CRISPR/Cas9 system to engineer modifications within mouse brains [89]. The ability of CRISPR/Cas9 to induce permanent genetic changes means that these alterations can potentially be inherited by subsequent generations. However, the application of CRISPR/Cas9 raises important societal and ethical questions, affecting not just humans but also animals and ecosystems. Concerns include the potential for ecological harm, safety risks, and debates over the use of CRISPR for genetic enhancement purposes. It is essential to carefully consider these risks, particularly regarding unintended effects on living organisms and the environment. Furthermore, there are significant ethical debates about editing the human germline — the genetic material in eggs, sperm, or early embryos that is passed on to descendants [90]. Up to this point, all genome editing therapies in humans have targeted somatic cells, which do not transmit genetic changes to offspring. Nonetheless, the work of Liang and colleagues has highlighted growing apprehension about the possibility of germline modifications in humans.

So far, CRISPR/Cas9 has not been implemented in clinical trials specifically to counteract resistance to anticancer medications. However, preliminary clinical investigations indicate that gene-editing methods could be both safe and effective for human use. Teams in the United States and China are preparing to apply CRISPR/Cas9 in similar ways, though they are focusing on different cancer types. The Chinese researchers are targeting non-small-cell lung cancer, while the American group is concentrating on melanoma, sarcoma, and myeloid cancers. Notably, scientists in China are close to being the first to administer CRISPR/Cas9-edited cells to patients [91]. At the University of Pennsylvania, a pilot study is underway where scientists aim to modify patients' immune cells so they can better recognize and attack cancer at its earliest stages [92]. Traditional drug development models may not be well-suited for these innovative targeted therapies. Resistance to both established and newer drugs continues to be a major hurdle in cancer care. Utilizing advanced gene-editing tools like CRISPR/Cas9 can provide deeper insights into the signaling pathways that define the "genomic landscape" of breast cancer. A better understanding of the molecular mechanisms behind resistance will improve our ability to target specific genes or pathways, potentially overcoming drug resistance and leading to better clinical outcomes. Although technical barriers remain for using CRISPR/Cas9 to edit cancer-related genes in patients, the outlook for gene therapy is very promising. CRISPR-based genome editing is expected to become a vital resource in both laboratory and clinical environments. The effectiveness of CRISPR/Cas9 therapies will rely on the precise design of single-guide RNAs, careful control of off-target effects, and efficient delivery systems. As this technology moves from research to clinical practice, it opens up exciting new opportunities for understanding and addressing drug resistance. In the era of personalized medicine, CRISPR/Cas9 is anticipated to offer improved strategies for managing the complexity of cancer and overcoming drug resistance, which is a central goal of precision medicine [91, 92].

2.9 Conclusion

CRISPR/Cas9 has shifted breast cancer research from descriptive genomics to actionable editing, enabling causative testing of drivers, systematic discovery of druggable vulnerabilities, and programmable modulation of immune and epigenetic circuits. Proof-of-concept studies support therapeutic editing to overcome resistance and suppress invasion, particularly in aggressive subtypes where targeted options are limited. Real-world impact now hinges on three pillars: engineering precision (optimized guides, high-fidelity/base/prime editors, robust off-target surveillance), effective and safe delivery (tumor-selective, repeat-dose-capable vectors and nanoparticles), and rigorous clinical frameworks (biomarker-guided patient selection, ethical and regulatory governance). With these advances, CRISPR/Cas9 is poised to complement endocrine, HER2-directed, and immunotherapies, accelerating a personalized treatment paradigm that converts genomic insight into durable clinical benefit for patients with breast cancer.

References

1. Siegel RL, Miller KD, Fuchs HE, Jemal A. Cancer statistics, 2022. CA Cancer J Clin. 2022;72(1):7–33.
2. Curigliano G. New drugs for breast cancer subtypes: targeting driver pathways to overcome resistance. Cancer Treat Rev. 2012;38(4):303–10.
3. Giuliano M, Hu H, Wang YC, Fu X, Nardone A, Herrera S, et al. Upregulation of ER Signaling as an Adaptive Mechanism of Cell Survival in HER2-Positive Breast Tumors Treated with Anti-HER2 Therapy. Clin Cancer Res. 2015;21(17):3995–4003.
4. Minicozzi P, Bella F, Toss A, Giacomin A, Fusco M, Zarcone M, et al. Relative and disease-free survival for breast cancer in relation to subtype: a population-based study. J Cancer Res Clin Oncol. 2013; 139(9):1569–77.
5. Toss A, Venturelli M, Peterle C, Piacentini F, Cascinu S, Cortesi L. Molecular Biomarkers for Prediction of Targeted Therapy Response in Metastatic Breast Cancer: Trick or Treat? Int J Mol Sci. 2017;18(1):85.
6. Paterson R, Phillips KA. Genetic testing in women with breast cancer: implications for treatment. Expert Rev Anticancer Ther. 2017; 17(11):991–1002.
7. Havas KM, Milchevskaya V, Radic K, Alladin A, Kafkia E, Garcia M, et al. Metabolic shifts in residual breast cancer drive tumor recurrence. J Clin Invest. 2017;127(6):2091–105.
8. Banerjee B, Sherwood RI. A CRISPR view of gene regulation. Curr Opin Syst Biol. 2017;1:1–8.
9. Bombonati A, Sgroi DC. The molecular pathology of breast cancer progression. J Pathol. 2011;223(2):307–17.
10. Huen MS, Sy SM, Chen J. BRCA1 and its toolbox for the maintenance of genome integrity. Nat Rev Mol Cell Biol. 2010;11(2):138–48.

11. Kostecka A, Nowikiewicz T, Olszewski P, Koczkowska M, Horbacz M, Heinzl M, et al. High prevalence of somatic PIK3CA and TP53 pathogenic variants in the normal mammary gland tissue of sporadic breast cancer patients revealed by duplex sequencing. NPJ Breast Cancer. 2022;8(1):76.
12. Bakhoum SF, Ngo B, Laughney AM, Cavallo JA, Murphy CJ, Ly P, et al. Chromosomal instability drives metastasis through a cytosolic DNA response. Nature. 2018;553(7689):467–72.
13. Bailey C, Black JRM, Reading JL, Litchfield K, Turajlic S, McGranahan N, et al. Tracking Cancer Evolution through the Disease Course. Cancer Discov. 2021;11(4):916–32.
14. López S, Lim EL, Horswell S, Haase K, Huebner A, Dietzen M, et al. Interplay between whole-genome doubling and the accumulation of deleterious alterations in cancer evolution. Nat Genet. 2020; 52(3):283–93.
15. Pedroza DA, Subramani R, Tiula K, Do A, Rashiraj N, Galvez A, et al. Crosstalk between progesterone receptor membrane component 1 and estrogen receptor α promotes breast cancer cell proliferation. Lab Invest. 2021;101(6):733–44.
16. Stoica GE, Franke TF, Moroni M, Mueller S, Morgan E, Iann MC, et al. Effect of estradiol on estrogen receptor-alpha gene expression and activity can be modulated by the ErbB2/PI 3-K/Akt pathway. Oncogene. 2003;22(39):7998–8011.
17. Schiff R, Massarweh S, Shou J, Osborne CK. Breast cancer endocrine resistance: how growth factor signaling and estrogen receptor coregulators modulate response. Clin Cancer Res. 2003;9(1 Pt 2):447s-54s.
18. Gómez V, Eykyn TR, Mustapha R, Flores-Borja F, Male V, Barber PR, et al. Breast cancer-associated macrophages promote tumorigenesis by suppressing succinate dehydrogenase in tumor cells. Sci Signal. 2020;13(652):eaax4585.
19. Sammut SJ, Galson JD, Minter R, Sun B, Chin SF, De Mattos-Arruda L, et al. Predictability of B cell clonal persistence and immunosurveillance in breast cancer. Nat Immunol. 2024;25(5):916–24.
20. Onkar SS, Carleton NM, Lucas PC, Bruno TC, Lee AV, Vignali DAA, Oesterreich S. The Great Immune Escape: Understanding the Divergent Immune Response in Breast Cancer Subtypes. Cancer Discov. 2023;13(1):23–40.

21. Li Y, Huang M, Wang M, Wang Y, Deng P, Li C, et al. Tumor cells impair immunological synapse formation via central nervous system-enriched metabolite. Cancer Cell. 2024;42(6):985–1002.e18.
22. Ji P, Gong Y, Jin ML, Wu HL, Guo LW, Pei YC, et al. In vivo multidimensional CRISPR screens identify Lgals2 as an immunotherapy target in triple-negative breast cancer. Sci Adv. 2022;8(26):eabl8247.
23. Cong L, Zhang F. Genome engineering using CRISPR-Cas9 system. Methods Mol Biol. 2015;1239:197–217.
24. Schuijers J, Manteiga JC, Weintraub AS, Day DS, Zamudio AV, Hnisz D, et al. Transcriptional Dysregulation of MYC Reveals Common Enhancer-Docking Mechanism. Cell Rep. 2018;23(2):349–60.
25. Yang M, Zeng C, Li P, Qian L, Ding B, Huang L, et al. Impact of CXCR4 and CXCR7 knockout by CRISPR/Cas9 on the function of triple-negative breast cancer cells. Onco Targets Ther. 2019; 12:3849–58.
26. Wu W, Qian L, Chen X, Ding B. Prognostic significance of CXCL12, CXCR4, and CXCR7 in patients with breast cancer. Int J Clin Exp Pathol. 2015;8(10):13217–24.
27. Hannafon BN, Cai A, Calloway CL, Xu YF, Zhang R, Fung KM, Ding WQ. miR-23b and miR-27b are oncogenic microRNAs in breast cancer: evidence from a CRISPR/Cas9 deletion study. BMC Cancer. 2019;19(1):642.
28. Álvarez-Fernández M, Sanz-Flores M, Sanz-Castillo B, Salazar-Roa M, Partida D, Zapatero-Solana E, et al. Therapeutic relevance of the PP2A-B55 inhibitory kinase MASTL/Greatwall in breast cancer. Cell Death Differ. 2018;25(5):828–40.
29. Wurzenberger C, Gerlich DW. Phosphatases: providing safe passage through mitotic exit. Nat Rev Mol Cell Biol. 2011;12(8):469–82.
30. Hardwicke MA, Rendina AR, Williams SP, Moore ML, Wang L, Krueger JA, et al. A human fatty acid synthase inhibitor binds β-ketoacyl reductase in the keto-substrate site. Nat Chem Biol. 2014;10(9):774–9.
31. Gonzalez-Salinas F, Rojo R, Martinez-Amador C, Herrera-Gamboa J, Trevino V. Transcriptomic and cellular analyses of CRISPR/Cas9-mediated edition of FASN show inhibition of aggressive characteristics in breast cancer cells. Biochem Biophys Res Commun. 2020;529(2):321–7.

32. Wang H, Sun W. CRISPR-mediated targeting of HER2 inhibits cell proliferation through a dominant negative mutation. Cancer Lett. 2017;385:137–43.
33. Bernardo GM, Keri RA. FOXA1: a transcription factor with parallel functions in development and cancer. Biosci Rep. 2012;32(2):113–30.
34. Zhang G, Zhao Y, Liu Y, Kao LP, Wang X, Skerry B, Li Z. FOXA1 defines cancer cell specificity. Sci Adv. 2016;2(3):e1501473.
35. Yang H, Jaeger M, Walker A, Wei D, Leiker K, Weitao T. Break Breast Cancer Addiction by CRISPR/Cas9 Genome Editing. J Cancer. 2018;9(2):219–31.
36. Wang Y, Zhang T, Kwiatkowski N, Abraham BJ, Lee TI, Xie S, et al. CDK7-dependent transcriptional addiction in triple-negative breast cancer. Cell. 2015;163(1):174–86.
37. Sun B, Mason S, Wilson RC, Hazard SE, Wang Y, Fang R, et al. Inhibition of the transcriptional kinase CDK7 overcomes therapeutic resistance in HER2-positive breast cancers. Oncogene. 2020;39(1):50–63.
38. Bolt MJ, Stossi F, Callison AM, Mancini MG, Dandekar R, Mancini MA. Systems level-based RNAi screening by high content analysis identifies UBR5 as a regulator of estrogen receptor-α protein levels and activity. Oncogene. 2015;34(2):154–64.
39. Liao L, Song M, Li X, Tang L, Zhang T, Zhang L, et al. E3 Ubiquitin Ligase UBR5 Drives the Growth and Metastasis of Triple-Negative Breast Cancer. Cancer Res. 2017;77(8):2090–101.
40. Luo S, Chen J, Mo X. The association of PTEN hypermethylation and breast cancer: a meta-analysis. Onco Targets Ther. 2016;9:5643–50.
41. Zuo T, Wang L, Morrison C, Chang X, Zhang H, Li W, et al. FOXP3 is an X-linked breast cancer suppressor gene and an important repressor of the HER-2/ErbB2 oncogene. Cell. 2007;129(7):1275–86.
42. Cui X, Zhang C, Xu Z, Wang S, Li X, Stringer-Reasor E, et al. Dual CRISPR interference and activation for targeted reactivation of X-linked endogenous FOXP3 in human breast cancer cells. Mol Cancer. 2022;21(1):38.
43. Dekkers JF, Whittle JR, Vaillant F, Chen HR, Dawson C, Liu K, et al. Modeling Breast Cancer Using CRISPR-Cas9-Mediated Engineering of Human Breast Organoids. J Natl Cancer Inst. 2020;112(5):540–4.
44. Azangou-Khyavy M, Ghasemi M, Khanali J, Boroomand-Saboor M, Jamalkhah M, Soleimani M, Kiani J. CRISPR/Cas: From Tumor Gene Editing to T Cell-Based Immunotherapy of Cancer. Front Immunol. 2020;11:2062.

45. Grenier JM, Yeung ST, Khanna KM. Combination Immunotherapy: Taking Cancer Vaccines to the Next Level. Front Immunol. 2018;9:610.
46. Eyquem J, Mansilla-Soto J, Giavridis T, van der Stegen SJ, Hamieh M, Cunanan KM, et al. Targeting a CAR to the TRAC locus with CRISPR/Cas9 enhances tumour rejection. Nature. 2017;543(7643):113–7.
47. Fan P, He Z-Y, Xu T, Phan K, Chen GG, Wei Y-Q. Exposing cancer with CRISPR-Cas9: from genetic identification to clinical therapy. Translational Cancer Research. 2018;7(3):817–27.
48. Gurusamy D, Henning AN, Yamamoto TN, Yu Z, Zacharakis N, Krishna S, et al. Multi-phenotype CRISPR-Cas9 Screen Identifies p38 Kinase as a Target for Adoptive Immunotherapies. Cancer Cell. 2020;37(6):818–33.e9.
49. Deng H, Tan S, Gao X, Zou C, Xu C, Tu K, et al. Cdk5 knocking out mediated by CRISPR-Cas9 genome editing for PD-L1 attenuation and enhanced antitumor immunity. Acta Pharm Sin B. 2020;10(2):358–73.
50. Russ A, Hua AB, Montfort WR, Rahman B, Riaz IB, Khalid MU, et al. Blocking "don't eat me" signal of CD47-SIRPα in hematological malignancies, an in-depth review. Blood Rev. 2018;32(6):480–9.
51. Chao MP, Weissman IL, Majeti R. The CD47-SIRPα pathway in cancer immune evasion and potential therapeutic implications. Curr Opin Immunol. 2012;24(2):225–32.
52. Wang G, Chow RD, Bai Z, Zhu L, Errami Y, Dai X, et al. Multiplexed activation of endogenous genes by CRISPRa elicits potent antitumor immunity. Nat Immunol. 2019;20(11):1494–505.
53. Bukowski K, Kciuk M, Kontek R. Mechanisms of Multidrug Resistance in Cancer Chemotherapy. Int J Mol Sci. 2020;21(9):3233.
54. Haider T, Pandey V, Banjare N, Gupta PN, Soni V. Drug resistance in cancer: mechanisms and tackling strategies. Pharmacol Rep. 2020;72(5):1125–51.
55. Vaghari-Tabari M, Hassanpour P, Sadeghsoltani F, Malakoti F, Alemi F, Qujeq D, et al. CRISPR/Cas9 gene editing: a new approach for overcoming drug resistance in cancer. Cell Mol Biol Lett. 2022;27(1):49.
56. Shalem O, Sanjana NE, Zhang F. High-throughput functional genomics using CRISPR-Cas9. Nat Rev Genet. 2015;16(5):299–311.
57. Ogbu SC, Rojas S, Weaver J, Musich PR, Zhang J, Yao ZQ, Jiang Y. DSTYK Enhances Chemoresistance in Triple-Negative Breast Cancer Cells. Cells. 2021;11(1):97.
58. Wang X, Yu J, Liu X, Luo D, Li Y, Song L, et al. PSMG2-controlled proteasome-autophagy balance mediates the tolerance for

MEK-targeted therapy in triple-negative breast cancer. Cell Rep Med. 2022;3(9):100741.

59. Shu S, Wu HJ, Ge JY, Zeid R, Harris IS, Jovanović B, et al. Synthetic Lethal and Resistance Interactions with BET Bromodomain Inhibitors in Triple-Negative Breast Cancer. Mol Cell. 2020;78(6):1096–113.e8.
60. Ge JY, Shu S, Kwon M, Jovanović B, Murphy K, Gulvady A, et al. Acquired resistance to combined BET and CDK4/6 inhibition in triple-negative breast cancer. Nat Commun. 2020;11(1):2350.
61. Shaath H, Vishnubalaji R, Elango R, Khattak S, Alajez NM. Single-cell long noncoding RNA (lncRNA) transcriptome implicates MALAT1 in triple-negative breast cancer (TNBC) resistance to neoadjuvant chemotherapy. Cell Death Discov. 2021;7(1):23.
62. Fugger K, Bajrami I, Silva Dos Santos M, Young SJ, Kunzelmann S, Kelly G, et al. Targeting the nucleotide salvage factor DNPH1 sensitizes BRCA-deficient cells to PARP inhibitors. Science. 2021;372(6538):156–65.
63. Tiwari PK, Ko TH, Dubey R, Chouhan M, Tsai LW, Singh HN, et al. CRISPR/Cas9 as a therapeutic tool for triple negative breast cancer: from bench to clinics. Front Mol Biosci. 2023;10:1214489.
64. Abd El-Aziz YS, Spillane AJ, Jansson PJ, Sahni S. Role of ABCB1 in mediating chemoresistance of triple-negative breast cancers. Biosci Rep. 2021;41(2):BSR20204092.
65. Famta P, Shah S, Chatterjee E, Singh H, Dey B, Guru SK, et al. Exploring new Horizons in overcoming P-glycoprotein-mediated multidrug-resistant breast cancer via nanoscale drug delivery platforms. Curr Res Pharmacol Drug Discov. 2021;2:100054.
66. Palasuberniam P, Yang X, Kraus D, Jones P, Myers KA, Chen B. ABCG2 transporter inhibitor restores the sensitivity of triple negative breast cancer cells to aminolevulinic acid-mediated photodynamic therapy. Sci Rep. 2015;5:13298.
67. Deepak Singh D, Han I, Choi EH, Yadav DK. CRISPR/Cas9 based genome editing for targeted transcriptional control in triple-negative breast cancer. Comput Struct Biotechnol J. 2021;19:2384–97.
68. Moiseenko F, Volkov N, Bogdanov A, Dubina M, Moiseyenko V. Resistance mechanisms to drug therapy in breast cancer and other solid tumors: An opinion. F1000Res. 2017;6:288.

69. Oppel F, Schürmann M, Goon P, Albers AE, Sudhoff H. Specific Targeting of Oncogenes Using CRISPR Technology. Cancer Res. 2018;78(19):5506–12.
70. Schmelas C, Grimm D. Split Cas9, Not Hairs — Advancing the Therapeutic Index of CRISPR Technology. Biotechnol J. 2018;13(9):e1700432.
71. Kühn R, Chu VT. Pop in, pop out: a novel gene-targeting strategy for use with CRISPR-Cas9. Genome Biol. 2015;16:244.
72. Chew WL. Immunity to CRISPR Cas9 and Cas12a therapeutics. Wiley Interdiscip Rev Syst Biol Med. 2018;10(1):e1408.
73. Hochheiser K, Kueh AJ, Gebhardt T, Herold MJ. CRISPR/Cas9: A tool for immunological research. Eur J Immunol. 2018;48(4):576–83.
74. Mollanoori H, Shahraki H, Rahmati Y, Teimourian S. CRISPR/Cas9 and CAR-T cell, collaboration of two revolutionary technologies in cancer immunotherapy, an instruction for successful cancer treatment. Hum Immunol. 2018;79(12):876–82.
75. Modell JW, Jiang W, Marraffini LA. CRISPR-Cas systems exploit viral DNA injection to establish and maintain adaptive immunity. Nature. 2017;544(7648):101–4.
76. Liang C, Li F, Wang L, Zhang ZK, Wang C, He B, et al. Tumor cell-targeted delivery of CRISPR/Cas9 by aptamer-functionalized lipopolymer for therapeutic genome editing of VEGFA in osteosarcoma. Biomaterials. 2017;147:68–85.
77. Wang HX, Song Z, Lao YH, Xu X, Gong J, Cheng D, et al. Nonviral gene editing via CRISPR/Cas9 delivery by membrane-disruptive and endosomolytic helical polypeptide. Proc Natl Acad Sci U S A. 2018;115(19):4903–8.
78. Gong S, Yu HH, Johnson KA, Taylor DW. DNA Unwinding Is the Primary Determinant of CRISPR-Cas9 Activity. Cell Rep. 2018;22(2):359–71.
79. Iyer V, Boroviak K, Thomas M, Doe B, Riva L, Ryder E, Adams DJ. No unexpected CRISPR-Cas9 off-target activity revealed by trio sequencing of gene-edited mice. PLoS Genet. 2018;14(7):e1007503.
80. Kimberland ML, Hou W, Alfonso-Pecchio A, Wilson S, Rao Y, Zhang S, Lu Q. Strategies for controlling CRISPR/Cas9 off-target effects and biological variations in mammalian genome editing experiments. J Biotechnol. 2018;284:91–101.

81. Xiao A, Cheng Z, Kong L, Zhu Z, Lin S, Gao G, Zhang B. CasOT: a genome-wide Cas9/gRNA off-target searching tool. Bioinformatics. 2014;30(8):1180–2.
82. Liu C, Zhang L, Liu H, Cheng K. Delivery strategies of the CRISPR-Cas9 gene-editing system for therapeutic applications. J Control Release. 2017;266:17–26.
83. Zhao C, Zhao Y, Zhang J, Lu J, Chen L, Zhang Y, et al. HIT-Cas9: A CRISPR/Cas9 Genome-Editing Device under Tight and Effective Drug Control. Mol Ther Nucleic Acids. 2018;13:208–19.
84. Kleinstiver BP, Pattanayak V, Prew MS, Tsai SQ, Nguyen NT, Zheng Z, Joung JK. High-fidelity CRISPR-Cas9 nucleases with no detectable genome-wide off-target effects. Nature. 2016;529(7587):490–5.
85. Chira S, Gulei D, Hajitou A, Zimta AA, Cordelier P, Berindan-Neagoe I. CRISPR/Cas9: Transcending the Reality of Genome Editing. Mol Ther Nucleic Acids. 2017;7:211–22.
86. Hay EA, Khalaf AR, Marini P, Brown A, Heath K, Sheppard D, MacKenzie A. An analysis of possible off target effects following CAS9/CRISPR targeted deletions of neuropeptide gene enhancers from the mouse genome. Neuropeptides. 2017;64:101–7.
87. Havlicek S, Shen Y, Alpagu Y, Bruntraeger MB, Zufir NB, Phuah ZY, et al. Re-engineered RNA-Guided FokI-Nucleases for Improved Genome Editing in Human Cells. Mol Ther. 2017;25(2):342–55.
88. Zhang XH, Tee LY, Wang XG, Huang QS, Yang SH. Off-target Effects in CRISPR/Cas9-mediated Genome Engineering. Mol Ther Nucleic Acids. 2015;4(11):e264.
89. Zuo E, Cai Y-J, Li K, Wei Y, Wang B-A, Sun Y, et al. One-step generation of complete gene knockout mice and monkeys by CRISPR/Cas9-mediated gene editing with multiple sgRNAs. Cell research. 2017;27(7):933–45.
90. Mo O. CRISPR-Cas9 human genome editing: challenges, ethical concerns and implications. J Clin Res Bioeth. 2015;6(6):1000253.
91. Cyranoski D. First trial of CRISPR in people. Nature. 2016;535(7613):476–7.
92. Castagnini A, Foldager L, Caffo E, Thomsen PH. Early-adult outcome of child and adolescent mental disorders as evidenced by a national-based case register survey. European Psychiatry. 2016;38:45–50.

https://doi.org/10.1142/9789819826759_0003

CHAPTER 3

CRISPR/Cas9 in the Treatment of Glioblastoma

Mehrdad Hashemi[1,2], *Alireza Khosravinejad*[1,3], *Mina Alimohammadi*[4], *Reza Mohajer Shirazi*[1,3], *Behdokht Jamali*[5], *Ali Shirazi*[1,3], *Kimia Sadat Esfahani*[1,3], *Rojin Ghannad Zadeh*[1,6], *Faranak Jamshidian*[1,7], *Neda Zali*[3], *Najma Farahani*[1,*], *Afshin Taheriazam*[1,8,*], *Payman Rahimzadeh*[9,*], *Maliheh Entezari*[1,2,*]

[1]Farhikhtegan Medical Convergent Sciences Research Center, Farhikhtegan Hospital, Faculty of Medicine, TeMs. C., Islamic Azad University, Tehran, Iran
[2]Department of Genetics, Faculty of Advanced Sciences and Technology, TeMs. C, Islamic Azad University, Tehran, Iran
[3]Basic and Molecular Epidemiology of Gastrointestinal Disorders Research Center, Research Institute for Gastroenterology and Liver Diseases, Shahid Beheshti University of Medical Sciences, Tehran, Iran
[4]Department of Immunology, School of Medicine, Shahid Beheshti University of Medical Sciences, Tehran, Iran
[5]Department of Microbiology and Genetics, Kherad Institute of Higher Education, Bushehr, Iran

* **Corresponding authors:** Najmafarahani@gmail.com (N.F.); a.taheriazam@iautmu.ac.ir (A.T.); P.rahimzadeh76@gmail.com (P.R.); mentezari@iautmu.ac.ir (M.E.)

[6]Department of Art & Sciences, Faculty of Biology, University of North Florida, Jacksonville, Florida, USA
[7]Department of Biology, ET.C., Islamic Azad University, Tehran, Iran
[8]Department of Orthopedics, Faculty of Medicine, TeMs. C, Islamic Azad University, Tehran, Iran
[9]Surgical Research Society (SRS), Students' Scientific Research Center, Tehran University of Medical Sciences, Tehran, Iran

Abstract

Glioblastoma is the most common and lethal primary malignant brain tumor in adults, marked by profound histologic and molecular heterogeneity that drives therapeutic resistance and poor survival. Canonical alterations, including TERT-promoter mutation, EGFR amplification, PTEN and CDKN2A loss, chromosome +7/−10 aneuploidy, and divergent evolutionary routes in primary versus secondary glioblastoma, create complex, target-rich but treatment-refractory biology. CRISPR/Cas9, an RNA-guided nuclease platform, has emerged as a versatile engine for precision oncology in glioblastoma: it enables modeling of patient-specific genotypes, functional dissection of driver pathways, genome and epigenome editing of oncogenic nodes, and discovery of synthetic-lethal vulnerabilities. Preclinical studies demonstrate proof-of-concept for disrupting EGFR/EGFRvIII, restoring tumor-suppressor functions, resensitizing tumors to temozolomide, and reprogramming glioblastoma stem-like cells; parallel advances in brain-targeted delivery (viral, nanoparticle, and convection-enhanced) are improving translational feasibility. Nonetheless, key barriers remain: off-target editing, p53-linked DNA-damage responses, intratumoral heterogeneity, immune and stromal constraints in the brain microenvironment, and safety/ethical considerations. This chapter synthesizes current applications and emerging strategies for CRISPR/Cas9 in glioblastoma, highlighting design principles for high-fidelity editors, rational combinations with radio-chemotherapy and immunotherapy, and clinically scalable delivery platforms to translate genome engineering into durable patient benefit.

Keywords: glioblastoma; CRISPR/Cas9; genome editing; EGFR/EGFRvIII; tumor heterogeneity; temozolomide; cancer stem cells

3.1 Introduction

Among adults, glioblastoma represents the most common and aggressive type of primary brain tumor, making up about 45.2% of all brain and central nervous system (CNS) malignancies [1]. As a grade IV diffuse astrocytic glioma, it is characterized by dense cellular growth, nuclear irregularities, blood vessel proliferation, tissue death, and infiltrative behavior. The key molecular signatures of glioblastoma include alterations in the TERT promoter, enhanced EGFR gene expression, and specific chromosomal modifications (+7/−10) [2]. The diverse cellular and molecular characteristics of glioblastoma make it particularly challenging to treat effectively and contribute to its poor survival rates [3].

The classification of glioblastoma includes two main subtypes — primary and secondary — each with unique genetic profiles, age distributions, and clinical outcomes. Primary glioblastoma develops spontaneously in elderly patients and is marked by increased EGFR gene activity, PTEN mutations, CDKN2A gene loss, and sometimes MDM2 gene amplification [1]. In contrast, secondary glioblastoma develops progressively from lower-grade astrocytomas in younger individuals. These cases frequently display TP53 gene mutations as their initial genetic change. These distinctions highlight the fundamental differences between primary and secondary glioblastoma variants.

Current treatment protocols for newly diagnosed glioblastoma patients typically involve maximizing tumor removal surgically, followed by combined radiation and temozolomide chemotherapy, and then maintenance temozolomide treatment [4]. However, even with this intensive therapeutic approach, improvements in patient survival remain limited [1].

The urgent need for effective glioblastoma treatments has become increasingly apparent. While the last 20 years have seen growing research into targeted therapies and immunological approaches, as noted by Begagić et al. [1], these efforts have not significantly extended patient survival. Glioblastoma continues to be an untreatable condition, representing one of neuro-oncology's greatest therapeutic challenges [5]. The field requires new treatment strategies that offer both enhanced effectiveness and reduced toxicity, specifically designed to target glioblastoma's distinct biological features [6].

The identification of specific genetic alterations in glioblastoma, including losses in chromosomes 10 and 9p, along with gains in chromosomes 7 and 19, points to gene therapy as a promising treatment avenue [7]. The CRISPR-Cas9 system, which enables precise genetic modification [8], has emerged as a revolutionary tool across various medical fields over the past ten years [9]. This technology stands out for its speed, cost-effectiveness, adaptability, and reliability in genetic manipulation, making it widely used in studying genetic changes, cancer targets, and epigenetic control mechanisms. For various cancers, including glioblastoma, CRISPR-Cas9 has become the preferred genetic editing method [10, 11]. Given the current focus on developing more accessible medical treatments [12], particularly for regions with limited resources [13], CRISPR-based gene editing shows promise for glioblastoma treatment. While numerous studies have explored this approach for glioblastoma therapy, the findings remain scattered across various research papers. This chapter aims to provide a comprehensive review and analysis of CRISPR-Cas9's capabilities and applications in developing precise gene therapies for glioblastoma.

3.2 Genetic and Molecular Alterations in Glioblastoma

Traditional histopathological classification, while valuable for glioblastoma diagnosis, fails to capture the tumor's complex heterogeneity and provides insufficient guidance for treatment decisions. The 2016 WHO classification of CNS tumors (CNS 4) addressed this limitation by integrating molecular characteristics with histopathological features. Notably, isocitrate dehydrogenase (IDH) mutation status became a key factor in categorizing glioblastoma into two subtypes: IDH-wild-type and IDH-mutant. Primary glioblastoma, corresponding to IDH-wild-type, develops spontaneously without prior lesions, affects approximately 90% of cases, typically occurs in older patients, and shows more aggressive progression. In contrast, IDH-mutant or secondary glioblastoma evolves from existing astrocytomas, represents about 10% of cases, typically affects younger patients (median age 44), and generally has a better outcome.

The 2021 WHO classification (CNS 5) further emphasized molecular-based categorization by incorporating additional genetic markers [14]. These include CDKN2A/B homozygous deletion, TERT promoter mutation, EGFR amplification, and chromosome modifications (+7/−10) as diagnostic criteria for IDH-wild-type glioblastoma [14]. This update strengthens the role of molecular diagnostics in glioblastoma classification.

Glioblastoma's genetic landscape includes several key alterations [15, 16]. Primary glioblastoma (IDH-wild-type) frequently exhibits TERT promoter mutations, PTEN deletions, and EGFR amplification, while secondary glioblastoma (IDH-mutant) commonly shows ATRX and TP53 mutations [15]. Additional genetic changes include modifications in NF1, PDGFRA, PIK3R1, PIK3CA, RB1, CDKN2A/B, MDM2, MDM4, CDK4, and H3F3A [17–20]. These genetic abnormalities typically influence three crucial biological processes: tumor initiation, senescence evasion, and continuous growth [15].

Epigenetic changes, encompassing DNA methylation, histone modifications, and chromatin restructuring, are now recognized as crucial factors in glioblastoma development and progression [21–23]. These modifications serve dual roles as potential diagnostic markers for patient classification and as therapeutic targets due to their reversible nature [21, 22]. A prime example is MGMT promoter methylation, which helps predict treatment response to alkylating agents and assess patient prognosis [24, 25].

Large-scale genome studies have revealed significant epigenetic patterns in glioblastoma [26]. Analysis of DNA methylation in 272 glioblastoma samples from The Cancer Genome Atlas (TCGA) identified a distinct subset showing widespread CpG Island hypermethylation [27]. Such patients demonstrated unique clinical characteristics and outcomes, suggesting epigenetic markers could improve patient classification [27]. DNA methylation patterns have proven valuable in categorizing various CNS tumors, including glioblastoma [28], and show dynamic changes during disease progression [29]. Recent research has also linked epigenetic modifications to the tumor microenvironment, affecting immune responses within glioblastoma [30].

In treatment applications, epigenetic-targeting drugs have shown promise in various cancers, including glioblastoma [23, 30, 31]. For instance, the HDAC inhibitor Vorinostat underwent Phase II trials for recurrent glioblastoma [32]. Histone methyltransferase inhibitors, particularly those targeting PRMT5, have demonstrated ability to trigger cell death and halt glioblastoma cell reproduction in laboratory and animal studies [33]. These epigenetic modifications influence various cellular processes, including cell division, differentiation, blood vessel formation, and programmed cell death, ultimately affecting glioblastoma tumor growth [21, 31]. Detailed reviews of epigenetic-based therapies for glioblastoma can be found in recent publications [22, 23, 31].

Advanced transcriptome analysis techniques have revealed glioblastoma's extensive transcriptional diversity [17, 18, 20, 34–37]. Glioblastoma was among the first cancers comprehensively studied through major international research initiatives like TCGA. Initial microarray studies by Phillips et al. identified three distinct glioblastoma subtypes: proneural, proliferative, and mesenchymal, each with different survival outcomes [38]. Verhaak et al. later expanded this research using a larger TCGA dataset, confirming these findings and adding a fourth subtype: neural [39]. These studies validated transcriptome-based classification as a reliable method for glioblastoma categorization, improving upon traditional histopathological approaches for predicting patient outcomes. Furthermore, they revealed connections between transcriptomic changes and other molecular alterations, enhancing our understanding of glioblastoma development and progression.

However, these bulk tissue analyses had limitations in capturing intra-tumor heterogeneity [40, 41] and understanding the tumor microenvironment's influence [42–44]. Recent single-cell RNA sequencing studies have addressed these shortcomings [41, 45].

This advanced technology has revealed the complex cellular composition within glioblastoma tumors [45–47]. Research now shows that glioblastoma heterogeneity exists both within tumor cells and their surrounding microenvironment, with significant differences between initial and recurring tumors a factor considered crucial in treatment resistance [45–51].

3.3 CRISPR-Cas9-based Genome-Wide Screens in Glioblastoma

CRISPR-Cas9 screening technology has emerged as a valuable tool for glioblastoma research, enabling identification of new biomarkers, cancer-driving genes, chemotherapy resistance mechanisms, and therapeutic response factors. These screens employ either knockout or interference methods, primarily using glioblastoma cell lines and glioma stem cells (GSCs), with some applications in cerebral organoids and mouse models. The genetic modifications are typically introduced through viral vectors carrying either coding or non-coding guide RNA libraries.

Several significant discoveries have been made using this technology. Research using CRISPR-Cas9 genome-wide knockouts identified ribosomal protein subunits 11, 16, and 18 as key biomarkers for glioblastoma response to topoisomerase II inhibitors [52]. This study also revealed that ribosomal subunit 11 deletion contributed to resistance against common chemotherapy drugs like etoposide and doxorubicin [52]. Another investigation found that NF-κB and E2F6 genes play crucial roles in temozolomide resistance in EGFRvIII-expressing U87MG cells [53].

Additional CRISPR-Cas9 applications include the identification of glioblastoma suppressor genes through *in vivo* screening in mice [54], the discovery of MAP4K4 as a key invasion regulator in U138MG cells [55], and the identification of genetic modifications affecting CD8+ T cell surface proteins that influence immunotherapy effectiveness in glioblastoma [56].

CRISPR-Cas9 screening has made significant contributions to understanding glioblastoma stem cell biology. Researchers employed this technology to identify key transcription factors governing growth, stemness characteristics, and temozolomide resistance in GSCs [57]. Using three-dimensional bioprinted systems, genome-wide CRISPR-Cas9 screening revealed new molecular regulators of cancer stem cells, highlighting the importance of tumor-microenvironment interactions [58]. Another notable discovery through CRISPR-Cas9 knockout screening showed that GSCs, unlike neural stem cells (NSCs), lose redundancy between mitosis regulators PKMYT1 and WEE1, resulting in enhanced growth [59].

The technology has also proven valuable in studying non-coding genomic regions in glioblastoma. CRISPR-Cas9 interference screening identified specific long non-coding RNAs that influence U87MG cell growth and radiation sensitivity [60]. Additionally, this approach revealed amplified non-coding DNA regions that regulate co-amplified cancer-causing genes in glioblastoma [61]. These findings have enhanced our understanding of the functional relationships among diverse glioblastoma mutations, potentially leading to new therapeutic strategies.

3.4 Mechanism and Rationale of CRISPR/Cas9 in Glioblastoma Therapy: Targeting Oncogenes or Restoring Tumor Suppressors

The development of glioblastoma is primarily driven by several factors, including specific genetic variations, exposure to ionizing radiation, and the effects of chemical carcinogens on brain tissue [61]. CRISPR/Cas9 technology is emerging as a promising tool in glioblastoma immunotherapy research. This innovative approach continues to gain attention in various studies and shows potential to become a crucial element in advancing both gene research and therapeutic strategies for glioma treatment [62].

While earlier studies lacked a systematic classification of precise gene therapy approaches for glioblastoma, Begagić et al. [1] identified three main therapeutic targets: protein kinase pathways, cell cycle mechanisms, and microenvironmental/immunomodulatory factors. In examining CRISPR/Cas9 applications in glioblastoma treatment, this chapter organizes specific gene targets into four main categories: cell cycle control, microenvironment regulation, interphase regulation, and mechanisms for reducing therapy resistance.

3.4.1 *CRISPR/Cas9 in Cell Cycle Control*

The cell cycle represents a crucial biological mechanism that controls organismal growth and development through precisely regulated events [1]. This process ensures accurate genetic information transfer between cell generations. When mutations occur, these genetic alterations are transmitted to daughter cells during division. This mechanism is particularly significant in glioblastoma, where cell cycle disruptions caused by genetic changes lead to abnormal cell proliferation.

Genetic control of the cell cycle is paramount, and mutations in regulatory genes can result in unrestricted glioblastoma cell division and growth. Research has identified several key mutations linked to glioblastoma development, affecting genes including EGFR, ERBB2, IDH1, NF1, PIK3CA, PIK3R1, and PTEN, among others.

Studies using glioblastoma cell lines and *in vitro* models have demonstrated CRISPR-Cas9's effectiveness in promoting cell death and autophagy. Researchers have targeted various genes, including PDPN, C14orf166, IGFBP3, IGFBP5, ERN1, ATF4, ATG5, CHAF1A, FAT1, CIS, ATG7, and PIN1.

In CRISPR-Cas9 applications, three distinct approaches are utilized: knockout (complete gene elimination, as shown in FAT1 gene studies enhancing apoptosis susceptibility), knockdown (reducing gene expression, demonstrated in PDPN studies affecting cell death and proliferation), and knock-in strategies. Each approach serves specific research and therapeutic purposes in glioblastoma treatment.

Wang et al. [63] conducted a study utilizing PDPN gene knockdown to investigate mechanisms of cell death and growth regulation, with a particular focus on surface-membrane molecules. Mutations in PDPN are closely linked to the aggressive and invasive behavior of glioblastoma multiforme. Their findings demonstrated that PDPN overexpression enhances macrophage M2 polarization and neutrophil degranulation, underscoring its pivotal role in reshaping the tumor microenvironment. This immunomodulatory activity suggests that PDPN contributes significantly to the establishment of an immunosuppressive niche, especially in IDH-wild-type gliomas, thereby promoting immune evasion and tumor progression [63].

In parallel, several notable CRISPR-Cas9-based investigations have further elucidated key molecular pathways in glioblastoma. Knockout studies targeting IGFBP3 and IGFBP5 revealed their involvement in apoptosis initiation via the unfolded protein response mechanism [64]. Research on ATG5 gene disruption highlighted its dual impact on apoptosis and autophagy [65]. CHAF1A knockout experiments shed light on its regulatory influence over the AKT/FOXO3a/Bim signaling axis, affecting both cell proliferation and DNA repair processes [66]. FAT1 gene ablation was shown to mediate apoptosis through activation of the death-inducing signaling complex [67]. Investigations into the CIS gene uncovered its role in modulating NK-cell activation, apoptotic pathways, and broader immune responses [68]. Moreover, combined knockouts of ATG5 and ATG7 provided insights into their cooperative function in autophagosome membrane formation [69].

Further CRISPR-Cas9 studies have delved into additional dimensions of glioblastoma cell cycle regulation. PIN1 knockout experiments revealed its multifaceted role in glioblastoma pathogenesis, influencing cell death, migration, and progression through the cell cycle. Targeted disruption of ATM, PTEN, p85α, and XIAP genes highlighted their tumor-suppressive functions, offering deeper insights into the molecular control of cell cycle dynamics in glioblastoma [70]. Investigations into RGS4 gene knockout elucidated its involvement in apoptosis via G protein-coupled signaling pathways, while GLI1-targeted studies demonstrated its regulatory effect on cell death through the PI3K/Akt axis [71].

Collectively, the expanding landscape of CRISPR-Cas9 applications in glioblastoma research has unveiled a spectrum of gene manipulation strategies, each contributing to our understanding of tumor biology. These include gene knockouts [e.g., FAT1, ATM, PTEN, GLI1], gene expression modulation [e.g., PDPN, IGFBP3, CHAF1A], and knock-in approaches. Such interventions have significantly advanced our comprehension of cell death regulation, proliferation control, and immune system interactions within the glioblastoma microenvironment. Importantly, these findings challenge prevailing models of gene function and open new avenues for therapeutic innovation through precise molecular targeting. As CRISPR-Cas9 technology continues to evolve, its integration into glioblastoma research holds promise for the development of more effective and personalized treatment strategies against this highly aggressive malignancy.

CRISPR/Cas9 gene therapy research in glioblastoma multiforme has extensively focused on cell interphase-related targets to elucidate gene regulation during critical phases of the cell cycle. This emphasis on interphase — comprising the G1, S, and G2 phases — is essential for understanding glioblastoma development and identifying potential therapeutic strategies [35]. Recent CRISPR-Cas9 investigations have targeted a range of genes with diverse functional implications. Fierro et al. [72] studied the effects of PD-L1 knockout on cell proliferation, invasion, and macrophage behavior, highlighting its immunomodulatory role. Lumibao et al. [73] explored CHCHD2 knockout, demonstrating its impact on mitochondrial function and cell growth, particularly in EGFRvIII-mutant glioblastoma contexts. Toledano et al. [74] examined Plexin-A2 knockout, revealing its influence on cellular morphology, flattening, and cycle arrest, with mechanistic links to β-galactosidase, MAPK, and FARP2 signaling pathways. Gallo et al. [75] investigated 14-3-3β knockout, identifying its regulatory interactions with Bad, FBI1, Raf-1, and Cdc25b, and its role in cell growth modulation. Guda et al. [76] analyzed RGS4 knockout, showing its impact on MMP2 expression and tumor cell proliferation. Zhang et al. [77] utilized Nanos3 knockdown to assess its effects on stemness markers such as CD133 and Oct4, as well as its.

Recent investigations utilizing CRISPR/Cas9 techniques have examined various genes and their functions in cell renewal regulation. Research conducted by Bulstrode and colleagues [78] examined Foxo3's influence on differentiation through knockdown experiments, while also examining FOXG1, SOX2, EGFR, and EGFRvIII's involvement in renewal mechanisms. In another study, researchers [79] evaluated SRR2's function in self-renewal capabilities, particularly regarding SOX2, through deletion methods. Further research by Song and collaborators explored SRSF3's role in alternative splicing processes related to glioma through knockout approaches.

Research into cellular migration using CRISPR/Cas9 has enhanced our understanding of its molecular mechanisms. Scientists [80] investigated TP53's role in migration through recombination studies. Additional research [81] examined migration regulation through knockout studies of NRP2, Plexin-A4, Plexin-D1, and Semaphorin-3C. MAP4K4's impact on migration and invasion was revealed through knockout experiments [55], while BRG1's influence on migration, proliferation, and temozolomide resistance was demonstrated through similar methods [82]. Further investigations [83] revealed PIK3CD, PAK3, and PLEK2's contributions to migration and invasion processes. Research teams also explored THBS1 and TNF's effects on proliferation and migration [84], as well as ASH2L and SET1/MLL's involvement in these processes [85]. Studies on miR21 and SOX2 [86] provided insights into migration, invasion, and proliferation, while examination of GFAP variants [87] illuminated their role in invasion.

These collective findings using CRISPR/Cas9 technology have expanded our knowledge of glioblastoma cellular processes. The research has revealed intricate molecular networks controlling cell cycle progression, growth, and differentiation. Studies on renewal mechanisms have clarified how Foxo3, SRR2, and SRSF3 influence cellular regeneration and splicing patterns. Additionally, migration studies targeting various genes like TP53, NRP2, MAP4K4, and others have enhanced our understanding of glioblastoma cell movement and proliferation dynamics (**Table 3.1**).

Table 3.1 CRISPR-Cas9 applications in glioblastoma cell cycle research.

Gene Target	CRISPR-based Strategy	Primary Function/ Pathway	Impact on Cell Cycle Processes	Reference
PDPN	Knockdown	Surface-membrane cell molecules, immunomodulation	Modulates apoptosis, cell proliferation, macrophage M2 polarization	[63]
IGFBP3/ IGFBP5	Knockout	Unfolded protein response mechanism	Influences cell cycle dynamics, initiates apoptosis	[64]
ATG5	Knockout	Autophagy regulation	Dual impact on apoptosis and autophagy in cell cycle processes	[65]
CHAF1A	Knockout	AKT/FOXO3a/Bim pathway	Affects proliferation and DNA repair mechanisms	[66]
FAT1	Knockout	Death-inducing signaling complex	Active involvement in apoptosis during glioblastoma progression	[67]
CIS	Knockout	NK cell activation	Links immune responses to molecular mechanisms influencing cell cycle	[68]
ATG5/ ATG7	Knockout	Autophagosome membrane formation	Significance in autophagy regulation of cell cycle	[69]

(*Continued*)

Table 3.1 (*Continued*)

Gene Target	CRISPR-based Strategy	Primary Function/ Pathway	Impact on Cell Cycle Processes	Reference
PIN1	Knockout	Peptidylprolyl isomerase activity	Influences apoptosis, migration, and cell cycle progression	[88]
ATM/ PTEN/ p85α/ XIAP	Knockout	Tumor suppression	Regulatory mechanisms governing cell cycle in glioblastoma	[70]
RGS4	Knockout	G protein signaling	Impact on apoptosis and potential therapeutic implications	[76]
GLI1	Knockout	PI3K/Akt pathway	Involvement in apoptosis and cell cycle regulation	[71]
PD-L1	Knockout	Immune checkpoint regulation	Impacts proliferation, invasion, and macrophage polarization	[72]
CHCHD2	Knockout	Mitochondrial respiration	Influences cell growth inhibition in EGFRvIII context	[73]
Plexin-A2	Knockout	Cytoskeletal organization	Involved in cell cycle arrest through MAPK and FARP2	[74]
14-3-3β	Knockout	Protein interactions (Bad, FBI1, Raf-1, Cdc25b)	Affects proliferation and spheroid formation	[75]

Table 3.1 (*Continued*)

Gene Target	CRISPR-based Strategy	Primary Function/ Pathway	Impact on Cell Cycle Processes	Reference
CDK7	Knockout	Cell cycle regulation	Role in cellular growth processes	
Nanos3	Knockdown	Stem cell regulation (CD133, Oct4)	Implications for proliferation, migration, chemoresistance	[77]
NRF2	Knockdown	Oxidative stress response	Role in self-renewal and cell proliferation	[89]
Dazl	Knockout	Regulatory axis (CD133/Oct4/ Nanog/Sox2)	Impact on proliferation processes	[90]
ERβ	Knockout	Estrogen receptor signaling	Effects on proliferation and apoptosis through mTOR/ STAT-3	[91]

3.4.2 *CRISPR/Cas9 and Microenvironmental Targets*

Glioblastoma investigations have increasingly concentrated on understanding and manipulating the tumor's surrounding environment, with special attention to blood vessel formation. A key investigation [92] focused on reducing Notch1 gene expression to examine its effects on oxygen deprivation, blood vessel development, and tumor expansion. Notch1, which plays multiple roles in cell functions, was targeted using CRISPR/Cas9 technology. This approach aimed to understand how reducing Notch1 levels affects the complex relationship between low oxygen conditions, blood vessel formation, and glioblastoma cell growth patterns.

Further research [93] examined PDPN's function through elimination studies, exploring how it affects blood vessel development and structural integrity in mouse brain tissue. PDPN interacts with platelet receptors (C-type lectin-like receptor 2) and contributes to blood vessel formation. The researchers used CRISPR/Cas9 to remove PDPN, aiming to disrupt normal blood vessel development processes. This intervention targeted systems that support glioblastoma growth and spread. Through this focused examination of PDPN, researchers gained valuable insights into how this molecule influences the vascular environment surrounding glioblastoma tumors.

Research [94] investigated DDX39B's influence on the extracellular matrix and blood vessel formation through NF-κB signaling. Using gene reduction techniques, scientists examined how DDX39B affects the complex signaling networks involved in blood vessel development and extracellular matrix regulation. The study focused on the NF-κB pathway, which is crucial for inflammation and blood vessel formation, to better understand its role in the glioblastoma environment. This research enhanced our knowledge of how specific genes can be modified to affect pro-angiogenic factors in glioblastoma.

In related work, researchers [95] studied BIG1 and BIG2 genes in 2019, focusing on reducing VEGF expression. VEGF plays a central role in forming new blood vessels that support tumor growth. The scientists used CRISPR/Cas9 to decrease BIG1 and BIG2 expression, thereby reducing VEGF levels, with the goal of disrupting blood vessel formation in glioblastoma tumors. This gene manipulation revealed important regulatory mechanisms controlling blood vessel development and suggested new therapeutic approaches.

These combined studies highlight CRISPR/Cas9's importance in understanding glioblastoma's complex environment. Through precise modification of genes controlling blood vessel formation (including Notch1, PDPN, DDX39B, BIG1, and BIG2), scientists have revealed molecular mechanisms governing blood vessel development, identifying potential treatment targets. Research targeting genes like CIS, OPN, and AIM2 has shown how CRISPR/Cas9 can enhance immune cell function, modify macrophage behavior, and trigger cell death, contributing to glioblastoma immune regulation. CRISPR/Cas9's versatility in modifying these environmental factors offers promising directions for developing targeted glioblastoma treatments, demonstrating its potential as a revolutionary tool in glioblastoma therapy development (**Figure 3.1**).

3.5 CRISPR/Cas9 in Overcoming Treatment Resistance

Recent research has explored various genetic approaches to combat treatment resistance in glioblastoma. A study [96] focused on reducing ALDH1A3 expression to decrease temozolomide resistance. In 2023, researchers [97] targeted the MGMT gene through reduction techniques to address temozolomide resistance. Another 2023 investigation [98] decreased MUC1 expression, which is linked to EGFRvIII, also aiming to overcome temozolomide resistance. Scientists [99] eliminated the GSS gene to tackle radiation therapy resistance, particularly examining its relationship with Angiopep-2. A 2020 study [100] targeted several membrane proteins — MSH2, PTCH2, CLCA2, FZD6, CTNNB1, and NRF2 — using CRISPR/Cas9 elimination to combat temozolomide resistance. Additional research [101] focused on eliminating HPRT1 to address temozolomide resistance through AMPK pathways.

Several of these approaches showed promising results. The ALDH1A3 targeting study [96] effectively reduced temozolomide resistance, particularly at concentrations up to 300 μM. Research [97] successfully increased temozolomide effectiveness by reducing MGMT expression. The MUC1 study [98] revealed this gene's importance in repairing DNA damage during cancer treatments.

However, some approaches proved less effective. Despite targeting multiple genes [MSH2, PTCH2, CLCA2, FZD6, CTNNB1, and NRF2], the study by Rocha and colleagues [100] found that reducing expression of the three main target genes did not increase glioblastoma cells' sensitivity to temozolomide.

3.6 CRISPR/Cas9 and Glioblastoma Stem Cells

GSCs represent a distinct tumor cell subset with self-renewal abilities that drive glioblastoma progression, growth maintenance,

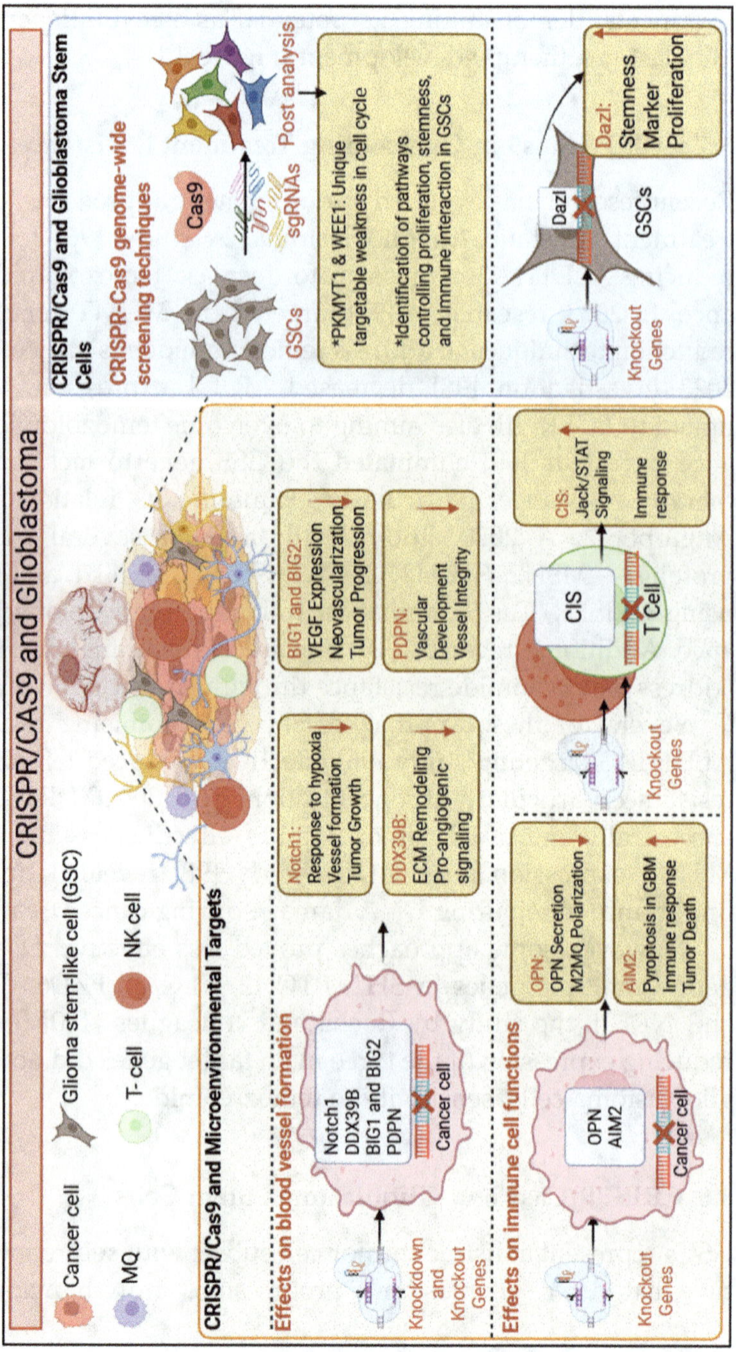
CRISPR/CAS9 and Glioblastoma
Cancer cell
MQ
Glioma stem-like cell (GSC)
T-cell
NK cell
CRISPR/Cas9 and Microenvironmental Targets
Effects on blood vessel formation
Knockdown and Knockout Genes
Notch1
DDX39B
BIG1 and BIG2
PDPN
Cancer cell
Notch1:
Response to hypoxia
Vessel formation
Tumor Growth
BIG1 and BIG2:
VEGF Expression
Neovascularization
Tumor Progression
DDX39B:
ECM Remodeling
Pro-angiogenic signaling
PDPN:
Vascular Development
Vessel Integrity
Effects on immune cell functions
Knockout Genes
OPN
AIM2
Cancer cell
OPN:
OPN Secretion
M2MQ Polarization
AIM2:
Pyroptosis in GBM
Immune response
Tumor Death
Knockout Genes
CIS
T Cell
CIS:
Jack/STAT Signaling
Immune response
CRISPR/Cas9 and Glioblastoma Stem Cells
CRISPR-Cas9 genome-wide screening techniques
GSCs
Cas9
sgRNAs
Post analysis
*PKMYT1 & WEE1: Unique targetable weakness in cell cycle
*Identification of pathways controlling proliferation, stemness, and immune interaction in GSCs
Knockout Genes
Dazl
GSCs
Dazl:
Stemness
Marker
Proliferation

Figure 3.1 CRISPR/Cas9 applications in targeting glioblastoma and its microenvironment. The illustration demonstrates the multifaceted utility of CRISPR/Cas9 genome editing technologies for investigating and therapeutically targeting glioblastoma and its tumor microenvironment. **Microenvironmental targets: Effects on blood vessel formation:** CRISPR/Cas9-mediated knockout of cancer cell genes such as Notch1, DDX39B, BIG1, BIG2, and PDPN modulates key processes in vasculature and angiogenesis. Notch1 drives vessel formation and tumor growth in response to hypoxia; DDX39B participates in extracellular matrix remodeling and pro-angiogenic signaling; BIG1 and BIG2 promote VEGF expression and neovascularization, contributing to tumor progression; and PDPN is crucial for vascular development and vessel integrity. Disruption of these genes impairs tumor neovascularization and progression. **Effects on immune cell functions:** Targeting OPN and AIM2 genes in cancer cells using CRISPR/Cas9 influences tumor-immune interactions. OPN knockout impairs osteopontin secretion and shifts macrophage polarization, while AIM2 knockout impacts pyroptosis, immune response, and tumor cell death. In immune cells, the knockout of CIS in T cells enhances JAK/STAT pathway activation, boosting anti-tumor immunity. **Glioblastoma stem cells:** CRISPR-Cas9 genome-wide screening techniques are employed with GSCs to identify vulnerabilities in cell cycle regulation (e.g., PKMYT1 and WEE1 pathways) and pathways regulating proliferation, stemness, and immune interactions unique to GSCs. **Stemness and proliferation:** Knockout studies targeting Dazl in GSCs highlight its critical role as a stemness marker and regulator of tumor cell proliferation. Together, the figure underscores the power of CRISPR/Cas9 platforms for functional genomics, drug target validation, and the development of novel therapeutic strategies that simultaneously disrupt tumor growth, vascularization, immune escape, and cancer stem cell maintenance in glioblastoma.

treatment resistance, and tumor recurrence [102, 103]. When these specialized cells become active and multiply, they lead to more aggressive forms of cancer that do not respond well to standard treatments [102, 103]. These cells differ both genetically and in their characteristics from the original tumor. They resist radiation and chemotherapy treatments by activating specific genetic and molecular pathways that prevent cell death, enhance DNA repair, control cell growth, or temporarily pause growth with the ability to resume later [102, 103].

Laboratory findings suggest that combining different therapeutic approaches synergistically could effectively reduce self-renewal capabilities and trigger programmed cell death in human GSCs. Currently, CRISPR-Cas9 genetic modification has become a widely adopted tool for comprehensive genetic screening, gene insertion, removal, and reduction of stem cell-related genes to better understand their roles in glioblastoma development and recurrence.

CRISPR-Cas9 genome-wide screening techniques have helped identify molecular signals crucial for maintaining glioblastoma growth and stem cell characteristics. Additionally, these screening methods, applied to both patient-derived GSCs and NSCs, have identified genes typically present in developing nerve cells that become reactivated in glioblastoma. Genome-wide screening of patient-derived GSCs using CRISPR-Cas9 technology has identified key mutations in genes regulating cell division, notably PKMYT1 and WEE1 [59]. The study revealed that GSCs lack the normal redundancy observed between these mitosis-regulating genes in NSCs, suggesting a unique vulnerability in glioblastoma cell cycle control [59]. Complementary research employed comprehensive genome-wide approaches to investigate signaling pathways governing GSC proliferation, stemness, and their interactions with macrophages, further illuminating the complexity of the tumor microenvironment [58].

CRISPR-Cas9 has also proven instrumental in dissecting the genetic regulation of stem cell characteristics in glioblastoma. For example, deletion of the Dazl gene — known to influence both cell division and stemness — resulted in reduced expression of stem cell markers, diminished cell proliferation, and increased sensitivity to chemotherapeutic agents such as doxorubicin and temozolomide [90].

3.7 Challenges, Risks, and Safety Considerations

While CRISPR/Cas9 shows great promise for genome modification and enhancing cancer immunotherapy, particularly in CAR-T cell function, several challenges remain before widespread clinical implementation. Key concerns include accuracy of targeting, potential DNA alterations, and safety considerations. Current research shows that Cas9 protein and sgRNA can reduce PD-1 in EvCAR T cells, effectively targeting EGFRvIII glioblastoma cells without affecting other checkpoint receptors, though further *in vivo* studies are needed. The technology's ability to modify multiple checkpoint signals offers promising therapeutic potential, but requires additional clinical evaluation to confirm safety and effectiveness.

The relationship between p53 and CRISPR editing presents specific challenges [104]. As a genetic guardian, p53 detects DNA damage and controls cell division and death responses. During CRISPR editing, which involves DNA strand breaks, p53's protective response can reduce editing efficiency by eliminating modified cells [104]. The situation becomes more complex as cells that survive CRISPR modification may have defective p53 function [104, 105]. This creates a concerning scenario where the editing process might preferentially preserve cells with impaired p53 function, reducing their ability to maintain genetic stability. Such cells face increased risks of mutation accumulation and potential cancer development [106].

This complex interaction between cellular defense mechanisms and gene editing technology highlights the need for careful consideration in therapeutic applications, particularly in cancer treatment contexts where genomic stability is crucial.

Many CRISPR/Cas9 studies targeting glioblastoma have shown positive results. Research [72] successfully reduced PD-L1 protein levels by 64% in U87 cells through gene elimination. Scientists [73] removed CHCHD2 in EGFRvIII-expressing U87 cells, successfully altering mitochondrial function, glutathione levels, and reducing cell growth and invasion. Another study [74] eliminated Plexin-A2, revealing its growth-promoting effects through FARP2, FYN, and GAP domain interactions. Additional successful interventions included RGS4 elimination [76], which decreased cell multiplication, and Nanos3 reduction [77], which limited cancer cell growth, movement, and spread, while also making cells more sensitive to doxorubicin and temozolomide treatments.

However, some genetic modifications produced unexpected or limited results. Research targeting TP53 [80] through genetic recombination had unclear effects on cell movement. Studies eliminating NRP2, Plexin-A4, Plexin-D1, and Semaphorin-3C [81] showed that Sema3D and Sema3G required neuropilins for signaling. MAP4K4 elimination [55] achieved only a 41% reduction in cell invasion compared to control groups. While BRG1 elimination [82] successfully reduced glioblastoma cell movement and invasion while increasing temozolomide effectiveness, other gene modifications did not achieve their expected outcomes, highlighting glioblastoma's complex nature and the need for continued research to develop effective treatments.

Studies targeting angiogenesis and tumor growth showed varied results. Research reducing Notch1 [92] found that modified tumors grew more slowly, taking 18.3 days versus 13.4 days to reach six times their initial size. PDPN elimination studies [93] showed no significant changes in cell growth, death rates, blood vessel formation, or tumor spread compared to untreated tumors. When DDX39B was reduced [94], researchers observed increased p65 phosphorylation and greater temozolomide resistance in U87 cells. Studies reducing BIG1 and BIG2 [95] successfully decreased VEGF levels in both U251 glioblastoma cells and HUVECs. ANGPT2 elimination [107] combined with 4E2 antibody treatment improved blood vessel structure throughout glioblastoma tissues.

Inflammation-focused studies produced some unexpected outcomes. CIS elimination [68], aimed at enhancing natural killer cell function, led to longer survival in the NK dCIS group compared to controls, though not as anticipated. OPN elimination studies [108] successfully reduced M2 macrophages but unexpectedly increased T-lymphocyte activity in tumor tissue. AIM2 reduction research [109] showed unusual results, with AIM2 concentrating in tumor cores and showing unexpected patterns without PCNA detection.

These mixed results highlight the intricate nature of glioblastoma's biological responses to genetic modification and emphasize the need for additional research to improve treatment approaches.

3.8 Future Perspectives

The clinical implementation of CRISPR/Cas9 for glioblastoma treatment faces several key challenges. A major concern involves the possible increase in new mutations when using viral Cas9 nucleases [110, 111]. The system's lack of perfect precision may create unintended DNA changes that could either kill cells or transform them into cancer cells [112–114]. Another significant challenge involves delivering CRISPR-Cas9 effectively to target cells, complicated by Cas9's size and packaging difficulties. This necessitates developing precise delivery methods, such as nanoparticles or exosomes, capable of crossing the blood-brain barrier. Patent regulations for these delivery systems present additional complications, raising ethical questions about balancing corporate profits and rapid immunotherapy development with patient benefits.

Individualized cancer treatment shows promise across various cancers by targeting specific genomic or epigenomic mutations in tumor cells. Glioblastoma patients show various mutations including TP53, INK4A/ARF, PTEN, and NF-1 [10, 115], which drive tumor development and growth in brain tissue. Glioblastoma surgical samples show significant variation in cellular composition, explaining why standard treatments often fail, contributing to poor outcomes and aggressive disease progression [116]. Personalized treatments targeting specific molecular changes and mutations offer hope for glioblastoma patients. New treatments must address both tumor variation and immune system characteristics. However, understanding tumor cell diversity remains challenging for drug development. Using multiple treatments might help prevent glioblastoma recurrence by targeting specific cancer-initiating cells, though this requires further study [117].

Since 2015, CRISPR/Cas9 gene editing has demonstrated promising progress in clinical investigations aimed at treating glioblastoma multiforme [118]. Despite its therapeutic potential, the considerable molecular size of Cas9 presents significant delivery challenges. Current research efforts are directed toward developing lipid nanoparticle-based delivery systems to suppress tumor growth and circumvent the limited permeability of the blood-brain barrier to conventional cancer therapeutics [119, 120].

However, several key limitations remain. Off-target effects due to imperfect targeting specificity pose risks to adjacent healthy cells, and proposed solutions include the use of multiple siRNAs in combination with CRISPR-Cas9 to enhance precision [114]. Additionally, the lack of high-fidelity DNA cleavage [121] may introduce deleterious mutations in non-targeted genomic regions. Another major concern is the immune system's recognition of bacterial Cas9 as a foreign protein, which can trigger adverse immune reactions and restrict the feasibility of repeated administrations.

Toxicological concerns further complicate clinical translation. There is limited understanding of CRISPR-Cas9's effects on the human CNS [122, 123], alongside the risk of unintended genetic alterations that may impair neuronal function. Inflammatory responses to bacterial Cas9 protein have also been reported [124, 125], along with systemic toxicity [126] and broader immune activation. These challenges underscore the urgent need for delivery platforms that minimize immunogenicity and enhance biocompatibility [127, 128].

3.9 Conclusion

Glioblastoma remains an incurable disease despite maximal surgery and chemoradiation, largely because of its genetic diversity, adaptive resistance, and the constraints of the brain microenvironment. CRISPR/Cas9 offers a unifying toolkit to interrogate and therapeutically remodel this complexity by validating drivers, engineering loss or gain-of-function states, and revealing actionable synthetic-lethal partners, while enabling direct correction or disruption of pathogenic alleles. The path to clinical impact will depend on integrating high-fidelity editors (including base and prime editors), rigorous off-target surveillance, and brain-appropriate, tumor-selective delivery systems, coupled with combination strategies that align editing with standard therapy and immunooncology. With these advances, CRISPR/Cas9 can evolve from a discovery workhorse to a therapeutic modality that meaningfully extends survival and quality of life for patients with glioblastoma.

References

1. Begagić E, Pugonja R, Bečulić H, Čeliković A, Tandir Lihić L, Kadić Vukas S, et al. Molecular Targeted Therapies in Glioblastoma Multiforme: A Systematic Overview of Global Trends and Findings. Brain Sci. 2023;13(11):1602.
2. Stoyanov GS, Lyutfi E, Georgieva R, Georgiev R, Dzhenkov DL, Petkova L, et al. Reclassification of Glioblastoma Multiforme According to the 2021 World Health Organization Classification of Central Nervous System Tumors: A Single Institution Report and Practical Significance. Cureus. 2022;14(2):e21822.
3. Jain KK. A Critical Overview of Targeted Therapies for Glioblastoma. Front Oncol. 2018;8:419.
4. Angom RS, Nakka NMR, Bhattacharya S. Advances in Glioblastoma Therapy: An Update on Current Approaches. Brain Sci. 2023;13(11):1536.
5. Agosti E, Zeppieri M, De Maria L, Tedeschi C, Fontanella MM, Panciani PP, Ius T. Glioblastoma Immunotherapy: A Systematic Review of the Present Strategies and Prospects for Advancements. Int J Mol Sci. 2023;24(20):15037.

6. Riemenschneider MJ, Jeuken JW, Wesseling P, Reifenberger G. Molecular diagnostics of gliomas: state of the art. Acta Neuropathol. 2010;120(5):567–84.
7. Senhaji N, Squalli Houssaini A, Lamrabet S, Louati S, Bennis S. Molecular and Circulating Biomarkers in Patients with Glioblastoma. Int J Mol Sci. 2022;23(13):7474.
8. Peixoto J, Príncipe C, Pestana A, Osório H, Pinto MT, Prazeres H, et al. Using a Dual CRISPR/Cas9 Approach to Gain Insight into the Role of LRP1B in Glioblastoma. Int J Mol Sci. 2023;24(14):11285.
9. Khlidj Y. What did CRISPR-Cas9 accomplish in its first 10 years? Biochem Med (Zagreb). 2023;33(3):030601.
10. Brennan CW, Verhaak RG, McKenna A, Campos B, Noushmehr H, Salama SR, et al. The somatic genomic landscape of glioblastoma. Cell. 2013;155(2):462–77.
11. Ding S, Liu J, Han X, Tang M. CRISPR/Cas9-Mediated Genome Editing in Cancer Therapy. Int J Mol Sci. 2023;24(22):16325.
12. Begagić E, Pugonja R, Bečulić H, Selimović E, Skomorac R, Saß B, Pojskić M. The New Era of Spinal Surgery: Exploring the Use of Exoscopes as a Viable Alternative to Operative Microscopes-A Systematic Review and Meta-Analysis. World Neurosurg. 2024;182:144–58.e1.
13. Begagić E, Bečulić H, Skomorac R, Pojskić M. Accessible Spinal Surgery: Transformation Through the Implementation of Exoscopes As Substitutes for Conventional Microsurgery in Low- and Middle-Income Settings. Cureus. 2023;15(9):e45350.
14. Louis DN, Perry A, Wesseling P, Brat DJ, Cree IA, Figarella-Branger D, et al. The 2021 WHO Classification of Tumors of the Central Nervous System: a summary. Neuro Oncol. 2021;23(8):1231–51.
15. del Pilar Guillermo Prieto M, de La Fuente MI. The role of molecular genetics of glioblastoma in the clinical setting. Precision Molecular Pathology of Glioblastoma: Springer; 2021. p. 21–33.
16. Delgado-Martín B, Medina M. Advances in the Knowledge of the Molecular Biology of Glioblastoma and Its Impact in Patient Diagnosis, Stratification, and Treatment. Adv Sci (Weinh). 2020;7(9):1902971.
17. D'Alessio A, Proietti G, Sica G, Scicchitano BM. Pathological and Molecular Features of Glioblastoma and Its Peritumoral Tissue. Cancers (Basel). 2019;11(4):469.

18. Ludwig K, Muthukrishnan SD, Alvarado AG, Kornblum HI. Overview of glioblastoma biological hallmarks and molecular pathology. Glioblastoma Resistance to Chemotherapy: Molecular Mechanisms and Innovative Reversal Strategies: Elsevier; 2021. p. 1–15.
19. Reifenberger G, Wirsching HG, Knobbe-Thomsen CB, Weller M. Advances in the molecular genetics of gliomas — implications for classification and therapy. Nat Rev Clin Oncol. 2017;14(7):434–52.
20. Verdugo E, Puerto I, Medina M. An update on the molecular biology of glioblastoma, with clinical implications and progress in its treatment. Cancer Commun (Lond). 2022;42(11):1083–111.
21. Montella L, Cuomo M, Del Gaudio N, Buonaiuto M, Costabile D, Visconti R, et al. Epigenetic alterations in glioblastomas: Diagnostic, prognostic and therapeutic relevance. Int J Cancer. 2023;153(3):476–88.
22. Phillips RE, Soshnev AA, Allis CD. Epigenomic Reprogramming as a Driver of Malignant Glioma. Cancer Cell. 2020;38(5):647–60.
23. Uddin MS, Mamun AA, Alghamdi BS, Tewari D, Jeandet P, Sarwar MS, Ashraf GM. Epigenetics of glioblastoma multiforme: From molecular mechanisms to therapeutic approaches. Semin Cancer Biol. 2022;83:100–20.
24. Hegi ME, Diserens AC, Gorlia T, Hamou MF, de Tribolet N, Weller M, et al. MGMT gene silencing and benefit from temozolomide in glioblastoma. N Engl J Med. 2005;352(10):997–1003.
25. Mansouri A, Hachem LD, Mansouri S, Nassiri F, Laperriere NJ, Xia D, et al. MGMT promoter methylation status testing to guide therapy for glioblastoma: refining the approach based on emerging evidence and current challenges. Neuro Oncol. 2019;21(2):167–78.
26. Della Monica R, Cuomo M, Buonaiuto M, Costabile D, Franca RA, Del Basso De Caro M, et al. MGMT and Whole-Genome DNA Methylation Impacts on Diagnosis, Prognosis and Therapy of Glioblastoma Multiforme. Int J Mol Sci. 2022;23(13):7148.
27. Noushmehr H, Weisenberger DJ, Diefes K, Phillips HS, Pujara K, Berman BP, et al. Identification of a CpG island methylator phenotype that defines a distinct subgroup of glioma. Cancer Cell. 2010;17(5):510–22.
28. Capper D, Jones DTW, Sill M, Hovestadt V, Schrimpf D, Sturm D, et al. DNA methylation-based classification of central nervous system tumours. Nature. 2018;555(7697):469–74.

29. Klughammer J, Kiesel B, Roetzer T, Fortelny N, Nemc A, Nenning KH, et al. The DNA methylation landscape of glioblastoma disease progression shows extensive heterogeneity in time and space. Nat Med. 2018;24(10):1611–24.
30. McClellan BL, Haase S, Nunez FJ, Alghamri MS, Dabaja AA, Lowenstein PR, Castro MG. Impact of epigenetic reprogramming on antitumor immune responses in glioma. J Clin Invest. 2023;133(2):e163450.
31. Romani M, Pistillo MP, Banelli B. Epigenetic Targeting of Glioblastoma. Front Oncol. 2018;8:448.
32. Ghiaseddin A, Reardon D, Massey W, Mannerino A, Lipp ES, Herndon JE, 2nd, et al. Phase II Study of Bevacizumab and Vorinostat for Patients with Recurrent World Health Organization Grade 4 Malignant Glioma. Oncologist. 2018;23(2):157-e21.
33. Banasavadi-Siddegowda YK, Welker AM, An M, Yang X, Zhou W, Shi G, et al. PRMT5 as a druggable target for glioblastoma therapy. Neuro Oncol. 2018;20(6):753–63.
34. Aldape K, Zadeh G, Mansouri S, Reifenberger G, von Deimling A. Glioblastoma: pathology, molecular mechanisms and markers. Acta Neuropathol. 2015;129(6):829–48.
35. Esemen Y, Awan M, Parwez R, Baig A, Rahman S, Masala I, et al. Molecular Pathogenesis of Glioblastoma in Adults and Future Perspectives: A Systematic Review. Int J Mol Sci. 2022;23(5):2607.
36. Lieberman F. Glioblastoma update: molecular biology, diagnosis, treatment, response assessment, and translational clinical trials. F1000Res. 2017;6:1892.
37. Molinaro AM, Taylor JW, Wiencke JK, Wrensch MR. Genetic and molecular epidemiology of adult diffuse glioma. Nat Rev Neurol. 2019;15(7):405–17.
38. Phillips HS, Kharbanda S, Chen R, Forrest WF, Soriano RH, Wu TD, et al. Molecular subclasses of high-grade glioma predict prognosis, delineate a pattern of disease progression, and resemble stages in neurogenesis. Cancer Cell. 2006;9(3):157–73.
39. Verhaak RG, Hoadley KA, Purdom E, Wang V, Qi Y, Wilkerson MD, et al. Integrated genomic analysis identifies clinically relevant subtypes of glioblastoma characterized by abnormalities in PDGFRA, IDH1, EGFR, and NF1. Cancer Cell. 2010;17(1):98–110.

40. Becker AP, Sells BE, Haque SJ, Chakravarti A. Tumor Heterogeneity in Glioblastomas: From Light Microscopy to Molecular Pathology. Cancers (Basel). 2021;13(4):761.
41. Eisenbarth D, Wang YA. Glioblastoma heterogeneity at single cell resolution. Oncogene. 2023;42(27):2155–65.
42. Bikfalvi A, da Costa CA, Avril T, Barnier JV, Bauchet L, Brisson L, et al. Challenges in glioblastoma research: focus on the tumor microenvironment. Trends Cancer. 2023;9(1):9–27.
43. Di Nunno V, Franceschi E, Tosoni A, Gatto L, Bartolini S, Brandes AA. Glioblastoma Microenvironment: From an Inviolable Defense to a Therapeutic Chance. Front Oncol. 2022;12:852950.
44. Pombo Antunes AR, Scheyltjens I, Duerinck J, Neyns B, Movahedi K, Van Ginderachter JA. Understanding the glioblastoma immune microenvironment as basis for the development of new immunotherapeutic strategies. Elife. 2020;9:e52176.
45. Patel AP, Tirosh I, Trombetta JJ, Shalek AK, Gillespie SM, Wakimoto H, et al. Single-cell RNA-seq highlights intratumoral heterogeneity in primary glioblastoma. Science. 2014;344(6190):1396–401.
46. LeBlanc VG, Trinh DL, Aslanpour S, Hughes M, Livingstone D, Jin D, et al. Single-cell landscapes of primary glioblastomas and matched explants and cell lines show variable retention of inter- and intratumor heterogeneity. Cancer Cell. 2022;40(4):379–92.e9.
47. Meyer M, Reimand J, Lan X, Head R, Zhu X, Kushida M, et al. Single cell-derived clonal analysis of human glioblastoma links functional and genomic heterogeneity. Proc Natl Acad Sci U S A. 2015; 112(3):851–6.
48. Darmanis S, Sloan SA, Croote D, Mignardi M, Chernikova S, Samghababi P, et al. Single-Cell RNA-Seq Analysis of Infiltrating Neoplastic Cells at the Migrating Front of Human Glioblastoma. Cell Rep. 2017;21(5):1399–410.
49. Meng Q, Zhang Y, Li G, Li Y, Xie H, Chen X. New insights for precision treatment of glioblastoma from analysis of single-cell lncRNA expression. J Cancer Res Clin Oncol. 2021;147(7):1881–95.
50. Neftel C, Laffy J, Filbin MG, Hara T, Shore ME, Rahme GJ, et al. An Integrative Model of Cellular States, Plasticity, and Genetics for Glioblastoma. Cell. 2019;178(4):835–49.e21.

51. Wu H, Guo C, Wang C, Xu J, Zheng S, Duan J, et al. Single-cell RNA sequencing reveals tumor heterogeneity, microenvironment, and drug-resistance mechanisms of recurrent glioblastoma. Cancer Sci. 2023;114(6):2609–21.
52. Awah CU, Chen L, Bansal M, Mahajan A, Winter J, Lad M, et al. Ribosomal protein S11 influences glioma response to TOP2 poisons. Oncogene. 2020;39(27):5068–81.
53. Huang K, Liu X, Li Y, Wang Q, Zhou J, Wang Y, et al. Genome-Wide CRISPR-Cas9 Screening Identifies NF-κB/E2F6 Responsible for EGFRvIII-Associated Temozolomide Resistance in Glioblastoma. Adv Sci (Weinh). 2019;6(17):1900782.
54. Chow RD, Guzman CD, Wang G, Schmidt F, Youngblood MW, Ye L, et al. AAV-mediated direct in vivo CRISPR screen identifies functional suppressors in glioblastoma. Nat Neurosci. 2017;20(10): 1329–41.
55. Prolo LM, Li A, Owen SF, Parker JJ, Foshay K, Nitta RT, et al. Targeted genomic CRISPR-Cas9 screen identifies MAP4K4 as essential for glioblastoma invasion. Sci Rep. 2019;9(1):14020.
56. Ye L, Park JJ, Dong MB, Yang Q, Chow RD, Peng L, et al. In vivo CRISPR screening in CD8 T cells with AAV-Sleeping Beauty hybrid vectors identifies membrane targets for improving immunotherapy for glioblastoma. Nat Biotechnol. 2019;37(11):1302–13.
57. MacLeod G, Bozek DA, Rajakulendran N, Monteiro V, Ahmadi M, Steinhart Z, et al. Genome-Wide CRISPR-Cas9 Screens Expose Genetic Vulnerabilities and Mechanisms of Temozolomide Sensitivity in Glioblastoma Stem Cells. Cell Rep. 2019;27(3):971–86.e9.
58. Tang M, Xie Q, Gimple RC, Zhong Z, Tam T, Tian J, et al. Three-dimensional bioprinted glioblastoma microenvironments model cellular dependencies and immune interactions. Cell Res. 2020; 30(10):833–53.
59. Toledo CM, Ding Y, Hoellerbauer P, Davis RJ, Basom R, Girard EJ, et al. Genome-wide CRISPR-Cas9 Screens Reveal Loss of Redundancy between PKMYT1 and WEE1 in Glioblastoma Stem-like Cells. Cell Rep. 2015;13(11):2425–39.
60. Liu SJ, Malatesta M, Lien BV, Saha P, Thombare SS, Hong SJ, et al. CRISPRi-based radiation modifier screen identifies long non-coding RNA therapeutic targets in glioma. Genome Biol. 2020;21(1):83.

61. Morton AR, Dogan-Artun N, Faber ZJ, MacLeod G, Bartels CF, Piazza MS, et al. Functional Enhancers Shape Extrachromosomal Oncogene Amplifications. Cell. 2019;179(6):1330–41.e13.
62. Qazi MA, Vora P, Venugopal C, Sidhu SS, Moffat J, Swanton C, Singh SK. Intratumoral heterogeneity: pathways to treatment resistance and relapse in human glioblastoma. Ann Oncol. 2017;28(7): 1448–56.
63. Wang X, Wang X, Li J, Liang J, Ren X, Yun D, et al. PDPN contributes to constructing immunosuppressive microenvironment in IDH wildtype glioma. Cancer Gene Ther. 2023;30(2):345–57.
64. Rodvold JJ, Xian S, Nussbacher J, Tsui B, Cameron Waller T, Searles SC, et al. IRE1α and IGF signaling predict resistance to an endoplasmic reticulum stress-inducing drug in glioblastoma cells. Sci Rep. 2020;10(1):8348.
65. Vu HT, Kobayashi M, Hegazy AM, Tadokoro Y, Ueno M, Kasahara A, et al. Autophagy inhibition synergizes with calcium mobilization to achieve efficient therapy of malignant gliomas. Cancer Sci. 2018;109(8):2497–508.
66. Peng H, Du B, Jiang H, Gao J. Over-expression of CHAF1A promotes cell proliferation and apoptosis resistance in glioblastoma cells via AKT/FOXO3a/Bim pathway. Biochem Biophys Res Commun. 2016;469(4):1111–6.
67. Kranz D, Boutros M. A synthetic lethal screen identifies FAT1 as an antagonist of caspase-8 in extrinsic apoptosis. Embo j. 2014;33(3): 181–97.
68. Nakazawa T, Morimoto T, Maeoka R, Matsuda R, Nakamura M, Nishimura F, et al. CIS deletion by CRISPR/Cas9 enhances human primary natural killer cell functions against allogeneic glioblastoma. J Exp Clin Cancer Res. 2023;42(1):205.
69. Zielke S, Meyer N, Mari M, Abou-El-Ardat K, Reggiori F, van Wijk SJL, et al. Loperamide, pimozide, and STF-62247 trigger autophagy-dependent cell death in glioblastoma cells. Cell Death Dis. 2018;9(10):994.
70. Ali R, Alabdullah M, Miligy I, Normatova M, Babaei-Jadidi R, Nateri AS, et al. ATM Regulated PTEN Degradation Is XIAP E3 Ubiquitin Ligase Mediated in p85α Deficient Cancer Cells and Influence Platinum Sensitivity. Cells. 2019;8(10):1271.

71. Ranjan A, Srivastava SK. Penfluridol suppresses glioblastoma tumor growth by Akt-mediated inhibition of GLI1. Oncotarget. 2017;8(20):32960–76.
72. Fierro J, Jr., DiPasquale J, Perez J, Chin B, Chokpapone Y, Tran AM, et al. Dual-sgRNA CRISPR/Cas9 knockout of PD-L1 in human U87 glioblastoma tumor cells inhibits proliferation, invasion, and tumor-associated macrophage polarization. Sci Rep. 2022;12(1):2417.
73. Lumibao JC, Haak PL, Kolossov VL, Chen JE, Stutchman J, Ruiz A, et al. CHCHD2 mediates glioblastoma cell proliferation, mitochondrial metabolism, hypoxia-induced invasion and therapeutic resistance. Int J Oncol. 2023;63(5):117.
74. Toledano S, Sabag AD, Ilan N, Liburkin-Dan T, Kessler O, Neufeld G. Plexin-A2 enables the proliferation and the development of tumors from glioblastoma derived cells. Cell Death Dis. 2023; 14(1):41.
75. Gallo K, Srinageshwar B, Ward A, Diola C, Dunbar G, Rossignol J, Bakke J. Inducible Knockout of 14-3-3β Attenuates Proliferation and Spheroid Formation in a Human Glioblastoma Cell Line U87MG. Brain Sci. 2023;13(6):868.
76. Guda MR, Velpula KK, Asuthkar S, Cain CP, Tsung AJ. Targeting RGS4 Ablates Glioblastoma Proliferation. Int J Mol Sci. 2020;21(9):3300.
77. Zhang F, Liu R, Liu C, Zhang H, Lu Y. Nanos3, a cancer-germline gene, promotes cell proliferation, migration, chemoresistance, and invasion of human glioblastoma. Cancer Cell Int. 2020;20:197.
78. Bulstrode H, Johnstone E, Marques-Torrejon MA, Ferguson KM, Bressan RB, Blin C, et al. Elevated FOXG1 and SOX2 in glioblastoma enforces neural stem cell identity through transcriptional control of cell cycle and epigenetic regulators. Genes Dev. 2017;31(8):757–73.
79. Saenz-Antoñanzas A, Moncho-Amor V, Auzmendi-Iriarte J, Elua-Pinin A, Rizzoti K, Lovell-Badge R, Matheu A. CRISPR/Cas9 Deletion of SOX2 Regulatory Region 2 (SRR2) Decreases SOX2 Malignant Activity in Glioblastoma. Cancers (Basel). 2021;13(7):1574.
80. Ogawa J, Pao GM, Shokhirev MN, Verma IM. Glioblastoma Model Using Human Cerebral Organoids. Cell Rep. 2018;23(4):1220–9.
81. Smolkin T, Nir-Zvi I, Duvshani N, Mumblat Y, Kessler O, Neufeld G. Complexes of plexin-A4 and plexin-D1 convey semaphorin-3C signals to induce cytoskeletal collapse in the absence of neuropilins. J Cell Sci. 2018;131(9):jcs208298.

82. Wang Y, Yang CH, Schultz AP, Sims MM, Miller DD, Pfeffer LM. Brahma-Related Gene-1 (BRG1) promotes the malignant phenotype of glioblastoma cells. J Cell Mol Med. 2021;25(6):2956–66.
83. Shao W, Azam Z, Guo J, To SST. Oncogenic potential of PIK3CD in glioblastoma is exerted through cytoskeletal proteins PAK3 and PLEK2. Lab Invest. 2022;102(12):1314–22.
84. Chen L, Fang W, Chen W, Wei Y, Ding J, Li J, et al. Deciphering the molecular mechanism of the THBS1 gene in the TNF signaling axis in glioma stem cells. Cell Signal. 2023;106:110656.
85. Ozyerli-Goknar E, Kala EY, Aksu AC, Bulut I, Cingöz A, Nizamuddin S, Biniossek M, Seker-Polat F, Morova T, Aztekin C, Kung SHY, Syed H, Tuncbag N, Gönen M, Philpott M, Cribbs AP, Acilan C, Lack NA, Onder TT, Timmers HTM, Bagci-Onder T. Epigenetic-focused CRISPR/Cas9 screen identifies (absent, small, or homeotic)2-like protein (ASH2L) as a regulator of glioblastoma cell survival. Cell Commun Signal. 2023;21(1):328.
86. Nieland L, van Solinge TS, Cheah PS, Morsett LM, El Khoury J, Rissman JI, et al. CRISPR-Cas knockout of miR21 reduces glioma growth. Mol Ther Oncolytics. 2022;25:121–36.
87. Uceda-Castro R, van Asperen JV, Vennin C, Sluijs JA, van Bodegraven EJ, Margarido AS, et al. GFAP splice variants fine-tune glioma cell invasion and tumour dynamics by modulating migration persistence. Sci Rep. 2022;12(1):424.
88. Maggio J, Cardama GA, Armando RG, Balcone L, Sobol NT, Gomez DE, Mengual Gómez DL. Key role of PIN1 in telomere maintenance and oncogenic behavior in a human glioblastoma model. Oncol Rep. 2023;49(5):91.
89. Godoy P, Pour Khavari A, Rizzo M, Sakamoto-Hojo ET, Haghdoost S. Targeting NRF2, Regulator of Antioxidant System, to Sensitize Glioblastoma Neurosphere Cells to Radiation-Induced Oxidative Stress. Oxid Med Cell Longev. 2020;2020:2534643.
90. Zhang F, Liu R, Zhang H, Liu C, Liu C, Lu Y. Suppressing Dazl modulates tumorigenicity and stemness in human glioblastoma cells. BMC Cancer. 2020;20(1):673.
91. Liu J, Sareddy GR, Zhou M, Viswanadhapalli S, Li X, Lai Z, et al. Differential Effects of Estrogen Receptor β Isoforms on Glioblastoma Progression. Cancer Res. 2018;78(12):3176–89.
92. Han N, Hu G, Shi L, Long G, Yang L, Xi Q, et al. Notch1 ablation radiosensitizes glioblastoma cells. Oncotarget. 2017;8(50):88059–68.

93. Eisemann T, Costa B, Harter PN, Wick W, Mittelbronn M, Angel P, Peterziel H. Podoplanin expression is a prognostic biomarker but may be dispensable for the malignancy of glioblastoma. Neuro Oncol. 2019;21(3):326–36.
94. Szymura SJ, Bernal GM, Wu L, Zhang Z, Crawley CD, Voce DJ, et al. DDX39B interacts with the pattern recognition receptor pathway to inhibit NF-κB and sensitize to alkylating chemotherapy. BMC Biol. 2020;18(1):32.
95. Lu FI, Wang YT, Wang YS, Wu CY, Li CC. Involvement of BIG1 and BIG2 in regulating VEGF expression and angiogenesis. Faseb j. 2019;33(9):9959–73.
96. Wu W, Wu Y, Mayer K, von Rosenstiel C, Schecker J, Baur S, et al. Lipid Peroxidation Plays an Important Role in Chemotherapeutic Effects of Temozolomide and the Development of Therapy Resistance in Human Glioblastoma. Transl Oncol. 2020;13(3):100748.
97. Han X, Abdallah MOE, Breuer P, Stahl F, Bakhit Y, Potthoff AL, et al. Downregulation of MGMT expression by targeted editing of DNA methylation enhances temozolomide sensitivity in glioblastoma. Neoplasia. 2023;44:100929.
98. Tong F, Zhao JX, Fang ZY, Cui XT, Su DY, Liu X, et al. MUC1 promotes glioblastoma progression and TMZ resistance by stabilizing EGFRvIII. Pharmacol Res. 2023;187:106606.
99. Liu X, Cao Z, Wang W, Zou C, Wang Y, Pan L, et al. Engineered Extracellular Vesicle-Delivered CRISPR/Cas9 for Radiotherapy Sensitization of Glioblastoma. ACS Nano. 2023;17(17):16432–47.
100. Rocha CRR, Reily Rocha A, Molina Silva M, Rodrigues Gomes L, Teatin Latancia M, Andrade Tomaz M, et al. Revealing Temozolomide Resistance Mechanisms via Genome-Wide CRISPR Libraries. Cells. 2020;9(12):2573.
101. Yin J, Wang X, Ge X, Ding F, Shi Z, Ge Z, et al. Hypoxanthine phosphoribosyl transferase 1 metabolizes temozolomide to activate AMPK for driving chemoresistance of glioblastomas. Nat Commun. 2023;14(1):5913.
102. Auffinger B, Spencer D, Pytel P, Ahmed AU, Lesniak MS. The role of glioma stem cells in chemotherapy resistance and glioblastoma multiforme recurrence. Expert Rev Neurother. 2015;15(7):741–52.

103. Ortensi B, Setti M, Osti D, Pelicci G. Cancer stem cell contribution to glioblastoma invasiveness. Stem Cell Res Ther. 2013;4(1):18.
104. Álvarez MM, Biayna J, Supek F. TP53-dependent toxicity of CRISPR/Cas9 cuts is differential across genomic loci and can confound genetic screening. Nat Commun. 2022;13(1):4520.
105. Ihry RJ, Worringer KA, Salick MR, Frias E, Ho D, Theriault K, et al. p53 inhibits CRISPR-Cas9 engineering in human pluripotent stem cells. Nat Med. 2018;24(7):939–46.
106. Enache OM, Rendo V, Abdusamad M, Lam D, Davison D, Pal S, et al. Cas9 activates the p53 pathway and selects for p53-inactivating mutations. Nat Genet. 2020;52(7):662–8.
107. Lee E, Lee EA, Kong E, Chon H, Llaiqui-Condori M, Park CH, et al. An agonistic anti-Tie2 antibody suppresses the normal-to-tumor vascular transition in the glioblastoma invasion zone. Exp Mol Med. 2023;55(2):470–84.
108. Wei J, Marisetty A, Schrand B, Gabrusiewicz K, Hashimoto Y, Ott M, et al. Osteopontin mediates glioblastoma-associated macrophage infiltration and is a potential therapeutic target. J Clin Invest. 2019;129(1):137–49.
109. Chen PA, Shrivastava G, Balcom EF, McKenzie BA, Fernandes J, Branton WG, et al. Absent in melanoma 2 regulates tumor cell proliferation in glioblastoma multiforme. J Neurooncol. 2019;144(2):265–73.
110. Bečulić H, Begagić E, Skomorac R, Mašović A, Selimović E, Pojskić M. ChatGPT's contributions to the evolution of neurosurgical practice and education: a systematic review of benefits, concerns and limitations. Med Glas (Zenica). 2024;21(1):126–31.
111. Hwang WY, Fu Y, Reyon D, Maeder ML, Tsai SQ, Sander JD, et al. Efficient genome editing in zebrafish using a CRISPR-Cas system. Nat Biotechnol. 2013;31(3):227–9.
112. Ayanoğlu FB, Elçin AE, Elçin YM. Bioethical issues in genome editing by CRISPR-Cas9 technology. Turk J Biol. 2020;44(2):110–20.
113. Rodriguez E. Ethical issues in genome editing using Crispr/Cas9 system. Journal of Clinical Research and Bioethics. 2016;7(2):1000266.
114. Zuo E, Sun Y, Yuan T, He B, Zhou C, Ying W, et al. A rationally engineered cytosine base editor retains high on-target activity while

reducing both DNA and RNA off-target effects. Nat Methods. 2020;17(6):600–4.
115. Xu PF, Li C, Xi SY, Chen FR, Wang J, Zhang ZQ, et al. Whole exome sequencing reveals the genetic heterogeneity and evolutionary history of primary gliomas and matched recurrences. Comput Struct Biotechnol J. 2022;20:2235–46.
116. Bhat KPL, Balasubramaniyan V, Vaillant B, Ezhilarasan R, Hummelink K, Hollingsworth F, et al. Mesenchymal differentiation mediated by NF-κB promotes radiation resistance in glioblastoma. Cancer Cell. 2013;24(3):331–46.
117. Ene CI, Holland EC. Personalized medicine for gliomas. Surg Neurol Int. 2015;6(Suppl 1):S89–95.
118. Kang X, Wang Y, Liu P, Huang B, Zhou B, Lu S, et al. Progresses, challenges, and prospects of CRISPR/Cas9 gene-editing in glioma studies. Cancers. 2023;15(2):396.
119. Luo YL, Xu CF, Li HJ, Cao ZT, Liu J, Wang JL, et al. Macrophage-Specific in Vivo Gene Editing Using Cationic Lipid-Assisted Polymeric Nanoparticles. ACS Nano. 2018;12(2):994–1005.
120. Rosenblum D, Gutkin A, Kedmi R, Ramishetti S, Veiga N, Jacobi AM, et al. CRISPR-Cas9 genome editing using targeted lipid nanoparticles for cancer therapy. Sci Adv. 2020;6(47):eabc9450.
121. Ray U, Raghavan SC. Modulation of DNA double-strand break repair as a strategy to improve precise genome editing. Oncogene. 2020;39(41):6393–405.
122. Janik E, Niemcewicz M, Ceremuga M, Krzowski L, Saluk-Bijak J, Bijak M. Various Aspects of a Gene Editing System-CRISPR-Cas9. Int J Mol Sci. 2020;21(24):9604.
123. Tsuchida CA, Brandes N, Bueno R, Trinidad M, Mazumder T, Yu B, et al. Mitigation of chromosome loss in clinical CRISPR-Cas9-engineered T cells. Cell. 2023;186(21):4567–82.e20.
124. Crudele JM, Chamberlain JS. Cas9 immunity creates challenges for CRISPR gene editing therapies. Nat Commun. 2018;9(1):3497.
125. Mehta A, Merkel OM. Immunogenicity of Cas9 Protein. J Pharm Sci. 2020;109(1):62–7.
126. Yang S, Chang R, Yang H, Zhao T, Hong Y, Kong HE, et al. CRISPR/Cas9-mediated gene editing ameliorates neurotoxicity in mouse model of Huntington's disease. J Clin Invest. 2017;127(7):2719–24.

127. Lu Y, Xue J, Deng T, Zhou X, Yu K, Deng L, et al. Safety and feasibility of CRISPR-edited T cells in patients with refractory non-small-cell lung cancer. Nat Med. 2020;26(5):732–40.
128. Zha MJ, Cai CE, He PM. Outlook on the Security and Potential Improvements of CRISPR-Cas9. Mol Biotechnol. 2023;65(11): 1729–36.

https://doi.org/10.1142/9789819826759_0004

CHAPTER 4

CRISPR/Cas9 in the Treatment of Gastric Cancer

Mehrdad Hashemi[1,2], *Alireza Khosravinejad*[1,3], *Mina Alimohammadi*[4], *Reza Mohajer Shirazi*[1,3], *Behdokht Jamali*[5], *Kimia Sadat Esfahani*[1,3], *Amir Sadeghi*[6], *Ali Shirazi*[1,3], *Faranak Jamshidian*[1,7], *Neda Zali*[3], *Najma Farahani*[1,*], *Afshin Taheriazam*[1,8,*], *Payman Rahimzadeh*[9,*], *Maliheh Entezari*[1,2,*]

[1]Farhikhtegan Medical Convergent Sciences Research Center, Farhikhtegan Hospital, Faculty of Medicine, TeMs. C., Islamic Azad University, Tehran, Iran

[2]Department of Genetics, Faculty of Advanced Sciences and Technology, TeMs. C, Islamic Azad University, Tehran, Iran

[3]Basic and Molecular Epidemiology of Gastrointestinal Disorders Research Center, Research Institute for Gastroenterology and Liver Diseases, Shahid Beheshti University of Medical Sciences, Tehran, Iran

[4]Department of Immunology, School of Medicine, Shahid Beheshti University of Medical Sciences, Tehran, Iran

[5]Department of Microbiology and Genetics, Kherad Institute of Higher Education, Bushehr, Iran

* **Corresponding authors:** Najmafarahani@gmail.com (N.F.); a.taheriazam@iautmu.ac.ir (A.T.); P.rahimzadeh76@gmail.com (P.R.); mentezari@iautmu.ac.ir (M.E.)

[6]Gastroenterology and Liver Diseases Research Center, Research Institute for Gastroenterology and Liver Diseases, Shahid Beheshti University of Medical Sciences, Tehran, Iran
[7]Department of Biology, ET.C., Islamic Azad University, Tehran, Iran
[8]Department of Orthopedics, Faculty of Medicine, TeMs. C, Islamic Azad University, Tehran, Iran
[9]Surgical Research Society (SRS), Students' Scientific Research Center, Tehran University of Medical Sciences, Tehran, Iran

Abstract

Gastric cancer is the fifth most incident and fourth most lethal cancer globally, with mortality driven by late-stage diagnosis and limited curative options beyond gastrectomy and adjunctive therapies, which still carry high recurrence rates and benefit only a subset of patients. Biological complexity, spanning *Helicobacter pylori*-associated carcinogenesis, genetic instability, and diverse inactivation of tumor suppressor genes and activation of oncogenes, yields profound interpatient heterogeneity that constrains biomarker adoption and therapeutic precision in routine practice. CRISPR/Cas9, built upon earlier zinc finger nuclease and transcription activator-like effector nuclease platforms, has emerged as a comparatively efficient and accessible gene-editing system capable of modeling disease mechanisms, validating targets, correcting or ablating oncogenic drivers, and sensitizing tumors to therapy, thereby bridging basic discovery with translational applications in gastric cancer. Applications include functional screening to map vulnerabilities, disruption or repair of recurrently altered genes (e.g., TP53, CDH1, KRAS, ARID1A, PTEN), modulation of resistance pathways, and integration with immunotherapy and nanotechnology-enabled delivery to enhance anti-tumor efficacy in solid tumors. This chapter outlines CRISPR/Cas9 mechanisms, surveys current use in gastric cancer research, diagnostics, and therapeutic exploration, and discusses opportunities and challenges for clinical translation, including delivery, off-target effects, tumor heterogeneity, and durability of response.

Keywords: CRISPR/Cas9; gastric cancer; gene editing therapy; functional genomics screening; drug resistance modulation; precision oncology

4.1 Introduction

Stomach cancer, also known as gastric cancer, continues to be a significant global health concern, being the fifth most common cancer and the fourth leading cause of cancer-related deaths worldwide [1]. The disease's high mortality is primarily attributed to late-stage diagnosis when curative treatment becomes unfeasible, along with limited therapeutic alternatives [2]. While surgical removal of the stomach (gastrectomy) represents the primary treatment for localized gastric cancer [3], the prognosis remains unfavorable even after successful surgery combined with post-operative chemotherapy, with approximately one-third of patients experiencing disease recurrence [4]. Although treatment modalities have expanded to include various approaches such as chemotherapy, radiation treatment, surgical interventions, immune-based therapies, and targeted medications, these options prove beneficial for only certain patient populations [5].

The development of gastric cancer involves multiple complex steps and demonstrates significant variability among patients. Environmental influences play a crucial role, particularly infection with *H. pylori* bacteria. Additionally, various molecular changes contribute to its development, including chromosomal instability, loss of tumor-suppressing gene function, and enhanced activity of cancer-promoting genes.

The molecular characteristics of gastric cancer show considerable variation between individuals. Despite numerous research efforts identifying potential diagnostic and prognostic indicators, clinical practice currently utilizes only a limited selection of these markers [6]. The process of gastric cancer formation involves various epigenetic modifications that enhance cancer-promoting genes while suppressing tumor-preventing genes [7]. This highlights the crucial importance of comprehending both the molecular mechanisms driving gastric cancer development and its diverse manifestations to establish effective multi-approach treatment strategies [8].

Gene-editing technologies have emerged as promising tools in gastric cancer research, offering capabilities to modify gene expression patterns and repair genetic mutations. These techniques also facilitate the discovery of previously unknown gene functions in crucial biological pathways, potentially leading to the identification of novel biomarkers, treatment targets, and improved understanding of drug response mechanisms [8].

Following Kim and colleagues' pioneering work, early gene-editing approaches utilized zinc finger nuclease and transcription activator-like effector nucleases, which target specific DNA-binding protein domains [9, 10]. The more recent CRISPR-associated protein 9 system has revolutionized gene editing by offering superior cost-effectiveness, efficiency, and ease of implementation. This breakthrough technology, developed by Emmanuelle Charpentier and Jennifer Doudna, earned them the 2020 Nobel Prize in Chemistry [11].

This chapter begins with an explanation of the CRISPR/Cas9 system's operational principles and development history. It then explores the system's current applications in fundamental gastric cancer research, diagnostic approaches, and therapeutic interventions. The discussion concludes by examining potential future applications of CRISPR/Cas9 in gastric cancer treatment and addressing associated challenges.

4.2 Molecular Landscape of Gastric Cancer

According to GLOBOCAN 2018 statistics, gastric cancer ranks as the fifth most prevalent cancer diagnosis and stands as the third most common cause of cancer-related mortality, presenting a particularly significant health challenge in West Asian nations [2]. While primary risk factors include *H. pylori* infection [12], poor dietary habits [13], and lifestyle factors such as alcohol and tobacco use [14], it would be an oversimplification to view gastric cancer solely as an environmentally triggered disease, without considering its important genetic components.

Adenocarcinomas represent the vast majority (80–90%) of gastric cancer cases [15]. While the WHO classification system recognizes multiple gastric cancer subtypes (including papillary, tubular, mucinous, signet-ring cell, and mixed carcinomas), the widely adopted Laurén classification provides a simpler categorization into intestinal, diffuse, and indeterminate types [16].

Recent advances in diagnostic capabilities and enhanced understanding of cancer genetics have enabled a molecular-level approach to cancer analysis, particularly in gastric cancer. Research has revealed numerous dysregulated signaling pathways in gastric cancer, with Wnt [17] and miR-126 [18] serving as notable examples.

Although surgical intervention remains the primary treatment approach for gastric cancer, chemotherapy continues to play a crucial role, especially in cases where surgery is not feasible or when dealing with metastatic disease. However, the development of chemotherapy resistance frequently compromises treatment success.

The advent of increasingly precise and efficient genome editing technologies, particularly CRISPR, has opened new possibilities for targeted cancer therapies. While CRISPR enables effective gene knockout and correction of defective cancer-related pathways, its *in vivo* efficiency remains a challenge. More promising results have been achieved in cancer immunotherapy, where T cells can be engineered to enhance their anti-cancer properties [19], a strategy that has shown potential in gastric cancer treatment [20].

For normal cells to transform into cancer cells, they must acquire several capabilities, including the ability to evade immune recognition that can occur following DNA alterations. Various immunotherapy approaches can enhance immune surveillance or prevent immune evasion in gastric cancer. Adoptive therapy using CAR-T cells involves modifying patient lymphocytes to express chimeric receptors targeting tumor antigens. Immune checkpoint inhibitor therapy targets negative regulatory pathways in immune responses. Cancer vaccines are designed to stimulate antigen-presenting cells (like dendritic cells) to present tumor antigens.

Some immunotherapy approaches could be considered indirect gene therapy, utilizing DNA editing technologies and comprehensive transcriptome analysis, though their effectiveness in solid tumors remains to be fully established [21]. CRISPR/Cas9 technology shows particular promise in T cell-based immunotherapy for generating CAR-T cells [22].

Looking ahead, highly efficient gene-editing techniques are expected to play a crucial role in gastric cancer treatment. Another promising avenue involves restoring tumor suppressor function that has been silenced by epigenetic modifications. Researchers have developed engineered artificial transcription factors with repressor or activator molecules, demonstrating successful gene expression control in mammalian cells [23]. Using these tools in combination with CRISPR, Garcia-Bloj et al. have successfully reactivated tumor suppressor genes like MASPIN and REPRIMO in gastric cancer cell lines, providing proof-of-concept for these therapeutic approaches [24].

Molecular-level studies of gastric cancer continue to reveal new opportunities for gene therapy interventions. For instance, researchers used CRISPR/Cas9 to knockout PANDAR, a long non-coding RNA that inhibits CDKN1A expression through p53 binding, resulting in successful inhibition of gastric cancer growth *in vivo* [25].

4.3 Mechanistic Insights: CRISPR/Cas9 in Gastric Cancer

CRISPR/Cas9 has emerged as a highly adaptable technology with applications spanning from understanding cancer development mechanisms to diagnosing and treating various conditions, including gastric cancer [11].

The first application of CRISPR/Cas9 in gastric cancer research was conducted by Gannom and colleagues in 2015 [26]. Their groundbreaking research investigated the effects of suppressing MAP2K1 (dual-specificity mitogen-activated protein kinase 1) and explored its relationship with MEK-inhibitory medications in various cancer cell lines, including gastric cancer. This work provided crucial insights into how MAP2K1 depletion drives RAS/MAPK activation in gastric cancer.

Since uncontrolled cell proliferation is fundamental to gastric cancer development, understanding the underlying biological mechanisms and genetic factors is crucial for identifying potential treatment targets. One significant study demonstrated that using CRISPR/Cas9 to eliminate ASC (apoptosis-associated speck-like protein containing a C-terminal caspase recruitment domain) inhibited IL18 and enhanced apoptosis in gastric cancer cells. This research revealed a previously unknown pro-tumorigenic ASC/IL18 signaling pathway crucial for gastric cancer cell survival, suggesting a potential therapeutic target [27].

Another important study employed CRISPR/Cas9 to suppress 15-PGDH (15-hydroxyprostaglandin dehydrogenase) in gastric cancer cells, demonstrating accelerated cell proliferation [28]. This research contributed to understanding how mir-21-induced loss of 15-PGDH affects early gastric cancer development. The findings suggest that maintaining 15-PGDH enzyme activity could serve as a preventive strategy against gastric cancer, particularly in cases of tubular adenocarcinoma.

4.4 CRISPR/Cas9-based Targeting of Genes Related to Gastric Cancer Hallmarks

Understanding genes that regulate the cell cycle is crucial for identifying the key cellular processes that distinguish cancer cells from normal cells. These include autonomous growth independent of external signals, resistance to programmed cell death, and suppression of tumor-controlling genes — characteristics that help identify specific biomarkers and potential therapeutic targets in gastric cancer.

Lai and colleagues [29] investigated DNA hypermethylation's role in regulating REPRIMO (RPRM), a TP53-dependent G2 arrest mediator and tumor suppressor gene in gastric cancer. Using CRISPR/Cas9 to suppress DNA methyltransferases (DNMTs), they found that reducing DNMT3A and DNMT3B increased RPRM mRNA levels by decreasing promoter methylation in gastric cancer cells, revealing an inverse relationship between DNMT activity and

RPRM expression. To verify RPRM's tumor-suppressing properties, they created RPRM-deficient gastric cancer cell lines using CRISPR/Cas9 and tested them in mice. Enhanced tumor formation in RPRM-deficient cells confirmed RPRM's role as a tumor suppressor in gastric cancer, suggesting potential therapeutic applications [29].

Another study restored tumor suppressor function by reactivating RPRM expression using CRISPR/dCas9 combined with VP64 and SAM effector domains in gastric cancer cells with heavily methylated RPRM promoters and low gene expression [24]. This intervention significantly reduced gastric cancer cell proliferation, demonstrating the potential of epigenome editing for reactivating methylation-silenced tumor suppressor genes as a gastric cancer treatment strategy.

Hu and colleagues [30] revealed another promising tumor suppressor through CRISPR/Cas9-mediated knockout of MRFAP1 (Morf4-family-associated protein 1) in gastric cancer cell lines. Their research showed that MRFAP1 deletion promoted interaction between MLN4924 substrate and tumor-suppressing proteins like p27, leading to reduced cell viability, increased cell cycle arrest, and enhanced apoptosis. These findings provide important insights into gene-substrate interactions that could improve cancer treatment approaches.

Liu and colleagues [25] investigated the effects of eliminating PANDAR (promoter of CDKN1A antisense DNA damage-activated RNA) using CRISPR/Cas9 in gastric cancer cell lines. Their findings showed that PANDAR elimination reduced both proliferation and colony formation in gastric cancer cells. Flow cytometry analysis revealed that removing PANDAR halted cell cycle progression at the G1/S checkpoint. Through its distinct transcriptional modification pattern, PANDAR was found to significantly enhance cancer cell proliferation, clone formation, and chemotherapy resistance.

In a separate study, Zhang and colleagues [31] used CRISPR/Cas9 to eliminate LMX1A (LIM homeobox transcription factor 1 α) in gastric cancer cell lines, identifying it as a primary miR-9 target. Their research demonstrated that LMX1A elimination led to increased cell viability and proliferation, supporting LMX1A's role as a tumor suppressor in gastric cancer.

The process of metastasis involves complex cellular mechanisms, including cells' ability to separate from the primary tumor and establish colonies at distant sites [32]. Given the challenges of early gastric cancer detection and limited treatment options, understanding metastatic processes is crucial. Zhou and colleagues [33] contributed to this understanding by using CRISPR/Cas9 to eliminate GMAN (gastric cancer metastasis-associated long non-coding RNA). Their research showed that removing GMAN reduced cellular invasion capabilities. The study also revealed an important relationship between GMAN and ephrin A1, where GMAN elimination led to decreased ephrin A1 expression. Further investigation showed that eliminating ephrin A1 in gastric cancer cell lines diminished both invasion and metastatic potential in living organisms.

Zhang et al. [34] found that eliminating PDEF (SAM-pointed domain-containing Ets transcription factor) using CRISPR/Cas9 reduced multiple cancer-related processes including apoptosis, colony formation, and cell movement in gastric cancer cells, confirming PDEF's involvement across various stages of gastric cancer development [34].

Araújo et al. [35] demonstrated that removing the PIWIL1 (Piwi-like protein 1) gene reduced gastric cancer cells' ability to migrate and invade, establishing PIWIL1's role as an oncogene. Conversely, Chen Chen's research [36] showed that eliminating somatostatin (SST) enhanced gastric cancer cells' migration and invasion capabilities, suggesting SST's potential role as a tumor suppressor.

An additional study examined EphB2 (ephrin type-B receptor 2) through CRISPR/Cas9-mediated knockin, evaluating its potential as a prognostic indicator in gastric cancer patients [37]. The findings revealed that EphB2 activation in gastric cancer cells enhanced their malignant characteristics by reducing adhesion while increasing migration and invasion capabilities. These results suggest EphB2's pro-tumor role in gastric cancer and its potential as a therapeutic target.

For categorized and illustrative information on the role of CRISPR/Cas9-based targeting and manipulating the genes related to gastric cancer hallmarks, see **Table 4.1** and **Figure 4.1**.

Table 4.1 CRISPR/Cas9 studies of genes influencing cell cycle and tumor development in gastric cancer.

Gene/Study Focus	Function/Role	CRISPR/Cas9-based Approach	Key Findings in Gastric Cancer	Reference
RPRM	Tumor suppressor, TP53-dependent G2 arrest mediator	Knockdown of DNMTs; RPRM-deficient cell lines	Inverse correlation between DNMT functions and RPRM expression; Loss enhanced tumor formation	[29]
MRFAP1	Tumor suppressor	Knockout	Promoted interaction with p27; Decreased vitality, increased cell cycle arrest and apoptosis	[30]
PANDAR	Oncogenic lncRNA	Knockout	Suppressed proliferative activity; Blocked cell cycle at G1/S checkpoint	[25]
LMX1A	Tumor suppressor, miR-9 target	Knockout	Increased cell viability and proliferation	[31]
GMAN lncRNA	Metastasis-associated	Knockout	Delayed invasive activity; Induced ephrin A1 reduction	[33]
SPOCD1	Cancer risk gene	Knockout	Inhibited cell proliferation and colony formation; Reduced tumor growth	[38]
BTN3A2	Susceptibility gene	Knockout	Inhibited cell proliferation and colony formation	[38]
PDEF	Oncogenic transcription factor	Deletion	Inhibited apoptosis, colony formation, migration, and invasion	[34]
PIWIL1	Oncogene	Elimination	Decreased migration and invasion abilities	[35]
SST	Tumor suppressor	Knockout	Promoted migration and invasion capabilities	[36]
EphB2	Pro-tumor receptor	Knockin	Increased malignant properties; Reduced adhesion but accelerated migration/invasion	[37]

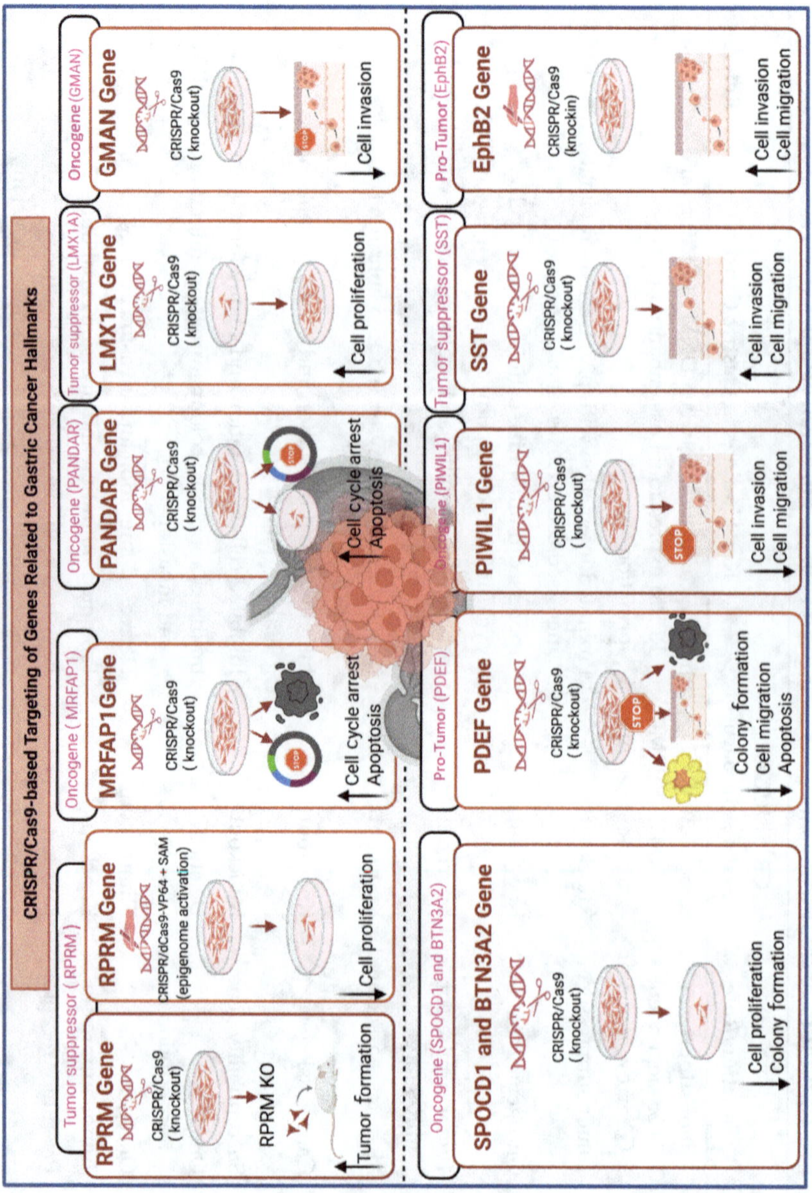

CRISPR/Cas9-based Targeting of Genes Related to Gastric Cancer Hallmarks
Tumor suppressor (RPRM)
RPRM Gene
CRISPR/Cas9 (knockout)
RPRM KO
Tumor formation
RPRM Gene
CRISPR/dCas9-VP64 + SAM (epigenome activation)
Cell proliferation
Oncogene (MRFAP1)
MRFAP1Gene
CRISPR/Cas9 (knockout)
Cell cycle arrest
Apoptosis
Oncogene (PANDAR)
PANDAR Gene
CRISPR/Cas9 (knockout)
Cell cycle arrest
Apoptosis
Tumor suppressor (LMX1A)
LMX1A Gene
CRISPR/Cas9 (knockout)
Cell proliferation
Oncogene (GMAN)
GMAN Gene
CRISPR/Cas9 (knockout)
Cell invasion
Oncogene (SPOCD1 and BTN3A2)
SPOCD1 and BTN3A2 Gene
CRISPR/Cas9 (knockout)
Cell proliferation
Colony formation
Pro-Tumor (PDEF)
PDEF Gene
CRISPR/Cas9 (knockout)
Colony formation
Cell migration
Apoptosis
Oncogene (PIWIL1)
PIWIL1 Gene
CRISPR/Cas9 (knockout)
Cell invasion
Cell migration
Tumor suppressor (SST)
SST Gene
CRISPR/Cas9 (knockout)
Cell invasion
Cell migration
Pro-Tumor (EphB2)
EphB2 Gene
CRISPR/Cas9 (knockin)
Cell invasion
Cell migration

Figure 4.1 CRISPR/Cas9-based targeting of genes involved in gastric cancer hallmarks. This schematic highlights the application of CRISPR/Cas9 genome-editing technologies for functional interrogation and modulation of key oncogenes and tumor suppressor genes implicated in gastric cancer pathobiology. **Tumor suppressors:** RPRM: CRISPR/Cas9 knockout of RPRM in animal models accelerates tumor formation, while CRISPR/dCas9-VP64 and SAM (epigenome activation) approaches modulate its role in regulating cell proliferation; LMX1A: Disruption leads to increased cell proliferation; SST: Knockout enhances cell invasion and migration. **Oncogenes and pro-tumor genes:** MRFAP1 and PANDAR: CRISPR/Cas9-mediated knockout in these loci induces cell cycle arrest and apoptosis through inhibition of oncogenic activities; GMAN gene: Knockout reduces cancer cell invasion; SPOCD1 and BTN3A2: Deletion inhibits cell proliferation and colony formation; PDEF: Targeted disruption limits colony growth, cell migration, and induces apoptosis; PIWIL1: Manipulation suppresses cell invasion and migration; EphB2: CRISPR/Cas9 knockin models demonstrate its pro-tumor influence by promoting invasion and migration. These experimental strategies underscore the versatility of CRISPR/Cas9 (including gene knockout, gene knockin, and epigenome editing technologies) in elucidating the contributions of tumor suppressor and oncogenic networks to hallmark processes such as proliferation, apoptosis, invasion, migration, and colony formation in gastric cancer. The genetic editing approaches detailed here facilitate target validation and provide a framework for the development of precision therapeutics against gastric malignancies.

4.5 CRISPR/Cas9 and *Helicobacter pylori* Infection

Helicobacter pylori, a Gram-negative spiral bacterium, infects approximately 58% of the global population [39]. While most infections are asymptomatic, *H. pylori* increases the risk of ulcers and gastric adenocarcinoma [40]. Hu and colleagues investigated vitamin D3's role in host defense against *H. pylori* through autophagy promotion [41]. Using CRISPR/Cas9 to eliminate PDIA3, they discovered a novel pathogenic mechanism where *H. pylori* survives within gastric cancer cell autophagosomes. Their research revealed a new vitamin D3 signaling pathway that activates the PDIA3-STAT3-MCOLN3-Ca2+ axis to restore lysosome function [41].

The exact molecular mechanisms by which *H. pylori* causes peptic ulcers or gastric cancer remain unclear but likely involve both host genetic factors and bacterial virulence elements, particularly VacA and CagA proteins [39]. VacA induces various cellular responses, including vacuolization, autophagy, and necrosis [42]. Foegeding and colleagues [43] studied this process by using CRISPR/Cas9 to eliminate ATG16L1 in HeLa cells, demonstrating increased VacA levels and vacuolization compared to controls, while showing VacA degradation occurs independently of autophagy.

CagA, a key virulence factor for *H. pylori* detection, is considered a significant risk factor for severe gastric diseases including gastric cancer. Zhao and colleagues [44] investigated integrin receptors and CEACAM's role in CagA translocation through the cag-T4SS by creating multiple CEACAM receptor knockouts in gastric cancer cells. Their findings showed that neither direct cag-T4SS-integrin interactions nor integrin-mediated signaling are essential for CagA translocation.

In another study, researchers used CRISPR/Cas9 to delete miR-30a in *H. pylori*-infected mice. While the genetic modification did not affect mouse development or significantly impact *H. pylori* colonization rates, these mice showed increased rates of chronic gastritis, chronic atrophic gastritis, atypical hyperplasia, and other pre-cancerous conditions, as well as adenocarcinoma in the antral or gastric mucosa. These results establish miR-30a's role as a tumor suppressor in gastric cancer [45].

4.6 CRISPR/Cas9 in Overcoming Drug Resistance in Gastric Cancer

CRISPR technology has proven valuable in understanding tumor cell resistance to chemotherapy and identifying new therapeutic targets and drugs for gastric cancer treatment. Wang and colleagues [46] investigated the relationship between GSDME (gasdermin E) and 5-fluorouracil's mechanism of action by using CRISPR/Cas9 to eliminate GSDME in gastric cancer cells. They discovered that cells lacking GSDME responded to 5-fluorouracil treatment with apoptosis rather than pyroptosis, characterized by cell shrinkage, fragmentation into apoptotic bodies, and death without lysis.

Cui and collaborators [47] explored the role of legumain (AEP), a known oncogene associated with gastric cancer invasiveness and metastasis, by using CRISPR/Cas9 to eliminate it from gastric cancer cells. They found that AEP-deficient gastric cancer cells showed significantly reduced proliferation when treated with various chemotherapy agents including 5-fluorouracil, paclitaxel, docetaxel, and T-DM1. These findings suggest AEP could be a valuable therapeutic target in gastric cancer treatment.

4.7 CRISPR/Cas9 and Gastric Cancer in the Clinical Setting

While CRISPR/Cas9 has revolutionized gene editing and unlocked new possibilities for treating previously "incurable" diseases, its clinical application in gastric cancer therapy still faces substantial hurdles. Chief among these is the challenge of developing delivery systems capable of selectively targeting specific cell populations within complex tissue environments.

Currently, two clinical trials are investigating the therapeutic potential of CRISPR/Cas9 in gastric cancer treatment. The first, titled *"Phase I/II Trial in Patients with Metastatic Gastrointestinal Epithelial Cancer"* (NCT04426669), is a pioneering study evaluating genetically engineered neoantigen-specific tumor-infiltrating lymphocytes. In this trial, CRISPR/Cas9 is employed to disrupt the expression of CISH (cytokine-induced SH2 protein), an intracellular immune checkpoint, with the goal of enhancing anti-tumor immunity. The study aims to assess both the safety and therapeutic efficacy of this approach in gastrointestinal malignancies [48].

The second trial, *"PD-1 Knockout EBV-CTLs for Advanced-Stage Epstein-Barr Virus (EBV)-Associated Malignancies,"* focuses on patients with advanced-stage EBV-associated gastric cancer. It involves the collection of peripheral blood lymphocytes to generate PD-1 knockout cytotoxic T-lymphocytes, which are then reintroduced into the patient. This strategy is designed to improve progression-free survival and overall survival by enhancing the cytotoxic potential of the modified immune cells [49].

4.8 Future Perspectives

Current treatment options for gastric cancer primarily rely on surgical gastrectomy and chemotherapy, despite ongoing research into alternative approaches driven by emerging molecular technologies [50]. The increasing understanding of novel molecular targets and mutations is crucial, particularly since drug resistance remains the primary obstacle to successful treatment. This knowledge helps illuminate genetic variations among different ethnic groups, supporting the advancement of personalized therapeutic approaches [50].

Several challenges must be addressed to achieve progress in this field. The selection of an appropriate gene-editing technique is paramount, especially considering the limited success of gastric cancer gene therapy clinical trials and the current absence of approved therapies. Among available methods, CRISPR technology stands out for its cost-effectiveness and accessibility in treatment applications, offering straightforward single-guide RNA design capabilities and the ability to target genes in various genomic regions, including heterochromatic sites.

However, CRISPR presents certain limitations, including potential off-target modifications and the challenge of delivering the genetic components specifically to tumor sites while preserving healthy tissue. The identification of suitable surface antigens for targeted delivery of the CRISPR system is essential. Promising candidates include the Carcino-Embryonic Antigen (CEA), which shows frequent expression in various gastric cancer types [51], and the oncofetal antigen 5T4 [52], associated with disease advancement and unfavorable clinical outcomes. For delivery mechanisms, adenoviruses, adeno-associated viruses, and ribonucleoproteins represent the most viable options currently available [53].

While viral delivery systems offer superior infection efficiency and knockout effectiveness, their clinical utility is often limited by the induction of strong immune responses that may undermine therapeutic outcomes. In contrast, ribonucleoproteins are better tolerated immunologically but exhibit lower transfection rates, necessitating further optimization to improve their delivery and editing efficiency. Moreover, the overall limited efficacy of CRISPR-based interventions in human subjects underscores the need for continued research to enhance their translational viability.

Gene-editing strategies for gastric cancer treatment can be broadly classified into three principal approaches: (1) tumor-suppressor interventions, which involve permanent gene knockout to inhibit cellular proliferation or reduce metastatic potential; (2) suicide gene therapy, wherein therapeutic genes are introduced to convert non-toxic prodrugs into cytotoxic agents; and (3) immunomodulation, aimed at boosting the host's innate immune response against malignant cells.

Given that TP53 mutations are present in approximately 60% of gastric cancer cases, restoring wild-type p53 function has emerged as a promising therapeutic avenue. In a landmark study conducted in 1999, Ohashi and colleagues demonstrated that adenovirus-mediated p53 restoration significantly suppressed tumor growth, highlighting its clinical potential [54]. Common suicide gene therapy modalities include cytosine deaminase-mediated conversion of 5-fluorocytosine to 5-fluorouracil, and herpes simplex virus thymidine kinase-mediated phosphorylation of ganciclovir, both approaches leveraging on CEA promoters to ensure cancer-specific gene expression [55, 56].

Despite these advances, substantial progress in molecular research is still required before gene therapy can be routinely implemented in clinical settings. A key challenge lies in identifying precise surface molecular targets to enhance therapeutic selectivity and minimize off-target effects. In this context, genome-wide pooled CRISPR libraries have emerged as a powerful tool for biomarker discovery. These lentiviral-based platforms enable the simultaneous random knockout of thousands of genes, facilitating the identification of critical genetic determinants associated with specific phenotypes under selective pressures such as anoikis resistance, chemotherapeutic response, or hypoxic stress [57].

4.9 Conclusion

CRISPR/Cas9 is well positioned to address the biological heterogeneity and therapeutic gaps in gastric cancer by enabling targeted disruption or repair of key driver and resistance genes, systematic mapping of vulnerabilities, and combinatorial strategies that augment existing modalities. Real-world impact will depend on advancing safe and tumor-selective delivery, minimizing off-target editing, and stratifying patients with molecularly guided frameworks so that editing strategies align with actionable alterations and treatment context. As platform technologies mature from discovery to early translational applications, CRISPR/Cas9 can help convert complex gastric cancer biology into actionable precision interventions, with the potential to improve outcomes beyond what is achievable with current standards alone.

References

1. Sung H, Ferlay J, Siegel RL, Laversanne M, Soerjomataram I, Jemal A, Bray F. Global Cancer Statistics 2020: GLOBOCAN Estimates of Incidence and Mortality Worldwide for 36 Cancers in 185 Countries. CA Cancer J Clin. 2021;71(3):209–49.

2. Bray F, Ferlay J, Soerjomataram I, Siegel RL, Torre LA, Jemal A. Global cancer statistics 2018: GLOBOCAN estimates of incidence and mortality worldwide for 36 cancers in 185 countries. CA Cancer J Clin. 2018;68(6):394–424.
3. Dikken JL, van de Velde CJ, Coit DG, Shah MA, Verheij M, Cats A. Treatment of resectable gastric cancer. Therap Adv Gastroenterol. 2012;5(1):49–69.
4. Ito S, Ohashi Y, Sasako M. Survival after recurrence in patients with gastric cancer who receive S-1 adjuvant chemotherapy: exploratory analysis of the ACTS-GC trial. BMC Cancer. 2018;18(1):449.
5. Joshi SS, Badgwell BD. Current treatment and recent progress in gastric cancer. CA Cancer J Clin. 2021;71(3):264–79.
6. Matsuoka T, Yashiro M. Biomarkers of gastric cancer: Current topics and future perspective. World J Gastroenterol. 2018;24(26):2818–32.
7. Leal MF, Wisnieski F, de Oliveira Gigek C, do Santos LC, Calcagno DQ, Burbano RR, Smith MC. What gastric cancer proteomic studies show about gastric carcinogenesis? Tumour Biol. 2016;37(8): 9991–10010.
8. La Russa MF, Qi LS. The New State of the Art: Cas9 for Gene Activation and Repression. Mol Cell Biol. 2015;35(22):3800–9.
9. Kim YG, Cha J, Chandrasegaran S. Hybrid restriction enzymes: zinc finger fusions to Fok I cleavage domain. Proc Natl Acad Sci U S A. 1996;93(3):1156–60.
10. Miller JC, Tan S, Qiao G, Barlow KA, Wang J, Xia DF, et al. A TALE nuclease architecture for efficient genome editing. Nat Biotechnol. 2011;29(2):143–8.
11. Zhang H, Qin C, An C, Zheng X, Wen S, Chen W, et al. Application of the CRISPR/Cas9-based gene editing technique in basic research, diagnosis, and therapy of cancer. Mol Cancer. 2021;20(1):126.
12. Ishaq S, Nunn L. Helicobacter pylori and gastric cancer: a state of the art review. Gastroenterol Hepatol Bed Bench. 2015;8(Suppl 1):S6–S14.
13. Kim J, Cho YA, Choi WJ, Jeong SH. Gene-diet interactions in gastric cancer risk: a systematic review. World J Gastroenterol. 2014;20(28): 9600–10.
14. Clinton SK, Giovannucci EL, Hursting SD. The world cancer research fund/American institute for cancer research third expert report on diet, nutrition, physical activity, and cancer: impact and future directions. J Nutrition. 2020;150(4):663–71.

15. Casamayor M, Morlock R, Maeda H, Ajani J. Targeted literature review of the global burden of gastric cancer. Ecancermedicalscience. 2018;12:883.
16. Berlth F, Bollschweiler E, Drebber U, Hoelscher AH, Moenig S. Pathohistological classification systems in gastric cancer: diagnostic relevance and prognostic value. World J Gastroenterol. 2014;20(19): 5679–84.
17. Clements WM, Wang J, Sarnaik A, Kim OJ, MacDonald J, Fenoglio-Preiser C, et al. beta-Catenin mutation is a frequent cause of Wnt pathway activation in gastric cancer. Cancer Res. 2002;62(12):3503–6.
18. Feng R, Chen X, Yu Y, Su L, Yu B, Li J, et al. miR-126 functions as a tumour suppressor in human gastric cancer. Cancer Lett. 2010;298(1): 50–63.
19. Moses C, Garcia-Bloj B, Harvey AR, Blancafort P. Hallmarks of cancer: The CRISPR generation. Eur J Cancer. 2018;93:10–8.
20. Su S, Zou Z, Chen F, Ding N, Du J, Shao J, et al. CRISPR-Cas9-mediated disruption of PD-1 on human T cells for adoptive cellular therapies of EBV positive gastric cancer. Oncoimmunology. 2017;6(1): e1249558.
21. Deng X, Nakamura Y. Cancer Precision Medicine: From Cancer Screening to Drug Selection and Personalized Immunotherapy. Trends Pharmacol Sci. 2017;38(1):15–24.
22. Gao Q, Dong X, Xu Q, Zhu L, Wang F, Hou Y, Chao CC. Therapeutic potential of CRISPR/Cas9 gene editing in engineered T-cell therapy. Cancer Med. 2019;8(9):4254–64.
23. Cong L, Zhou R, Kuo YC, Cunniff M, Zhang F. Comprehensive interrogation of natural TALE DNA-binding modules and transcriptional repressor domains. Nat Commun. 2012;3:968.
24. Garcia-Bloj B, Moses C, Sgro A, Plani-Lam J, Arooj M, Duffy C, et al. Waking up dormant tumor suppressor genes with zinc fingers, TALEs and the CRISPR/dCas9 system. Oncotarget. 2016;7(37):60535–54.
25. Liu J, Ben Q, Lu E, He X, Yang X, Ma J, et al. Long noncoding RNA PANDAR blocks CDKN1A gene transcription by competitive interaction with p53 protein in gastric cancer. Cell Death Dis. 2018;9(2):168.
26. Gannon HS, Kaplan N, Tsherniak A, Vazquez F, Weir BA, Hahn WC, Meyerson M. Identification of an "Exceptional Responder" Cell Line to MEK1 Inhibition: Clinical Implications for MEK-Targeted Therapy. Mol Cancer Res. 2016;14(2):207–15.

27. Deswaerte V, Nguyen P, West A, Browning AF, Yu L, Ruwanpura SM, et al. Inflammasome Adaptor ASC Suppresses Apoptosis of Gastric Cancer Cells by an IL18-Mediated Inflammation-Independent Mechanism. Cancer Res. 2018;78(5):1293–307.
28. Park YS, Lee JH, Jung DB, Kim HB, Jung JH, Pak S, et al. MicroRNA-21 induces loss of 15-hydroxyprostaglandin dehydrogenase in early gastric tubular adenocarcinoma. Sci Rep. 2018;8(1):17717.
29. Lai J, Wang H, Luo Q, Huang S, Lin S, Zheng Y, Chen Q. The relationship between DNA methylation and Reprimo gene expression in gastric cancer cells. Oncotarget. 2017;8(65):108610–23.
30. Hu L, Bai ZG, Ma XM, Bai N, Zhang ZT. MRFAP1 plays a protective role in neddylation inhibitor MLN4924-mediated gastric cancer cell death. Eur Rev Med Pharmacol Sci. 2018;22(23):8273–80.
31. Zhang X, Qian Y, Li F, Bei S, Li M, Feng L. microRNA-9 selectively targets LMX1A to promote gastric cancer cell progression. Biochem Biophys Res Commun. 2018;505(2):405–12.
32. Machlowska J, Baj J, Sitarz M, Maciejewski R, Sitarz R. Gastric Cancer: Epidemiology, Risk Factors, Classification, Genomic Characteristics and Treatment Strategies. Int J Mol Sci. 2020;21(11):4012.
33. Zhuo W, Liu Y, Li S, Guo D, Sun Q, Jin J, et al. Long Noncoding RNA GMAN, Up-regulated in Gastric Cancer Tissues, Is Associated With Metastasis in Patients and Promotes Translation of Ephrin A1 by Competitively Binding GMAN-AS. Gastroenterology. 2019;156(3):676–91.e11.
34. Zhang YQ, Pei JH, Shi SS, Guo XS, Cui GY, Li YF, et al. CRISPR/Cas9-mediated knockout of the PDEF gene inhibits migration and invasion of human gastric cancer AGS cells. Biomed Pharmacother. 2019;111:76–85.
35. Araújo T, Khayat A, Quintana L, Calcagno D, Mourão R, Modesto A, et al. Piwi like RNA-mediated gene silencing 1 gene as a possible major player in gastric cancer. World J Gastroenterol. 2018; 24(47):5338–50.
36. Chen W, Ding R, Tang J, Li H, Chen C, Zhang Y, et al. Knocking Out SST Gene of BGC823 Gastric Cancer Cell by CRISPR/Cas9 Enhances Migration, Invasion and Expression of SEMA5A and KLF2. Cancer Manag Res. 2020;12:1313–21.
37. Yin J, Li Z, Ye L, Birkin E, Li L, Xu R, et al. EphB2 represents an independent prognostic marker in patients with gastric cancer and promotes tumour cell aggressiveness. J Cancer. 2020;11(10):2778–87.

38. Zhu M, Yan C, Ren C, Huang X, Zhu X, Gu H, et al. Exome Array Analysis Identifies Variants in SPOCD1 and BTN3A2 That Affect Risk for Gastric Cancer. Gastroenterology. 2017;152(8):2011–21.
39. Wang F, Meng W, Wang B, Qiao L. Helicobacter pylori-induced gastric inflammation and gastric cancer. Cancer Lett. 2014;345(2): 196–202.
40. Hooi JKY, Lai WY, Ng WK, Suen MMY, Underwood FE, Tanyingoh D, et al. Global Prevalence of Helicobacter pylori Infection: Systematic Review and Meta-Analysis. Gastroenterology. 2017;153(2):420–9.
41. Hu W, Zhang L, Li MX, Shen J, Liu XD, Xiao ZG, et al. Vitamin D3 activates the autolysosomal degradation function against Helicobacter pylori through the PDIA3 receptor in gastric epithelial cells. Autophagy. 2019;15(4):707–25.
42. Foegeding NJ, Caston RR, McClain MS, Ohi MD, Cover TL. An Overview of Helicobacter pylori VacA Toxin Biology. Toxins (Basel). 2016;8(6):173.
43. Foegeding NJ, Raghunathan K, Campbell AM, Kim SW, Lau KS, Kenworthy AK, et al. Intracellular Degradation of Helicobacter pylori VacA Toxin as a Determinant of Gastric Epithelial Cell Viability. Infect Immun. 2019;87(4):e00783–18.
44. Zhao Q, Busch B, Jiménez-Soto LF, Ishikawa-Ankerhold H, Massberg S, Terradot L, et al. Integrin but not CEACAM receptors are dispensable for Helicobacter pylori CagA translocation. PLoS Pathog. 2018;14(10):e1007359.
45. Liu X, Ji Q, Zhang C, Liu X, Liu Y, Liu N, et al. miR-30a acts as a tumor suppressor by double-targeting COX-2 and BCL9 in H. pylori gastric cancer models. Sci Rep. 2017;7(1):7113.
46. Wang Y, Yin B, Li D, Wang G, Han X, Sun X. GSDME mediates caspase-3-dependent pyroptosis in gastric cancer. Biochem Biophys Res Commun. 2018;495(1):1418–25.
47. Cui Y, Li Q, Li H, Wang Y, Wang H, Chen W, et al. Asparaginyl endopeptidase improves the resistance of microtubule-targeting drugs in gastric cancer through IQGAP1 modulating the EGFR/JNK/ERK signaling pathway. Onco Targets Ther. 2017;10:627–43.
48. Lou E, Choudhry MS, Starr TK, Folsom TD, Bell J, Rathmann B, et al. Targeting the intracellular immune checkpoint CISH with CRISPR-Cas9-edited T cells in patients with metastatic colorectal cancer: a first-in-human, single-centre, phase 1 trial. Lancet Oncol. 2025;26(5): 559–70.

49. Yang Y. PD-1 knockout EBV-CTLs for advanced stage Epstein–Barr virus (EBV) associated malignancies. 2017. https://clinicaltrials.gov/study/NCT03044743.
50. Marin JJ, Al-Abdulla R, Lozano E, Briz O, Bujanda L, Banales JM, Macias RI. Mechanisms of Resistance to Chemotherapy in Gastric Cancer. Anticancer Agents Med Chem. 2016;16(3):318–34.
51. Khare PD, Shao-Xi L, Kuroki M, Hirose Y, Arakawa F, Nakamura K, et al. Specifically targeted killing of carcinoembryonic antigen (CEA)-expressing cells by a retroviral vector displaying single-chain variable fragmented antibody to CEA and carrying the gene for inducible nitric oxide synthase. Cancer Res. 2001;61(1):370–5.
52. Shaw DM, Embleton MJ, Westwater C, Ryan MG, Myers KA, Kingsman SM, et al. Isolation of a high affinity scFv from a monoclonal antibody recognising the oncofoetal antigen 5T4. Biochim Biophys Acta. 2000;1524(2–3):238–46.
53. Biagioni A, Chillà A, Andreucci E, Laurenzana A, Margheri F, Peppicelli S, et al. Type II CRISPR/Cas9 approach in the oncological therapy. J Exp Clin Cancer Res. 2017;36(1):80.
54. Ohashi M, Kanai F, Ueno H, Tanaka T, Tateishi K, Kawakami T, et al. Adenovirus mediated p53 tumour suppressor gene therapy for human gastric cancer cells in vitro and in vivo. Gut. 1999;44(3):366–71.
55. Okino T, Onda M, Matsukura N, Inada KI, Tatematsu M, Suzuki S, Shimada T. Sequential histopathological changes in vivo after suicide gene therapy of gastric cancer induced by N-methyl-N′-nitro-N-nitrosoguanidine in rats. Jpn J Cancer Res. 2001;92(6):673–9.
56. Shimizu T, Shimada H, Ochiai T, Hamada H. Enhanced growth suppression in esophageal carcinoma cells using adenovirus-mediated fusion gene transfer (uracil phosphoribosyl transferase and herpes simplex virus thymidine kinase). Cancer Gene Ther. 2001;8(7):512–21.
57. Joung J, Konermann S, Gootenberg JS, Abudayyeh OO, Platt RJ, Brigham MD, et al. Genome-scale CRISPR-Cas9 knockout and transcriptional activation screening. Nat Protoc. 2017;12(4):828–63.

https://doi.org/10.1142/9789819826759_0005

CHAPTER 5

CRISPR/Cas9 in the Treatment of Pancreatic Cancer

Mehrdad Hashemi[1,2], *Alireza Khosravinejad*[1,3], *Mina Alimohammadi*[4], *Reza Mohajer Shirazi*[1,3], *Behdokht Jamali*[5], *Kimia Sadat Esfahani*[1,3], *Ali Shirazi*[1,3], *Faranak Jamshidian*[1,6], *Amir Sadeghi*[7], *Neda Zali*[3], *Najma Farahani*[1,*], *Afshin Taheriazam*[1,8,*], *Payman Rahimzadeh*[9,*], *Maliheh Entezari*[1,2,*]

[1]Farhikhtegan Medical Convergent Sciences Research Center, Farhikhtegan Hospital, Faculty of Medicine, TeMs. C., Islamic Azad University, Tehran, Iran
[2]Department of Genetics, Faculty of Advanced Sciences and Technology, TeMs. C, Islamic Azad University, Tehran, Iran
[3]Basic and Molecular Epidemiology of Gastrointestinal Disorders Research Center, Research Institute for Gastroenterology and Liver Diseases, Shahid Beheshti University of Medical Sciences, Tehran, Iran
[4]Department of Immunology, School of Medicine, Shahid Beheshti University of Medical Sciences, Tehran, Iran
[5]Department of Microbiology and Genetics, Kherad Institute of Higher Education, Bushehr, Iran

* **Corresponding authors:** Najmafarahani@gmail.com (N.F.); a.taheriazam@iautmu.ac.ir (A.T.); P.rahimzadeh76@gmail.com (P.R.); mentezari@iautmu.ac.ir (M.E.)

[6]Department of Biology, ET.C., Islamic Azad University, Tehran, Iran
[7]Gastroenterology and Liver Diseases Research Center, Research Institute for Gastroenterology and Liver Diseases, Shahid Beheshti University of Medical Sciences, Tehran, Iran
[8]Department of Orthopedics, Faculty of Medicine, TeMs. C, Islamic Azad University, Tehran, Iran
[9]Surgical Research Society (SRS), Students' Scientific Research Center, Tehran University of Medical Sciences, Tehran, Iran

Abstract

Pancreatic cancer remains one of the deadliest malignancies, ranking as the 12th most common cancer but the fifth leading cause of cancer-related mortality in the United States. Despite advances in medical oncology, the overall five-year survival rate for pancreatic cancer has only modestly improved, lingering around 9%. Standard therapeutic approaches such as surgical resection, radiotherapy, and systemic chemotherapy continue to dominate clinical practice, yet they provide limited benefits due to late-stage diagnosis, intrinsic resistance, and rapid disease progression. Consequently, novel and more effective strategies are urgently needed. In recent years, targeted therapies, immunomodulatory approaches, and gene-editing platforms have emerged as potential avenues for intervention. Among these, the CRISPR/Cas9 system has garnered considerable attention for its simplicity, efficiency, and versatility compared with earlier gene-editing technologies, including meganucleases, zinc finger nucleases, and transcription activator-like effector nucleases. Originally discovered as a microbial adaptive immune defense system, CRISPR/Cas9 has since been repurposed to enable precise genomic modifications, with compelling preclinical evidence supporting its application in pancreatic cancer research. This chapter highlights the growing potential of CRISPR/Cas9 as a therapeutic tool for pancreatic cancer, examining its advantages over conventional gene-editing platforms, its relevance for precision oncology, and its implications for future clinical translation.

Keywords: pancreatic cancer; CRISPR/Cas9; gene editing; precision oncology; targeted therapy; cancer therapeutics

5.1 Introduction

Based on statistics from the North American Association of Central Cancer Registries, pancreatic cancer ranks as the 12th most prevalent cancer type and holds the position of having the 5th poorest survival outlook in the United States. Projections for 2019 indicate approximately 56,770 new diagnoses and 45,750 fatalities attributed to pancreatic cancer in the United States [142]. Unlike advancements seen in other cancer types, pancreatic cancer treatment success rates have remained relatively stagnant, maintaining a mere 9% five-year survival rate [1]. While traditional approaches such as surgical intervention, radiotherapy, and chemical treatments remain the standard of care, researchers are actively pursuing novel therapeutic strategies, including precision-targeted treatments, immunological approaches, and potential genetic modifications using CRISPR/Cas9 technology.

The initial discovery of CRISPR sequences was made by researchers in 1987 [2], followed by a breakthrough in 2012 that demonstrated how a dual-RNA structure could guide an endonuclease to specific DNA targets [3]. This technology has since undergone rapid development, leading to significant advances in both research and clinical applications. When compared to alternative genetic modification methods like meganucleases, zinc finger nucleases, and transcription activator-like effector nucleases, the CRISPR/Cas9 system offers distinct advantages: it is more cost-effective, demonstrates superior efficiency, and requires less complex implementation procedures.

5.2 Genetic and Molecular Landscape of Pancreatic Cancer

Pancreatic ductal adenocarcinoma (PDAC) represents one of the most lethal malignancies, showing substantial resistance to existing treatments. Late detection means that surgical options are available to only 15–20% of diagnosed individuals [1]. Even with improvements in both surgical techniques and chemotherapy regimens, patients still face a dire prognosis, with fewer than 10%

surviving beyond five years [1]. The incidence of PDAC continues to rise by roughly 1% each year, and experts project it will rank second among cancer-related deaths by 2030 [4].

The molecular landscape of PDAC reveals consistent alterations in principal oncogenic drivers, with KRAS, TP53, SMAD4, and CDKN2A mutations appearing either alone or together in over 50% of cases. Additional genetic changes affecting ARID1A, KDM6A, MLL3, TGFBR2, RBM10, and BCORL1 occur less commonly, being present in less than 10% of tumors [5–7]. A limited group of PDAC cases shows genetic modifications that could respond to specific targeted treatments, including amplified ERBB2, altered BRAF, and variations in DNA damage repair (DDR) genes such as BRCA1, BRCA2, and PALB2 [8, 9]. Scientists are currently investigating several promising "actionable molecular phenotypes" in clinical trials [6].

An extensive review analyzing 21,842 PDAC genomes identified that DDR gene mutations leading to homologous recombination deficiency (HRD) are present in 14.5–16.5% of instances [10]. New research indicates that genomic instability, detected through structural variation examination and BRCA mutation patterns (BRCAness phenotype), may offer alternative methods for identifying HRD [7, 10]. This expanded HRD classification includes not just inherited mutation carriers but also encompasses patients with acquired DDR mutations or those exhibiting "BRCAness phenotype" characteristics [10]. Since HRD status can predict positive responses to DNA-damaging therapeutic agents, including platinum compounds and PARP inhibitors, as many as 44% of PDAC patients might respond to these treatment approaches [6, 10].

Research utilizing transcriptomic studies has revealed that PDAC can be categorized into two primary subtypes: Classical and Basal-like, with patients having the Basal-like subtype showing poorer survival rates [5, 11–14]. The key distinction between these subtypes lies in the expression patterns of specific pancreatic transcription factors, notably GATA6, PDX1, and HNF1A, which maintain their activity in Classical tumors but show no expression in

Basal-like cases [5, 11, 13, 14]. Modern analytical methods, particularly scRNAseq and snRNAseq, have provided deeper insights into cellular diversity within tumors and helped explain treatment resistance and spread [15].

Studies have demonstrated that the tumor microenvironment plays a vital role in both cancer advancement and treatment efficacy in PDAC [16, 17]. A distinctive feature of PDAC is its classification as an "immunologically cold" cancer, characterized by reduced numbers of CD8+ cytotoxic T cells and increased levels of immunosuppressive cells, which explains why most patients respond poorly to immune-based treatments [18, 19]. Immunotherapy has shown limited effectiveness, with positive outcomes restricted mainly to a subset of patients whose cancers exhibit MSI-high or dMMR characteristics [20, 21].

The implementation of cutting-edge technologies, such as spatially resolved transcriptomics and multiplexed imaging methods, has allowed researchers to gain unprecedented understanding of how tumor and immune cells interact, leading to new perspectives on PDAC's immunological landscape [15]. By examining bulk RNA data through established genetic markers, researchers have discovered that multiple immune cell populations — including T cells, B cells, and myeloid cells — create diverse immunological patterns within the PDAC tumor microenvironment.

Modern immune profiling methods including single-cell RNA sequencing, spatial transcriptomics, and advanced immunofluorescence have revealed specific immune landscapes linked to Classical and Basal-like PDAC subtypes [15]. Research shows that Basal-like tumors contain higher numbers of macrophages while having fewer cytotoxic T cells at both primary and metastatic locations [22]. This insight points to the potential effectiveness of macrophage-targeting therapies, particularly CSF1R inhibitors, in treating Basal-like tumors [23]. The interplay between DNA damage repair and microsatellite instability status and their effects on immune composition within different PDAC molecular subtypes requires further investigation.

Higher numbers of T cells within tumors have been linked to better survival outcomes in PDAC patients and could indicate potential success with immunotherapy [24, 25]. Analysis at the single-cell level has shown that when myeloid cells are abundant, CD8+ T cell infiltration tends to be lower [17]. These tumor-infiltrating CD8+ T cells frequently show signs of exhaustion, which becomes more pronounced as the cancer progresses [25].

Research has identified increased TIGIT expression as a key marker of exhausted CD8+ T cells [15]. Its binding partner PVR appears on various cell types, including cancerous, endocrine, endothelial, and myeloid cells, highlighting myeloid cells' contribution to immune suppression in PDAC [17]. Studies reveal that PD-1/PD-L1 checkpoint expression varies among PDAC patients and corresponds to specific immune environments [25]. Researchers have also noted differences in immune profiles between original tumors and their metastases [22, 23]. These observations suggest the need for customized checkpoint-targeted treatments based on individual immune characteristics [15, 17]. Our understanding of how immune environments change during treatment remains limited, emphasizing the value of ongoing longitudinal single-cell research.

Mutations in genes like KRAS and MYC have been demonstrated to shape the tumor microenvironment and increase its immunosuppressive nature [26–28]. While microsatellite instability, which often predicts immunotherapy success, is uncommon in PDAC (about 1%) [21], tumors with BRCA1/2 deficiencies typically show increased immune cell presence but limited response to immune checkpoint inhibitors (ICIs). Recent experimental studies with animals indicate that BRCA2-deficient tumors may respond better to ICIs than BRCA1-deficient ones [29, 30]. The frequent loss of CDKN2A in PDAC has been identified as a potential marker for ICI resistance across multiple cancer types [31]. These discoveries highlight how various factors affect immunotherapy outcomes and stress the importance of examining both genomic and biomarker profiles when developing immunotherapy strategies.

5.3 Mechanistic Basis of CRISPR/Cas9 in Pancreatic Cancer

Recent advancements in CRISPR knockout screening have revolutionized the identification of genes linked to metastasis progression [32, 33]. Research conducted by Bakke et al. utilized the Brunello human CRISPR knockout library in combination with Cas9-expressing PANC-1 cells to explore critical PDAC genes. Through next-generation sequencing, they identified PSMA6 (proteasome subunit alpha type 6) as a key target, with subsequent siRNA validation confirming its significance as a potential therapeutic avenue in PDAC treatment [34].

Building on this methodology, Oladimeji et al. employed comparable screening techniques with the same library and cellular model, leading to the discovery of two crucial modulators of pancreatic cancer cell invasion: MBNL3 (Muscleblind Like Splicing Regulator 3) and KANSL2 (KAT8 Regulatory NSL Complex Subunit 2). Their findings were substantiated through both CRISPR knockout and siRNA suppression techniques [35].

In 2024, Martinez and colleagues conducted innovative *in vivo* CRISPR/Cas9 screening to investigate lesser-studied PDAC genes and their relationships with oncogenic KRASG12D during cancer development. Their investigation uncovered USP15 (Ubiquitin Specific Peptidase 15) and SCAF1 (SR-Related CTD Associated Factor 1) as tumor-suppressing elements that modulate inflammatory responses and sensitivity to Olaparib [36]. Further *in vivo* CRISPR studies highlighted the significance of SREBPs (sterol regulatory element-binding proteins) and terpenoid backbone biosynthesis in PDAC development, pointing toward potential therapeutic interventions targeting lipid metabolism pathways [37].

The implementation of these comprehensive CRISPR screening methodologies has significantly enhanced our understanding of how cancer cells respond to various drug treatments [38].

Understanding gemcitabine resistance in pancreatic cancer treatment has advanced through Yang et al.'s extensive research using genome-scale CRISPR knockout GeCKO library screening in TB32047 mouse pancreatic cancer cells. Their investigation revealed that elimination of deoxycytidine kinase and cyclin L1 enhanced resistance to gemcitabine [39].

A comprehensive investigation by Ramaker et al. combined CRISPRa and CRISPR knockout genome-wide screenings, utilizing SAM and GeCKO pooled single-guide RNA (sgRNA) libraries in PDAC cells to examine drug resistance mechanisms. Their study identified ATP-binding cassette transporter (ABCG2) activation as a consistent factor in chemoresistance across all screenings. They discovered that activating transcriptional co-repressor complex genes, including HDAC1, through CRISPR enhanced promoter binding and activated epithelial-mesenchymal transition (EMT)-related genes and cell migration pathways. However, their validation efforts for VPS25, a promising candidate from their knockout screening, produced inconsistent outcomes [40].

Independent genome-wide CRISPR/Cas9 loss-of-function screening identified CDK7 as a vital target among various cell cycle checkpoint and DNA damage-related kinases in addressing drug resistance [41].

Further whole-genome CRISPR/Cas9 loss-of-function screening established PKMYT1 as both a genetic vulnerability and potential therapeutic target in PDAC [42]. Additional screening revealed that disrupting PI3K/AKT/mTOR pathway genes improved CDK4/6 inhibitor efficacy in pancreatic cancer [43]. Wang et al., employing GeCKOv2 and Avana libraries in KRAS-mutant pancreatic cancer cells [PATU8902 and PATU8988T], identified CIC and ATXN1L as crucial regulators of MEK1/2 inhibitor resistance [44]. A separate genome-wide study combining CRISPR interference and knockout screening identified several SAC genes — including BUB1B, BUB3, and TTK — that enhance cell survival during nab-paclitaxel treatment. These SAC genes, essential for chromosome segregation during cell division, were found to modulate nab-paclitaxel's cytotoxic effects when inhibited [45].

The role of CRISPR-based functional genomic screening has become crucial in discovering and confirming novel therapeutic targets for precision medicine applications [46]. Research by

Steinhart et al. employed CRISPR/Cas9 screening with a TKO gRNA library in RNF43-mutant PDAC cells, revealing key Wnt pathway elements (WLS, CTNNB1, TCF7L2, LRP5, PORCN) and specific genes (FZD5, WNT7B, WNT10A) essential for HPAFII cell growth. Their research confirmed the Wnt signaling pathway's fundamental role in driving pancreatic cancer progression [47].

Scientists have identified the RAS/RAF/MEK/ERK pathway as a fundamental driver of tumor development, providing vital survival signals to cancer cells [48]. A comprehensive study by Szlachta et al. in 2018 conducted both *in vivo* and *in vitro* CRISPR knockout screening using a specialized nuclear sgRNA library targeting 3,733 nuclear protein genes. Their investigation in a PDX model identified genes whose removal enhanced the effectiveness of the MEK inhibitor trametinib. Further validation of top candidates CENPE and RRM1 demonstrated that their suppression notably improved trametinib treatment response [49].

The applications of CRISPR-based screening have expanded beyond identifying tumorigenic or chemoresistance genes to explore genetic factors involved in immune evasion and immunotherapy resistance. A 2023 investigation utilized genome-scale CRISPR/Cas9 loss-of-function screens in mesothelin-expressing pancreatic cancer cells to examine CAR-T cell therapy resistance mechanisms. Through the use of the Brunello lentiviral library, followed by puromycin selection and co-culture with mesothelin-specific CAR-T cells, researchers discovered that disrupting glycosylphosphatidylinositol-anchor biosynthesis genes undermined CAR-T cell anti-tumor efficacy. Additionally, they found that TFAP4 elimination increased NFκB transcription factor p65, indicating that CAR-T cell therapy resistance involves changes in intrinsic tumor states [50].

Research by Gu et al. implemented genome-wide CRISPR/Cas9 knockout screening across both epithelial and mesenchymal-like pancreatic cancer cells, leading to the identification and confirmation of EGFR and MFGE8 as specific regulators of CTL-mediated killing in mesenchymal cells. Their findings revealed that elevated expression of these genes was linked to decreased survival rates and increased immune evasion from CD8+ T cells, while their elimination enhanced the vulnerability of mesenchymal-like cancer cells to CTL-mediated destruction [51].

In recent work from 2024, Sang and colleagues utilized *in vivo* CRISPR screening in orthotopic PDAC models to discover RIPK2's crucial role in regulating the immunosuppressive tumor microenvironment, demonstrating its impact on suppressing antigen presentation and cytotoxic T-cell function [52]. Complementary *in vivo* studies validated KDM3A as an epigenetic modulator influencing PDAC's immune landscape, with its removal leading to enhanced immune cell infiltration and improved immunotherapy response (**Table 5.1**) [53].

While these investigations highlight the value of CRISPR pooled library screening in uncovering new gene functions and therapeutic targets in pancreatic cancer, several technical considerations can impact screening reliability. The size of the library determines cell quantity requirements for sufficient coverage, and selection pressure intensity affects both data completeness and false-positive rates. Furthermore, varying selection methodologies may introduce experimental inconsistencies, while sequencing quality and analytical tool selection play vital roles in result accuracy. These challenges underscore the necessity of validating discoveries through multiple experimental approaches.

5.4 Targeting Oncogenes in Pancreatic Cancer with CRISPR/Cas9

Current research is extensively exploring CRISPR's potential to target cancer-associated oncogenic mutations [70] and eliminate mutant KRAS function across various cancer models [71]. CRISPR knockout offers advantages over RNA interference approaches, providing complete gene expression elimination with minimal off-target effects [72].

KRAS, a G-protein family member controlling cell survival and proliferation, becomes oncogenic when mutations disable its GTPase activity, leading to abnormal signaling and pancreatic cancer development [73]. Present in over 90% of pancreatic cancer cases, oncogenic KRAS mutations are primary drivers of poor

Table 5.1 CRISPR applications in pancreatic cancer research.

Target Gene or Protein	CRISPR-based System Used	Outcome	References
KRAS	CRISPR/Cas9	Knockout reduced cancer cell viability and tumor proliferation	[54, 55]
KRASG12D	CRISPR/Cas9	Successful knockout in human and mouse pancreatic cancer cell lines	[56]
KRASG12D	Exosomal CRISPR/Cas9	Oncogenic allele knockout using exosomal delivery approach	[57]
KRASG12S	CRISPR/Cas9 and dCas9-KRAB	Inhibition of cancer cell proliferation *in vitro* and *in vivo*	[54]
KRAS transcripts	CRISPR/Cas13a	Up to 94% knockdown efficiency without affecting wild-type mRNA	[58]
KRASG12D transcript	CRISPR/CasRx	Precise silencing with exceptional specificity in PDAC cells	[59]
SMAD2/SMAD3	CRISPR/Cas9	Restricted pancreatic cancer invasiveness	[60]
ASAP2	CRISPR/Cas9	Elevated in 72.3% of PDAC patients; knockout elucidated tumor growth role	[61]
Rab11-FIP4	CRISPR/Cas9	Knockout inhibited cell cycle progression and tumorigenesis	[62]
KLF5	CRISPR/Cas9	Knockout decreased acinar-to-ductal metaplasia and pancreatic intraepithelial neoplasia development	[63]
Amylase	CRISPR/Cas9	Knockout diminished autophagy, contributing to pancreatic cancer etiology	[64]
TERT	CRISPR/Cas9	Multi-exon targeting reduced cancer cell survival *in vitro* and *in vivo*	[65]
Annexin A1	CRISPR/Cas9	Knockout reversed EMT and reduced metastasis rate	[66]
CD73	CRISPR/Cas9	Knockout inhibited cell growth, migration, and induces cell cycle arrest	[67]
EIF4EBP3	CRISPR/Cas9	Knockout diminished inhibitory effects of mTOR inhibitors	[68]
SphK1	CRISPR/Cas9	Knockout enhanced proliferation and migration in pancreatic cancer	[69]
SphK2	CRISPR/Cas9	Knockout exhibited effects favoring pancreatic cancer inhibition	[69]

prognosis and therapy resistance, making KRAS silencing a crucial therapeutic strategy [74]. Traditional treatments have focused on targeting downstream KRAS effectors due to the challenges of directly targeting mutated KRAS [75].

Groundbreaking CRISPR research by Muzumdar et al. explored KRAS suppression resistance in pancreatic cancer, though they acknowledged limitations in sgRNA's ability to differentiate between wild-type and mutant KRAS due to Protospacer Adjacent Motif (PAM) site constraints [76]. Their research confirmed that KRAS knockdown significantly reduced viability only in KRAS-dependent cells [77].

Scientists have successfully applied CRISPR/Cas9 to target multiple KRAS mutant variants (G12V, G12D, G12S, G13D) for tumor control [54, 55, 75]. In 2018, Lee and colleagues showed that CRISPR/Cas9-mediated elimination of G12V and G12D mutations at KRAS codon-12, frequently found in pancreatic cancer, decreased cancer cell survival [75]. Following this, Lentsch et al. achieved successful heterozygous removal of KRASG12D in both human and mouse pancreatic cancer cells [56].

Innovation in delivery methods now includes exosome-based approaches for KRASG12D knockout [57], with systems delivering CRISPR/Cas9 components as plasmid DNA, mRNA, or ribonucleoprotein to reduce risks linked to extended bacterial Cas9 expression [78].

Gao et al. developed an innovative dual CRISPR strategy targeting oncogenic KRASG12S, combining traditional CRISPR/Cas9 genome editing with dCas9-KRAB transcriptional repression. The dCas9-KRAB system functions by binding to target sequences while suppressing mRNA production. Both approaches successfully targeted the mutation while preserving normal KRAS, leading to decreased cancer cell growth in both laboratory and animal models [54].

As an alternative to CRISPR/Cas9, Cas13a has emerged as a novel CRISPR effector specifically targeting RNA sequences [79]. Zhao et al. developed a CRISPR/Cas13a system targeting KRASG12D and KRASG12C transcripts in pancreatic cancer. Their approach, using bacterial Cas13a protein with CRISPR RNA, achieved 94% reduction in mutant KRAS mRNA while maintaining normal KRAS mRNA levels [58].

CasRx, a modified Cas13d variant with nuclear localization capability, represents a significant advance in post-transcriptional gene silencing, showing improved efficiency in targeting both coding and non-coding RNAs with enhanced specificity [80].

CasRx has demonstrated limited off-target activity in mammalian cells and possesses a more compact structure compared to Cas9 [81]. Research by Jiang and colleagues revealed that the CRISPR/CasRx platform could efficiently and selectively inhibit mutant KRASG12D expression in PDAC cells. Their experiments showed that when guided by KRASG12D-specific gRNA, CasRx effectively suppressed mutant KRASG12D expression in these cells. This suppression inhibited downstream signaling cascades activated by mutant KRASG12D, which ultimately decreased tumor progression and improved PDAC cells' response to gemcitabine treatment. These results demonstrate the potential of CRISPR/CasRx as a viable strategy for targeting and downregulating mutant KRASG12D transcripts to reduce PDAC malignancy [59].

The application of CRISPR for mutant KRAS targeting encounters several challenges. A key technical limitation is the limited availability of appropriate PAM sites near crucial point mutations, complicating selective modification of mutant alleles while maintaining wild-type sequences. This restriction hampers the development of precise gene-editing strategies for oncogenic KRAS variants, often resulting in non-selective KRAS suppression, which is typical of current CRISPR-based approaches under evaluation [76]. Although alternative enzymes such as Cas12a [Cpf1] recognize distinct PAM sequences and may address certain PAM constraints depending on the genetic context [82], the fundamental sequence-dependency issue remains across all PAM-dependent CRISPR systems. Advanced gene-editing technologies like base editors and prime editors, developed from modified Cas9 or Cas12 variants, provide greater precision by allowing specific nucleotide modifications without double-strand break formation. These innovative methods help circumvent some PAM-related limitations and reduce off-target effects [83, 84], showing promise for allele-specific modification of oncogenic mutations, including KRAS variants.

The inability of current therapeutic agents to target frequently mutated driver genes such as KRAS, TP53, CDKN2A, and SMAD4, which correlate with poor PDAC patient outcomes [85], emphasizes the necessity for identifying new targetable molecules. One notable example involves TGF-β signaling, which plays a crucial role in PDAC tumor progression through SMAD pathway activation. During cancer advancement, SMAD2 and SMAD3 enhance cell motility, and their removal via CRISPR-mediated knockout diminishes pancreatic cancer invasion [60]. This analysis synthesizes various research findings demonstrating the significance of CRISPR systems in eliminating novel targets in pancreatic cancer cells to comprehend their biological relevance and assess their impact on cancer development.

Analysis of clinical data reveals that ASAP2 (ankyrin repeat and PH domain 2) shows increased DNA copy numbers in 72.3% of PDAC cases, with these patients experiencing notably poorer outcomes. Through CRISPR/Cas9-mediated gene deletion, Fujii and colleagues investigated ASAP2's influence on tumor development, seeking to identify new therapeutic targets. Their research suggests ASAP2's potential as a valuable treatment target for PDAC [61]. In a related study, He and collaborators advanced the understanding of pancreatic cancer drivers by showing that eliminating Rab11-FIP4 (Rab11-family interacting protein 4) through CRISPR/Cas9 technology inhibited cellular proliferation and tumor formation in PANC-1 cells. Research indicates that Rab11-FIPs may act as cancer-promoting factors in certain malignancies, with increased expression observed across 60 pancreatic cancer specimens [62].

Immunohistochemistry evaluations have detected higher KLF5 (Krüppel-like factor 5) levels in 96 PDAC samples and mouse models compared to normal tissue. KLF5 appears to play a crucial role in the development of KRAS-induced pancreatic intraepithelial neoplasia. During PDAC development, acinar cells undergo a transformation, losing their original characteristics and acquiring duct cell features. Once KLF5 was removed using CRISPR/Cas9, researchers observed increased NDRG2 expression and reduced

STAT3 activation, leading to decreased acinar-to-ductal transformation and reduced pancreatic intraepithelial neoplasia formation in mouse studies [63]. Additionally, amylase, a key acinar cell marker, has been linked to pancreatic cancer progression when depleted; its removal through CRISPR technology results in reduced autophagy, contributing to pancreatic cancer development [64].

CRISPR technologies can be developed to simultaneously target multiple genes, including those involved in telomere maintenance (such as TERT), ALT pathway components, and other essential genes for cancer cell survival [65]. Most cancer cells achieve immortality by utilizing TERT to prevent continuous telomere shortening [86]. Various research groups have employed Cas9 to modify TERT promoter sequences or eliminate the TERT gene entirely [87–90]. One investigation utilized a CRISPR/Cas9 approach with three distinct gRNAs targeting different TERT exons in pancreatic, cervical, and breast cancer cells. This comprehensive editing strategy effectively reduced cancer cell viability in both laboratory and animal studies [65]. Additionally, CRISPR/Cas9-mediated elimination of annexin A1 has been shown to reverse EMT, resulting in reduced cancer aggressiveness and decreased metastasis in animal models, emphasizing annexin A1's significant role in pancreatic cancer advancement [66].

In recent work, Zhang and colleagues demonstrated that CRISPR/Cas9-mediated CD73 targeting inhibited cellular proliferation and movement while inducing G1 phase cell cycle arrest in both human and mouse cell lines. The removal of CD73 activated the E-cadherin pathway while suppressing ERK/STAT3 signaling [67]. Tsukumo and collaborators employed CRISPR technology to investigate mTOR inhibition effects on 4E-BPs in cancer-related genes. Their research revealed increased 4E-BP3 expression during prolonged mTORC1 inhibition, while CRISPR/Cas9 deletion of the EIF4EBP3 gene promoter reduced mTOR inhibitor effectiveness, suggesting 4E-BP3's crucial role in mTORC1 regulation [68]. A study examining sphingosine kinases [SphK1 and SphK2] in pancreatic cancer found that CRISPR/Cas9 elimination of SphK1 in PAN02 cells enhanced proliferation and migration while reducing survival in mice with pancreatic cancer peritoneal carcinomatosis. In contrast, SphK2 elimination produced opposite effects that suppressed pancreatic cancer, identifying it as a potential PDAC therapeutic target [69].

5.5 Restoring Tumor Suppressor Functions

In cancer development, the suppression of tumor suppressor genes carries equal importance to oncogene activation [91]. In pancreatic carcinomas, tumor suppressor genes like p16/CDKN2A, TP53, and SMAD4 frequently exhibit loss-of-function mutations in their promoter regions, with inactivation seen in more than half of all cases [92]. CRISPR systems aid in the restoration of normal tumor suppressor gene function and activity, which helps prevent tumor formation and progression [93]. A notable example involves PTEN tumor suppressor, which shows reduced or absent expression in many primary melanomas. Researchers found that enhancing PTEN expression using dCas9-VPR suppressed cancer-promoting pathways, limited cell movement, and decreased colony establishment in melanoma cells exposed to various targeted treatments [94].

CRISPR technology has also facilitated the discovery of new tumor suppressors relevant to cancer treatment, with research revealing several promising results [93]. Vorvis and colleagues demonstrated that pancreatic tumor xenografts lacking FOXA2 (forkhead box protein A2) in PANC-1 cells exhibited significantly greater mass and size compared to control groups [92]. Research has also identified Rnf43 (ring finger protein 43) as a tumor suppressor in pancreatic cancer, with its CRISPR/Cas9-mediated disruption as an E3 ubiquitin ligase accelerating KRASG12D-driven tumor growth [95]. Additionally, when FAM110C and RAC1B were eliminated through CRISPR/Cas9 knockout, PDAC cells showed increased invasive properties, suggesting these genes may function as tumor suppressors in PDAC [96, 97].

Figure 5.1 collectively illustrates pancreatic cancer-related oncogenes and tumor suppressive genes targeted by CRISPR/Cas9 systems.

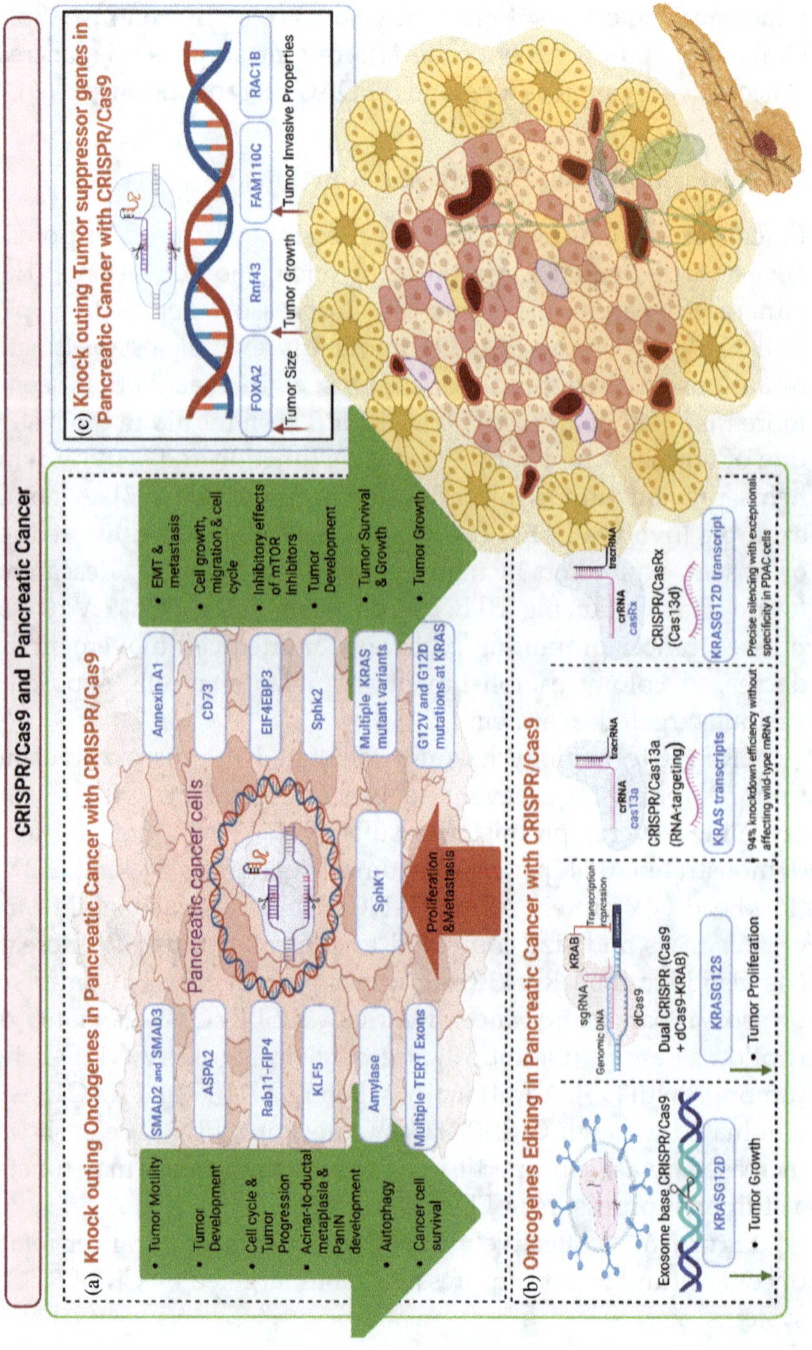

CRISPR/Cas9 and Pancreatic Cancer
(a) Knock outing Oncogenes in Pancreatic Cancer with CRISPR/Cas9
Tumor Motility
Tumor Development
Cell cycle & Tumor Progression
Acinar-to-ductal metaplasia & PanIN development
Autophagy
Cancer cell survival
SMAD2 and SMAD3
ASPA2
Rab11-FIP4
KLF5
Amylase
Multiple TERT Exons
Pancreatic cancer cells
SphK1
Proliferation &Metastasis
Annexin A1
CD73
EIF4EBP3
Sphk2
Multiple KRAS mutant variants
G12V and G12D mutations at KRAS
EMT & metastasis
Cell growth, migration & cell cycle
Inhibitory effects of mTOR inhibitors
Tumor Development
Tumor Survival & Growth
Tumor Growth
(b) Oncogenes Editing in Pancreatic Cancer with CRISPR/Cas9
Exosome base CRISPR/Cas9
KRASG12D
Tumor Growth
Genomic DNA
sgRNA
KRAB
Transcription repression
dCas9
Dual CRISPR (Cas9 + dCas9-KRAB)
KRASG12S
Tumor Proliferation
crRNA
cas13a
tracrRNA
CRISPR/Cas13a (RNA-targeting)
KRAS transcripts
94% knockdown efficiency without affecting wild-type mRNA
crRNA
casRx
tracrRNA
CRISPR/CasRx (Cas13d)
KRASG12D transcript
Precise silencing with exceptional specificity in PDAC cells
(c) Knock outing Tumor suppressor genes in Pancreatic Cancer with CRISPR/Cas9
FOXA2
Rnf43
FAM110C
RAC1B
Tumor Size
Tumor Growth
Tumor Invasive Properties

Figure 5.1 CRISPR/Cas9 applications in targeting key genes for pancreatic cancer therapy and research. This figure presents an overview of CRISPR/Cas9-based genome editing approaches tailored to disrupt oncogenes and tumor suppressor genes involved in the initiation and progression of pancreatic cancer. **(a) Knockout of oncogenes in pancreatic cancer cells:** CRISPR/Cas9-mediated knockouts target a spectrum of oncogenes — such as SMAD2/3, KLF5, Amylase, Sphk1, Annexin A1, CD73, EIF4EBP3, Sphk2, Rab11-FIP4, multiple TERT exons, and multiple KRAS mutant variants (including G12V and G12D) — affecting critical processes including tumor cell motility, development, cell cycle progression, tumor survival, autophagy, and metastasis. These interventions disrupt molecular pathways that drive acinar-to-ductal metaplasia, pancreatic intraepithelial neoplasia development, and the metastatic cascade. **(b) Editing oncogenes using diverse CRISPR platforms:** Innovative editing strategies are depicted, including exosome-based delivery of CRISPR/Cas9 components to inhibit KRASG12D and suppress tumor growth; dual CRISPR (Cas9/dCas9-KRAB) systems to repress KRASG12S and curtail tumor proliferation through targeted transcriptional repression; RNA-targeting CRISPR/Cas13a and Cas13d systems achieving highly efficient and specific knockdown of mutant KRAS transcripts — demonstrated by 94% knockdown efficiency for KRASG12D with exceptional selectivity, minimizing off-target effects in PDAC cells. **(c) Knockout of tumor suppressor genes in pancreatic cancer:** The knockout of tumor suppressors including FOXA2, Rnf43, FAM110C, and RAC1B using CRISPR/Cas9 results in increased tumor size, growth, and enhanced invasive properties, highlighting their critical role in restraining tumor aggressiveness.

5.6 CRISPR/Cas9 against Drug Resistance in Pancreatic Cancer

The progressive development of drug resistance presents a major challenge in cancer treatment [98]. CRISPR technology has been extensively applied to target genes associated with drug resistance through direct DNA modification, allowing researchers to alter cancer cell characteristics and identify new therapeutic targets [99]. While drug resistance develops through various mechanisms, genetic changes in cancer cells typically underlie these adaptations [100]. Many cancer cells show increased production of mucin glycoproteins, including MUC4, with studies linking this overproduction to treatment resistance [101]. Research by Skrypek and colleagues revealed that pancreatic cancer cells expressing MUC4 become resistant to gemcitabine, a key chemotherapeutic agent in pancreatic cancer treatment protocols [102]. Recent findings demonstrate that eliminating MUC4 through CRISPR/Cas9 significantly increases pancreatic cancer cells' responsiveness to gemcitabine [103].

Genetic studies have revealed that BRCA mutations appear in the germline DNA of 4–7% of pancreatic cancer patients, with mutations in either BRCA1 or BRCA2 linked to elevated risk of various cancers, including pancreatic cancer [104]. Research by Witz et al. demonstrated that CRISPR/Cas9-mediated introduction of specific mutations at Glu255 and Cys711 resulted in truncated forms of BRCA1 and BRCA2 proteins, respectively, enhancing olaparib sensitivity [105]. In a complementary investigation, scientists discovered that CRISPR/Cas9-based elimination of GPRC5a (G-protein-coupled receptor family C, member 5, group A), which shows elevated expression in PDAC, diminished resistance to several chemotherapeutic agents including gemcitabine, oxaliplatin, and fluorouracil in both human and mouse pancreatic cancer cell models [106].

5.7 CRISPR/Cas9 in Tumor Microenvironment and Immunotherapy

Cancer cells exhibit distinctive characteristics including apoptosis resistance, blood vessel formation, invasion and metastasis capability, inflammation promotion, and immune system evasion. These features are influenced by various components within the tumor microenvironment. The complex and diverse nature of this environment creates substantial barriers to treatment effectiveness. PDAC tumors typically show poor vascularization, primarily due to dense stromal tissue that captures and neutralizes signals promoting blood vessel growth [107].

Rapid cell division, a defining feature of cancer development, requires increased oxygen consumption, creating oxygen-deprived conditions within tumors that lead to specific abnormal changes [108, 109]. Under low-oxygen conditions, HIF-1α helps cancer cells adapt by coordinating cellular responses to oxygen level changes [110]. HIF-mediated responses to hypoxia enhance PDAC's malignant characteristics, suggesting that targeting HIFs and related pathways could improve treatment outcomes [111]. Li and colleagues conducted animal studies showing that a CRISPR/Cas9 delivery system using R8-dGR-modified cationic liposomes enhanced BxPC-3 pancreatic cancer cells' sensitivity to paclitaxel by reducing HIF-1α expression and its downstream targets VEGF and MMP9. Importantly, this liposomal delivery method showed minimal toxicity *in vivo*, as it had little effect on HIF-1α levels in normal liver cells [112]. Additionally, hypoxic conditions trigger various mediators including HO-1, which may protect pancreatic cancer cells from oxidative stress. Research by Abdalla and colleagues showed that targeting HO-1 in PDAC cells using various techniques, including CRISPR/Cas9 knockout, increased the effectiveness of gemcitabine treatment in pancreatic cancer cell lines [99].

Previous research has shown that p53 tumor suppressor inactivation correlates with increased invasiveness and worse patient outcomes. Recent work by Czaplinska and colleagues demonstrated that CRISPR-mediated TP53 deletion enhanced the cancer-promoting effects of acid adaptation, making PDAC cells more aggressive in acidic tumor environments [113]. Furthermore, researchers have identified a relationship between TP53 mutations and neutrophil presence, as evidenced by significant tumor-associated neutrophil infiltration in human PDAC squamous subtypes. To investigate this relationship in

PDAC, Siolas and team used CRISPR/Cas9 technology combined with single-strand DNA homology-directed repair templates to create TP53R172H mutations in mouse pancreatic ductal epithelial cells derived from KRASG12D mutant GEMMs. Their results showed that introducing the TP53R172H mutation led to increased neutrophil infiltration while reducing T-cell presence [114].

A distinctive characteristic of PDAC is its fibrotic stromal tissue, which creates an environment that restricts immune system function, primarily by limiting immune cell penetration [115]. This condition develops due to the presence of dense desmoplastic stroma, consisting of activated pancreatic stellate cells and extracellular matrix components, which forms a physical obstruction preventing effector T cells from reaching the tumor's core [116].

During PDAC development, the immune cell composition within tumors undergoes significant changes, characterized by a decrease in CD8+ cytotoxic T cells while CD4+ regulatory T cells become more prevalent [117]. The tumor microenvironment demonstrates limited functionality of CD8+ T cells, indicating compromised immune responses and T cell exhaustion. Various immunosuppressive myeloid populations, including tumor-associated macrophages, neutrophils, and myeloid-derived suppressor cells, contribute to this environment by releasing immunosuppressive cytokines like IL-10 and TGF-β, which suppress T cell activity [117].

These conditions create a protected environment where cancer cells can escape immune detection and continue to proliferate. This immune-privileged status poses a significant challenge for CRISPR-based immune interventions, potentially limiting their effectiveness [117]. Research has shown that when CRISPR is used to suppress oncogenic KRAS in PDAC, the effects extend beyond reducing tumor growth. The intervention actually disrupts immune evasion mechanisms that depend on KRAS signaling, making tumor cells more susceptible to immune clearance in hosts with functioning immune systems [27].

Studies have identified the CD40-CD40L pathway as a key therapeutic target for improving PDAC immunotherapy. This pathway enhances immune responses by activating antigen-presenting cells through NF-κB signaling and facilitating immune cell recruitment.

A groundbreaking study by Wang et al. in 2022 demonstrated the effectiveness of CRISPR/Cas9-engineered oncolytic viruses expressing membrane-bound CD40L [118]. This innovative approach significantly extended survival in mouse models by promoting dendritic cell maturation and enhancing cytotoxic T cell responses. The treatment also increased pro-inflammatory macrophages and lymphocytes in the tumor environment, leading to improved immunotherapy outcomes and sustained immune responses [118, 119].

Additionally, researchers found that CRISPR-based suppression of ISG15 resulted in increased CD8+ T cell infiltration into tumors and decreased PD-L1 expression, ultimately improving the effectiveness of anti-PD-1 immunotherapy [120].

5.8 CRISPR/Cas9 in Pancreatic Cancer Epigenetic Modulation

Among the defining features of cancer, epigenetic modifications play a vital role in promoting both cancer development and therapy resistance. The emergence of epigenome editing technologies, particularly CRISPR-based systems, has enabled researchers to examine specific epigenetic modifications and their influence on cancer progression and treatment outcomes [121].

At the molecular level, epigenetic mechanisms modify specific lysine residues on histone proteins through processes such as methylation, acetylation, and ubiquitination. These modifications regulate crucial cellular processes including DNA accessibility, chromatin structure, and gene expression patterns, which ultimately determine cellular identity and differentiation status [122].

In the context of pancreatic cancer, epigenetic regulation significantly influences cancer cell metastasis. Research has revealed that Ring1b functions as a catalyst for histone H2A lysine 119 monoubiquitylation, representing a key epigenetic modification that suppresses acinar cell transcription factors in both pancreatic cancer cells and during acinar-to-ductal metaplasia. Studies using CRISPR to eliminate ring1b expression in mouse models demonstrated reduced acinar cell dedifferentiation, resulting in tumor cells adopting an epigenetically altered state with decreased aggressiveness [123].

Separate investigations using a KRASG12D-driven mouse model of PDAC showed that suppressing p53 through CRISPRi technology led to reduced expression of differentiation markers [124].

The dCas9-effector system's ability to modulate endogenous gene expression through activation or repression has created novel possibilities for studying mutations in non-coding regions associated with cancer [121]. Research has shown that non-coding mutations can significantly impact enhancer cluster functionality, contributing to cancer development. For instance, Patel and colleagues demonstrated that using CRISPRi to disrupt an enhancer cluster containing non-coding mutations near the MIR100HG long non-coding RNA gene resulted in decreased MIR100HG expression, leading to significant downregulation of the TGF-β pathway and other crucial PDAC-related pathways [125].

An important advantage of epigenetic modification approaches is their reversible nature, contrasting with permanent alterations caused by traditional Cas9 genome engineering. This reversibility eliminates concerns about permanent DNA sequence changes, particularly beneficial when targeting tumors characterized by high genetic instability [126]. However, the persistence of dCas9-induced epigenetic and transcriptional changes may vary depending on the specific target sites and the combination of effectors employed. Current challenges in epigenome engineering research include optimizing the technology for different genomic locations across various cell types with distinct chromatin environments [127].

5.9 CRISPR/Cas9 and Pancreatic Cancer Therapy in Clinical Setting

Recent developments in CRISPR gene editing have led to its implementation in various cancer treatment clinical trials. While CRISPR-based treatments specifically for pancreatic cancer remain at the preclinical stage without direct clinical trials, ongoing research in solid tumors provides promising data regarding their potential application, safety, and effectiveness in pancreatic cancer management.

Current clinical research includes Intima Bioscience's Phase I/II trial (NCT04426669), investigating the effects of CRISPR/Cas9-based CISH gene deletion in tumor-infiltrating lymphocytes for metastatic gastrointestinal cancer treatment. CISH acts as an internal immune checkpoint, and its removal is expected to enhance T cells' cancer-fighting ability [128]. The study aims to determine whether CISH elimination improves tumor-infiltrating lymphocytes and T cells' anti-tumor effectiveness in patients with metastatic pancreatic and other gastrointestinal cancers, while evaluating clinical safety and efficacy.

CRISPR Therapeutics initiated a Phase I/II trial (NCT05795595) in 2023 studying CTX131, which uses CRISPR/Cas9-modified allogeneic T cells targeting CD70, in patients with resistant solid tumors including pancreatic adenocarcinoma [129]. Preliminary results demonstrate positive safety outcomes and dose-dependent therapeutic responses.

Mesothelin surface proteins are commonly expressed in various solid tumors, including pancreatic cancer. A Phase I trial (NCT03545815) evaluated CRISPR/Cas9 technology for eliminating both PD-1 and TCR in mesothelin-targeting CAR-T cells (MPTK-CAR-T) for treating mesothelin-expressing solid tumors. Simultaneously, another Phase I trial (NCT03747965) investigated PD-1-deleted CAR-T cells combined with paclitaxel and cyclophosphamide pretreatment. While initial findings from both trials indicate safety and feasibility, more research is required to understand their broader therapeutic impact [130], particularly for pancreatic cancer treatment.

Although CRISPR-based cancer therapies show promise, most are still in early clinical trials. Substantial research remains necessary to definitively establish their safety profiles, therapeutic efficacy, and optimal integration with existing cancer treatments. Furthermore, there remains an urgent need to develop specialized CRISPR-based approaches for pancreatic cancer to overcome current therapeutic limitations.

5.10 Future Perspectives

CRISPR/Cas technology is undergoing swift advancement, showing promising applications in pancreatic cancer studies and treatment approaches. A key focus area involves improving delivery mechanisms to increase targeting accuracy and biological compatibility [131–133]. Novel developments in non-viral delivery methods, particularly utilizing lipid-based nanoparticles and exosomal transport systems, could address existing challenges related to stability and immune response, facilitating safer clinical applications.

The introduction of enhanced Cas variants with improved accuracy, along with advanced editing techniques such as base and prime editing systems, presents opportunities to reduce unintended genomic modifications while accurately targeting cancer-associated mutations, particularly KRAS [134–138]. The integration of CRISPR technologies with established treatment protocols, including chemotherapeutic agents and immune-based therapies, could potentially yield improved therapeutic outcomes. Specifically, engineered CAR-T cells and modified oncolytic viruses incorporating immune modulators show promise in altering the tumor's immune-suppressive environment [51].

A notable research gap exists in exploring CRISPR applications for pancreatic cancer immunotherapy, particularly regarding CAR-T cell development and strategies to overcome immune suppression within pancreatic tumors. These research areas require dedicated investigation to advance treatment options.

The utilization of organoid models derived from patient samples and genetically engineered mouse models continues to be crucial for confirming therapeutic targets and developing individualized treatment approaches, especially for uncommon genetic variants [139, 140]. Broadening CRISPR screening to encompass non-coding genomic elements and epigenetic modifiers may reveal previously unknown therapeutic targets, including enhancer regions and long non-coding RNAs that influence tumor adaptation and treatment resistance [141].

5.11 Conclusion

Pancreatic cancer continues to pose a major clinical challenge due to its aggressive biology, high mortality rate, and limited therapeutic options. The advent of the CRISPR/Cas9 system offers an unprecedented opportunity to break new ground in the development of targeted, patient-specific interventions. By surpassing earlier gene-editing modalities in efficiency and accessibility, CRISPR/Cas9 provides a promising foundation for precision oncology strategies aimed at overcoming therapeutic resistance and improving survival outcomes in pancreatic cancer patients. While translational and ethical hurdles remain, the integration of CRISPR/Cas9 into future therapeutic paradigms may radically transform the landscape of pancreatic cancer treatment.

References

1. Siegel RL, Miller KD, Jemal A. Cancer statistics, 2019. CA Cancer J Clin. 2019;69(1):7–34.
2. Ishino Y, Shinagawa H, Makino K, Amemura M, Nakata A. Nucleotide sequence of the iap gene, responsible for alkaline phosphatase isozyme conversion in Escherichia coli, and identification of the gene product. J Bacteriol. 1987;169(12):5429–33.
3. Jinek M, Chylinski K, Fonfara I, Hauer M, Doudna JA, Charpentier E. A programmable dual-RNA-guided DNA endonuclease in adaptive bacterial immunity. Science. 2012;337(6096):816–21.
4. Park W, Chawla A, O'Reilly EM. Pancreatic cancer: a review. Jama. 2021;326(9):851–62.
5. Bailey P, Chang DK, Nones K, Johns AL, Patch AM, Gingras MC, et al. Genomic analyses identify molecular subtypes of pancreatic cancer. Nature. 2016;531(7592):47–52.
6. Collisson EA, Bailey P, Chang DK, Biankin AV. Molecular subtypes of pancreatic cancer. Nat Rev Gastroenterol Hepatol. 2019;16(4):207–20.
7. Waddell N, Pajic M, Patch AM, Chang DK, Kassahn KS, Bailey P, et al. Whole genomes redefine the mutational landscape of pancreatic cancer. Nature. 2015;518(7540):495–501.

8. Biankin AV, Waddell N, Kassahn KS, Gingras MC, Muthuswamy LB, Johns AL, et al. Pancreatic cancer genomes reveal aberrations in axon guidance pathway genes. Nature. 2012;491(7424):399–405.
9. Witkiewicz AK, McMillan EA, Balaji U, Baek G, Lin WC, Mansour J, et al. Whole-exome sequencing of pancreatic cancer defines genetic diversity and therapeutic targets. Nat Commun. 2015;6:6744.
10. Casolino R, Paiella S, Azzolina D, Beer PA, Corbo V, Lorenzoni G, et al. Homologous Recombination Deficiency in Pancreatic Cancer: A Systematic Review and Prevalence Meta-Analysis. J Clin Oncol. 2021;39(23):2617–31.
11. Integrated Genomic Characterization of Pancreatic Ductal Adenocarcinoma. Cancer Cell. 2017;32(2):185–203.e13.
12. Chan-Seng-Yue M, Kim JC, Wilson GW, Ng K, Figueroa EF, O'Kane GM, et al. Transcription phenotypes of pancreatic cancer are driven by genomic events during tumor evolution. Nat Genet. 2020;52(2):231–40.
13. Collisson EA, Sadanandam A, Olson P, Gibb WJ, Truitt M, Gu S, et al. Subtypes of pancreatic ductal adenocarcinoma and their differing responses to therapy. Nat Med. 2011;17(4):500–3.
14. Moffitt RA, Marayati R, Flate EL, Volmar KE, Loeza SG, Hoadley KA, et al. Virtual microdissection identifies distinct tumor- and stroma-specific subtypes of pancreatic ductal adenocarcinoma. Nat Genet. 2015;47(10):1168–78.
15. Schreyer D, Neoptolemos JP, Barry ST, Bailey P. Deconstructing Pancreatic Cancer Using Next Generation-Omic Technologies-From Discovery to Knowledge-Guided Platforms for Better Patient Management. Front Cell Dev Biol. 2021;9:795735.
16. Candido JB, Morton JP, Bailey P, Campbell AD, Karim SA, Jamieson T, et al. CSF1R(+) Macrophages Sustain Pancreatic Tumor Growth through T Cell Suppression and Maintenance of Key Gene Programs that Define the Squamous Subtype. Cell Rep. 2018;23(5):1448–60.
17. Steele NG, Carpenter ES, Kemp SB, Sirihorachai VR, The S, Delrosario L, et al. Multimodal Mapping of the Tumor and Peripheral Blood Immune Landscape in Human Pancreatic Cancer. Nat Cancer. 2020;1(11):1097–112.
18. Ho WJ, Jaffee EM, Zheng L. The tumour microenvironment in pancreatic cancer — clinical challenges and opportunities. Nat Rev Clin Oncol. 2020;17(9):527–40.

19. Karamitopoulou E. Tumour microenvironment of pancreatic cancer: immune landscape is dictated by molecular and histopathological features. Br J Cancer. 2019;121(1):5–14.
20. Le DT, Durham JN, Smith KN, Wang H, Bartlett BR, Aulakh LK, et al. Mismatch repair deficiency predicts response of solid tumors to PD-1 blockade. Science. 2017;357(6349):409–13.
21. Le DT, Uram JN, Wang H, Bartlett BR, Kemberling H, Eyring AD, et al. PD-1 Blockade in Tumors with Mismatch-Repair Deficiency. N Engl J Med. 2015;372(26):2509–20.
22. Raghavan S, Winter PS, Navia AW, Williams HL, DenAdel A, Lowder KE, et al. Microenvironment drives cell state, plasticity, and drug response in pancreatic cancer. Cell. 2021;184(25):6119–37.e26.
23. Ho WJ, Jaffee EM. Macrophage-Targeting by CSF1/1R Blockade in Pancreatic Cancers. Cancer Res. 2021;81(24):6071–3.
24. Carstens JL, Correa de Sampaio P, Yang D, Barua S, Wang H, Rao A, et al. Spatial computation of intratumoral T cells correlates with survival of patients with pancreatic cancer. Nat Commun. 2017;8:15095.
25. Karamitopoulou E, Andreou A, Pahud de Mortanges A, Tinguely M, Gloor B, Perren A. PD-1/PD-L1-Associated Immunoarchitectural Patterns Stratify Pancreatic Cancer Patients into Prognostic/Predictive Subgroups. Cancer Immunol Res. 2021;9(12):1439–50.
26. Dey P, Li J, Zhang J, Chaurasiya S, Strom A, Wang H, et al. Oncogenic KRAS-Driven Metabolic Reprogramming in Pancreatic Cancer Cells Utilizes Cytokines from the Tumor Microenvironment. Cancer Discov. 2020;10(4):608–25.
27. Ischenko I, D'Amico S, Rao M, Li J, Hayman MJ, Powers S, et al. KRAS drives immune evasion in a genetic model of pancreatic cancer. Nat Commun. 2021;12(1):1482.
28. Muthalagu N, Monteverde T, Raffo-Iraolagoitia X, Wiesheu R, Whyte D, Hedley A, et al. Repression of the Type I Interferon Pathway Underlies MYC- and KRAS-Dependent Evasion of NK and B Cells in Pancreatic Ductal Adenocarcinoma. Cancer Discov. 2020;10(6):872–87.
29. Samstein RM, Krishna C, Ma X, Pei X, Lee KW, Makarov V, et al. Mutations in BRCA1 and BRCA2 differentially affect the tumor microenvironment and response to checkpoint blockade immunotherapy. Nat Cancer. 2021;1(12):1188–203.

30. Zhou Z, Li M. Evaluation of BRCA1 and BRCA2 as Indicators of Response to Immune Checkpoint Inhibitors. JAMA Netw Open. 2021;4(5):e217728.
31. Adib E, Nassar AH, Akl EW, Abou Alaiwi S, Nuzzo PV, Mouhieddine TH, et al. CDKN2A Alterations and Response to Immunotherapy in Solid Tumors. Clin Cancer Res. 2021;27(14):4025–35.
32. Chen S, Sanjana NE, Zheng K, Shalem O, Lee K, Shi X, et al. Genome-wide CRISPR screen in a mouse model of tumor growth and metastasis. Cell. 2015;160(6):1246–60.
33. Li W, Xu H, Xiao T, Cong L, Love MI, Zhang F, et al. MAGeCK enables robust identification of essential genes from genome-scale CRISPR/Cas9 knockout screens. Genome Biol. 2014;15(12):554.
34. Bakke J, Wright WC, Zamora AE, Oladimeji P, Crawford JC, Brewer CT, et al. Genome-wide CRISPR screen reveals PSMA6 to be an essential gene in pancreatic cancer cells. BMC Cancer. 2019;19(1):253.
35. Oladimeji PO, Bakke J, Wright WC, Chen T. KANSL2 and MBNL3 are regulators of pancreatic ductal adenocarcinoma invasion. Sci Rep. 2020;10(1):1485.
36. Martinez S, Wu S, Geuenich M, Malik A, Weber R, Woo T, et al. In vivo CRISPR screens reveal SCAF1 and USP15 as drivers of pancreatic cancer. Nat Commun. 2024;15(1):5266.
37. Kubota CS, Myers SL, Seppälä TT, Burkhart RA, Espenshade PJ. In vivo CRISPR screening identifies geranylgeranyl diphosphate as a pancreatic cancer tumor growth dependency. Mol Metab. 2024;85:101964.
38. Sarr A, Bré J, Um IH, Chan TH, Mullen P, Harrison DJ, Reynolds PA. Genome-scale CRISPR/Cas9 screen determines factors modulating sensitivity to ProTide NUC-1031. Sci Rep. 2019;9(1):7643.
39. Yang H, Liu B, Liu D, Yang Z, Zhang S, Xu P, et al. Genome-Wide CRISPR Screening Identifies DCK and CCNL1 as Genes That Contribute to Gemcitabine Resistance in Pancreatic Cancer. Cancers (Basel). 2022;14(13):3152.
40. Ramaker RC, Hardigan AA, Gordon ER, Wright CA, Myers RM, Cooper SJ. Pooled CRISPR screening in pancreatic cancer cells implicates co-repressor complexes as a cause of multiple drug resistance via regulation of epithelial-to-mesenchymal transition. BMC Cancer. 2021;21(1):632.

41. Zeng S, Lan B, Ren X, Zhang S, Schreyer D, Eckstein M, et al. CDK7 inhibition augments response to multidrug chemotherapy in pancreatic cancer. J Exp Clin Cancer Res. 2022;41(1):241.
42. Wang S, Xiong Y, Luo Y, Shen Y, Zhang F, Lan H, et al. Genome-wide CRISPR screens identify PKMYT1 as a therapeutic target in pancreatic ductal adenocarcinoma. EMBO Mol Med. 2024;16(5):1115–42.
43. Goodwin CM, Waters AM, Klomp JE, Javaid S, Bryant KL, Stalnecker CA, et al. Combination Therapies with CDK4/6 Inhibitors to Treat KRAS-Mutant Pancreatic Cancer. Cancer Res. 2023;83(1):141–57.
44. Wang B, Krall EB, Aguirre AJ, Kim M, Widlund HR, Doshi MB, et al. ATXN1L, CIC, and ETS Transcription Factors Modulate Sensitivity to MAPK Pathway Inhibition. Cell Rep. 2017;18(6):1543–57.
45. Mondal P, Alyateem G, Mitchell AV, Gottesman MM. A whole-genome CRISPR screen identifies the spindle accessory checkpoint as a locus of nab-paclitaxel resistance in a pancreatic cancer cell line. Sci Rep. 2024;14(1):15912.
46. le Sage C, Lawo S, Cross BCS. CRISPR: A Screener's Guide. SLAS Discov. 2020;25(3):233–40.
47. Steinhart Z, Pavlovic Z, Chandrashekhar M, Hart T, Wang X, Zhang X, et al. Genome-wide CRISPR screens reveal a Wnt-FZD5 signaling circuit as a druggable vulnerability of RNF43-mutant pancreatic tumors. Nat Med. 2017;23(1):60–8.
48. Samatar AA, Poulikakos PI. Targeting RAS-ERK signalling in cancer: promises and challenges. Nat Rev Drug Discov. 2014;13(12):928–42.
49. Szlachta K, Kuscu C, Tufan T, Adair SJ, Shang S, Michaels AD, et al. CRISPR knockout screening identifies combinatorial drug targets in pancreatic cancer and models cellular drug response. Nat Commun. 2018;9(1):4275.
50. Hagel KR, Arafeh R, Gang S, Arnoff TE, Larson RC, Doench JG, et al. Systematic Interrogation of Tumor Cell Resistance to Chimeric Antigen Receptor T-cell Therapy in Pancreatic Cancer. Cancer Res. 2023;83(4):613–25.
51. Gu Y, Zhang Z, Camps MGM, Ossendorp F, Wijdeven RH, Ten Dijke P. Genome-wide CRISPR screens define determinants of epithelial-mesenchymal transition mediated immune evasion by pancreatic cancer cells. Sci Adv. 2023;9(28):eadf9915.

52. Sang W, Zhou Y, Chen H, Yu C, Dai L, Liu Z, et al. Receptor-interacting Protein Kinase 2 Is an Immunotherapy Target in Pancreatic Cancer. Cancer Discov. 2024;14(2):326–47.
53. Li J, Yuan S, Norgard RJ, Yan F, Sun YH, Kim IK, et al. Epigenetic and Transcriptional Control of the Epidermal Growth Factor Receptor Regulates the Tumor Immune Microenvironment in Pancreatic Cancer. Cancer Discov. 2021;11(3):736–53.
54. Gao Q, Ouyang W, Kang B, Han X, Xiong Y, Ding R, et al. Selective targeting of the oncogenic KRAS G12S mutant allele by CRISPR/Cas9 induces efficient tumor regression. Theranostics. 2020;10(11):5137–53.
55. Kim W, Lee S, Kim HS, Song M, Cha YH, Kim YH, et al. Targeting mutant KRAS with CRISPR-Cas9 controls tumor growth. Genome Res. 2018;28(3):374–82.
56. Lentsch E, Li L, Pfeffer S, Ekici AB, Taher L, Pilarsky C, Grützmann R. CRISPR/Cas9-Mediated Knock-Out of Kras(G12D) Mutated Pancreatic Cancer Cell Lines. Int J Mol Sci. 2019;20(22):5706.
57. McAndrews KM, Xiao F, Chronopoulos A, LeBleu VS, Kugeratski FG, Kalluri R. Exosome-mediated delivery of CRISPR/Cas9 for targeting of oncogenic Kras(G12D) in pancreatic cancer. Life Sci Alliance. 2021;4(9):e202000875.
58. Zhao X, Liu L, Lang J, Cheng K, Wang Y, Li X, et al. A CRISPR-Cas13a system for efficient and specific therapeutic targeting of mutant KRAS for pancreatic cancer treatment. Cancer Lett. 2018;431:171–81.
59. Jiang W, Li H, Liu X, Zhang J, Zhang W, Li T, et al. Precise and efficient silencing of mutant Kras(G12D) by CRISPR-CasRx controls pancreatic cancer progression. Theranostics. 2020;10(25):11507–19.
60. Bertrand-Chapel A, Caligaris C, Fenouil T, Savary C, Aires S, Martel S, et al. SMAD2/3 mediate oncogenic effects of TGF-β in the absence of SMAD4. Commun Biol. 2022;5(1):1068.
61. Fujii A, Masuda T, Iwata M, Tobo T, Wakiyama H, Koike K, et al. The novel driver gene ASAP2 is a potential druggable target in pancreatic cancer. Cancer Sci. 2021;112(4):1655–68.
62. He Y, Ye M, Zhou L, Shan Y, Lu G, Zhou Y, et al. High Rab11-FIP4 expression predicts poor prognosis and exhibits tumor promotion in pancreatic cancer. Int J Oncol. 2017;50(2):396–404.

63. He P, Yang JW, Yang VW, Bialkowska AB. Krüppel-like Factor 5, Increased in Pancreatic Ductal Adenocarcinoma, Promotes Proliferation, Acinar-to-Ductal Metaplasia, Pancreatic Intraepithelial Neoplasia, and Tumor Growth in Mice. Gastroenterology. 2018;154(5):1494–508.e13.
64. Yasunaga K, Ito T, Miki M, Ueda K, Fujiyama T, Tachibana Y, et al. Using CRISPR/Cas9 to Knock out Amylase in Acinar Cells Decreases Pancreatitis-Induced Autophagy. Biomed Res Int. 2018;2018: 8719397.
65. Wen L, Zhao C, Song J, Ma L, Ruan J, Xia X, et al. CRISPR/Cas9-Mediated TERT Disruption in Cancer Cells. Int J Mol Sci. 2020;21(2).
66. Belvedere R, Bizzarro V, Forte G, Dal Piaz F, Parente L, Petrella A. Annexin A1 contributes to pancreatic cancer cell phenotype, behaviour and metastatic potential independently of Formyl Peptide Receptor pathway. Sci Rep. 2016;6:29660.
67. Zhang J, Zhang S, Dörflein I, Ren X, Pfeffer S, Britzen-Laurent N, et al. Impact of CRISPR/Cas9-Mediated CD73 Knockout in Pancreatic Cancer. Cancers (Basel). 2023;15(19):4842.
68. Tsukumo Y, Alain T, Fonseca BD, Nadon R, Sonenberg N. Translation control during prolonged mTORC1 inhibition mediated by 4E-BP3. Nat Commun. 2016;7:11776.
69. Yuza K, Nakajima M, Nagahashi M, Tsuchida J, Hirose Y, Miura K, et al. Different Roles of Sphingosine Kinase 1 and 2 in Pancreatic Cancer Progression. J Surg Res. 2018;232:186–94.
70. Zhao Z, Li C, Tong F, Deng J, Huang G, Sang Y. Review of applications of CRISPR-Cas9 gene-editing technology in cancer research. Biol Proced Online. 2021;23(1):14.
71. Bender G, Fahrioglu Yamaci R, Taneri B. CRISPR and KRAS: a match yet to be made. J Biomed Sci. 2021;28(1):77.
72. Wang T, Wei JJ, Sabatini DM, Lander ES. Genetic screens in human cells using the CRISPR-Cas9 system. Science. 2014;343(6166):80–4.
73. Chen PY, Muzumdar MD, Dorans KJ, Robbins R, Bhutkar A, Del Rosario A, et al. Adaptive and Reversible Resistance to Kras Inhibition in Pancreatic Cancer Cells. Cancer Res. 2018;78(4):985–1002.
74. Takakura K, Kawamura A, Torisu Y, Koido S, Yahagi N, Saruta M. The Clinical Potential of Oligonucleotide Therapeutics against Pancreatic Cancer. Int J Mol Sci. 2019;20(13):3331.

75. Lee W, Lee JH, Jun S, Lee JH, Bang D. Selective targeting of KRAS oncogenic alleles by CRISPR/Cas9 inhibits proliferation of cancer cells. Sci Rep. 2018;8(1):11879.
76. Muzumdar MD, Chen PY, Dorans KJ, Chung KM, Bhutkar A, Hong E, et al. Survival of pancreatic cancer cells lacking KRAS function. Nat Commun. 2017;8(1):1090.
77. Singh A, Greninger P, Rhodes D, Koopman L, Violette S, Bardeesy N, Settleman J. A gene expression signature associated with "K-Ras addiction" reveals regulators of EMT and tumor cell survival. Cancer Cell. 2009;15(6):489–500.
78. Kim SM, Yang Y, Oh SJ, Hong Y, Seo M, Jang M. Cancer-derived exosomes as a delivery platform of CRISPR/Cas9 confer cancer cell tropism-dependent targeting. J Control Release. 2017;266:8–16.
79. Gootenberg JS, Abudayyeh OO, Lee JW, Essletzbichler P, Dy AJ, Joung J, et al. Nucleic acid detection with CRISPR-Cas13a/C2c2. Science. 2017;356(6336):438–42.
80. Larochelle S. CRISPR–Cas goes RNA. Nat Methods. 2018;15(5):312.
81. Konermann S, Lotfy P, Brideau NJ, Oki J, Shokhirev MN, Hsu PD. Transcriptome Engineering with RNA-Targeting Type VI-D CRISPR Effectors. Cell. 2018;173(3):665–76.e14.
82. Xuan Q, Wang J, Nie Y, Fang C, Liang W. Research Progress and Application of Miniature CRISPR-Cas12 System in Gene Editing. Int J Mol Sci. 2024;25(23):12686.
83. Anzalone AV, Randolph PB, Davis JR, Sousa AA, Koblan LW, Levy JM, et al. Search-and-replace genome editing without double-strand breaks or donor DNA. Nature. 2019;576(7785):149–57.
84. Rees HA, Liu DR. Publisher Correction: Base editing: precision chemistry on the genome and transcriptome of living cells. Nat Rev Genet. 2018;19(12):801.
85. Qian ZR, Rubinson DA, Nowak JA, Morales-Oyarvide V, Dunne RF, Kozak MM, et al. Association of Alterations in Main Driver Genes With Outcomes of Patients With Resected Pancreatic Ductal Adenocarcinoma. JAMA Oncol. 2018;4(3):e173420.
86. Barthel FP, Wei W, Tang M, Martinez-Ledesma E, Hu X, Amin SB, et al. Systematic analysis of telomere length and somatic alterations in 31 cancer types. Nat Genet. 2017;49(3):349–57.

87. Akıncılar SC, Khattar E, Boon PL, Unal B, Fullwood MJ, Tergaonkar V. Long-Range Chromatin Interactions Drive Mutant TERT Promoter Activation. Cancer Discov. 2016;6(11):1276–91.
88. Brane AC, Tollefsbol TO. Targeting Telomeres and Telomerase: Studies in Aging and Disease Utilizing CRISPR/Cas9 Technology. Cells. 2019;8(2):186.
89. Chiba K, Johnson JZ, Vogan JM, Wagner T, Boyle JM, Hockemeyer D. Cancer-associated TERT promoter mutations abrogate telomerase silencing. Elife. 2015;4:e07918.
90. Xi L, Schmidt JC, Zaug AJ, Ascarrunz DR, Cech TR. A novel two-step genome editing strategy with CRISPR-Cas9 provides new insights into telomerase action and TERT gene expression. Genome Biol. 2015;16:231.
91. Liu H, Sui T, Liu D, Liu T, Chen M, Deng J, et al. Multiple homologous genes knockout (KO) by CRISPR/Cas9 system in rabbit. Gene. 2018;647:261–7.
92. Vorvis C, Hatziapostolou M, Mahurkar-Joshi S, Koutsioumpa M, Williams J, Donahue TR, et al. Transcriptomic and CRISPR/Cas9 technologies reveal FOXA2 as a tumor suppressor gene in pancreatic cancer. Am J Physiol Gastrointest Liver Physiol. 2016;310(11):G1124–37.
93. Jiang C, Meng L, Yang B, Luo X. Application of CRISPR/Cas9 gene editing technique in the study of cancer treatment. Clin Genet. 2020;97(1):73–88.
94. Moses C, Nugent F, Waryah CB, Garcia-Bloj B, Harvey AR, Blancafort P. Activating PTEN Tumor Suppressor Expression with the CRISPR/dCas9 System. Mol Ther Nucleic Acids. 2019;14:287–300.
95. Mishra A, Emamgholi F, Erlangga Z, Hartleben B, Unger K, Wolff K, et al. Generation of focal mutations and large genomic deletions in the pancreas using inducible in vivo genome editing. Carcinogenesis. 2020;41(3):334–44.
96. Liu F, Gao A, Zhang M, Li Y, Zhang F, Herman JG, Guo M. Methylation of FAM110C is a synthetic lethal marker for ATR/CHK1 inhibitors in pancreatic cancer. J Transl Int Med. 2024;12(3):274–87.
97. Ungefroren H, Braun R, Lapshyna O, Konukiewitz B, Wellner UF, Lehnert H, Marquardt JU. Suppressive Role of ACVR1/ALK2 in Basal

and TGFβ1-Induced Cell Migration in Pancreatic Ductal Adenocarcinoma Cells and Identification of a Self-Perpetuating Autoregulatory Loop Involving the Small GTPase RAC1b. Biomedicines. 2022;10(10):2640.

98. Vaghari-Tabari M, Hassanpour P, Sadeghsoltani F, Malakoti F, Alemi F, Qujeq D, et al. CRISPR/Cas9 gene editing: a new approach for overcoming drug resistance in cancer. Cell Mol Biol Lett. 2022; 27(1):49.
99. Abdalla MY, Ahmad IM, Rachagani S, Banerjee K, Thompson CM, Maurer HC, et al. Enhancing responsiveness of pancreatic cancer cells to gemcitabine treatment under hypoxia by heme oxygenase-1 inhibition. Transl Res. 2019;207:56–69.
100. Chen Y, Zhang Y. Application of the CRISPR/Cas9 System to Drug Resistance in Breast Cancer. Adv Sci (Weinh). 2018;5(6):1700964.
101. Reynolds IS, Fichtner M, McNamara DA, Kay EW, Prehn JHM, Burke JP. Mucin glycoproteins block apoptosis; promote invasion, proliferation, and migration; and cause chemoresistance through diverse pathways in epithelial cancers. Cancer Metastasis Rev. 2019;38(1–2):237–57.
102. Skrypek N, Duchêne B, Hebbar M, Leteurtre E, van Seuningen I, Jonckheere N. The MUC4 mucin mediates gemcitabine resistance of human pancreatic cancer cells via the Concentrative Nucleoside Transporter family. Oncogene. 2013;32(13):1714–23.
103. Sagar S, Leiphrakpam PD, Thomas D, McAndrews KL, Caffrey TC, Swanson BJ, et al. MUC4 enhances gemcitabine resistance and malignant behaviour in pancreatic cancer cells expressing cancer-associated short O-glycans. Cancer Lett. 2021;503:91–102.
104. Wong W, Raufi AG, Safyan RA, Bates SE, Manji GA. BRCA Mutations in Pancreas Cancer: Spectrum, Current Management, Challenges and Future Prospects. Cancer Manag Res. 2020;12:2731–42.
105. Witz A, Dardare J, Francois A, Husson M, Rouyer M, Demange J, et al. CRISPR/Cas9-mediated knock-in of BRCA1/2 mutations restores response to olaparib in pancreatic cancer cell lines. Sci Rep. 2023;13(1):18741.
106. Liu B, Yang H, Pilarsky C, Weber GF. The Effect of GPRC5a on the Proliferation, Migration Ability, Chemotherapy Resistance, and Phosphorylation of GSK-3β in Pancreatic Cancer. Int J Mol Sci. 2018;19(7):1870.

107. Katsuta E, Qi Q, Peng X, Hochwald SN, Yan L, Takabe K. Pancreatic adenocarcinomas with mature blood vessels have better overall survival. Sci Rep. 2019;9(1):1310.
108. Erkan M, Kurtoglu M, Kleeff J. The role of hypoxia in pancreatic cancer: a potential therapeutic target? Expert Rev Gastroenterol Hepatol. 2016;10(3):301–16.
109. Li X, Pan Y, Chen C, Gao Y, Liu X, Yang K, et al. Hypoxia-Responsive Gene Editing to Reduce Tumor Thermal Tolerance for Mild-Photothermal Therapy. Angew Chem Int Ed Engl. 2021; 60(39):21200–4.
110. Jin X, Dai L, Ma Y, Wang J, Liu Z. Implications of HIF-1α in the tumorigenesis and progression of pancreatic cancer. Cancer Cell Int. 2020;20:273.
111. Tao J, Yang G, Zhou W, Qiu J, Chen G, Luo W, et al. Targeting hypoxic tumor microenvironment in pancreatic cancer. J Hematol Oncol. 2021;14(1):14.
112. Li M, Xie H, Liu Y, Xia C, Cun X, Long Y, et al. Knockdown of hypoxia-inducible factor-1 alpha by tumor targeted delivery of CRISPR/Cas9 system suppressed the metastasis of pancreatic cancer. J Control Release. 2019;304:204–15.
113. Czaplinska D, Ialchina R, Andersen HB, Yao J, Stigliani A, Dannesboe J, et al. Crosstalk between tumor acidosis, p53 and extracellular matrix regulates pancreatic cancer aggressiveness. Int J Cancer. 2023;152(6):1210–25.
114. Siolas D, Vucic E, Kurz E, Hajdu C, Bar-Sagi D. Gain-of-function p53(R172H) mutation drives accumulation of neutrophils in pancreatic tumors, promoting resistance to immunotherapy. Cell Rep. 2021;36(8):109578.
115. Chick RC, Pawlik TM. Updates in Immunotherapy for Pancreatic Cancer. J Clin Med. 2024;13(21):6419.
116. Masugi Y. The Desmoplastic Stroma of Pancreatic Cancer: Multilayered Levels of Heterogeneity, Clinical Significance, and Therapeutic Opportunities. Cancers (Basel). 2022;14(13):3293.
117. Goulart MR, Stasinos K, Fincham REA, Delvecchio FR, Kocher HM. T cells in pancreatic cancer stroma. World J Gastroenterol. 2021;27(46):7956–68.
118. Wang R, Chen J, Wang W, Zhao Z, Wang H, Liu S, et al. CD40L-armed oncolytic herpes simplex virus suppresses pancreatic ductal

adenocarcinoma by facilitating the tumor microenvironment favorable to cytotoxic T cell response in the syngeneic mouse model. J Immunother Cancer. 2022;10(1):e003809.

119. Raoufi A, Soleimani Samarkhazan H, Nouri S, Khaksari MN, Abbasi Sourki P, Sargazi Aval O, et al. Macrophages in graft-versus-host disease (GVHD): dual roles as therapeutic tools and targets. Clin Exp Med. 2025;25(1):73.
120. Burks J, Fleury A, Livingston S, Smith JP. ISG15 pathway knockdown reverses pancreatic cancer cell transformation and decreases murine pancreatic tumor growth via downregulation of PDL-1 expression. Cancer Immunol Immunother. 2019;68(12):2029–39.
121. Lampreht Tratar U, Horvat S, Cemazar M. Transgenic Mouse Models in Cancer Research. Front Oncol. 2018;8:268.
122. Flavahan WA, Gaskell E, Bernstein BE. Epigenetic plasticity and the hallmarks of cancer. Science. 2017;357(6348):eaal2380.
123. Benitz S, Straub T, Mahajan UM, Mutter J, Czemmel S, Unruh T, et al. Ring1b-dependent epigenetic remodelling is an essential prerequisite for pancreatic carcinogenesis. Gut. 2019;68(11):2007–18.
124. Twardowski JJ, Heist TI, Soares ZG, Berry ES, Ruffolo LI, Pröschel C, Mello SS. Drug-Induced p53 Activation Promotes Acinar Cell Identity and Prevents Pancreatic Cancer Initiation. bioRxiv. https://www.biorxiv.org/content/10.1101/2024.05.29.595146v2.abstract.
125. Patel MB, Maniati E, Atanur SS, Pal D, Rio-Machin A, Heward J, et al. Non-coding mutations at enhancer clusters contribute to pancreatic ductal adenocarcinoma. bioRxiv. https://www.biorxiv.org/content/10.1101/2023.06.28.546873v1.full.pdf.
126. Alves E, Taifour S, Dolcetti R, Chee J, Nowak AK, Gaudieri S, Blancafort P. Reprogramming the anti-tumor immune response via CRISPR genetic and epigenetic editing. Mol Ther Methods Clin Dev. 2021;21:592–606.
127. Li J, Mahata B, Escobar M, Goell J, Wang K, Khemka P, Hilton IB. Programmable human histone phosphorylation and gene activation using a CRISPR/Cas9-based chromatin kinase. Nat Commun. 2021;12(1):896.
128. Palmer DC, Guittard GC, Franco Z, Crompton JG, Eil RL, Patel SJ, et al. Cish actively silences TCR signaling in CD8+ T cells to maintain tumor tolerance. J Exp Med. 2015;212(12):2095–113.
129. Pal SK, Tran B, Haanen J, Hurwitz ME, Sacher A, Tannir NM, et al. CD70-Targeted Allogeneic CAR T-Cell Therapy for Advanced Clear Cell Renal Cell Carcinoma. Cancer Discov. 2024;14(7):1176–89.

130. Wang Z, Li N, Feng K, Chen M, Zhang Y, Liu Y, et al. Phase I study of CAR-T cells with PD-1 and TCR disruption in mesothelin-positive solid tumors. Cell Mol Immunol. 2021;18(9):2188–98.
131. Huang J, Zhou Y, Li J, Lu A, Liang C. CRISPR/Cas systems: Delivery and application in gene therapy. Front Bioeng Biotechnol. 2022;10:942325.
132. Kim S, Kim D, Cho SW, Kim J, Kim JS. Highly efficient RNA-guided genome editing in human cells via delivery of purified Cas9 ribonucleoproteins. Genome Res. 2014;24(6):1012–9.
133. Park J, Choe S. DNA-free genome editing with preassembled CRISPR/Cas9 ribonucleoproteins in plants. Transgenic Res. 2019;28(Suppl 2):61–4.
134. Jang G, Kweon J, Kim Y. CRISPR prime editing for unconstrained correction of oncogenic KRAS variants. Commun Biol. 2023;6(1):681.
135. Kantor A, McClements ME, MacLaren RE. CRISPR-Cas9 DNA Base-Editing and Prime-Editing. Int J Mol Sci. 2020;21(17):6240.
136. Murray JB, Harrison PT, Scholefield J. Prime editing: therapeutic advances and mechanistic insights. Gene Ther. 2025;32(2):83–92.
137. Noormohamadi H, Soleimani Samarkhazan H, Maroufi F, Servatian N, Davami F. CRISPR/Cas technologies in pancreatic cancer research and therapeutics: recent advances and future outlook. Discover Oncology. 2025;16(1):1–39.
138. Zhao Z, Shang P, Mohanraju P, Geijsen N. Prime editing: advances and therapeutic applications. Trends Biotechnol. 2023;41(8):1000–12.
139. Chen H, Zhuo Q, Ye Z, Xu X, Ji S. Organoid model: A new hope for pancreatic cancer treatment? Biochim Biophys Acta Rev Cancer. 2021;1875(1):188466.
140. Tiriac H, Plenker D, Baker LA, Tuveson DA. Organoid models for translational pancreatic cancer research. Curr Opin Genet Dev. 2019;54:7–11.
141. Hussen BM, Rasul MF, Abdullah SR, Hidayat HJ, Faraj GSH, Ali FA, et al. Targeting miRNA by CRISPR/Cas in cancer: advantages and challenges. Mil Med Res. 2023;10(1):32.
142. Yang H, Bailey P, Pilarsky C. CRISPR Cas9 in Pancreatic Cancer Research. Front Cell Dev Biol. 2019;7:239.

https://doi.org/10.1142/9789819826759_0006

CHAPTER 6

CRISPR/Cas9 in the Treatment of Colorectal Cancer

Mehrdad Hashemi[1,2], *Alireza Khosravinejad*[1,3], *Mina Alimohammadi*[4], *Kimia Sadat Esfahani*[1,3], *Reza Mohajer Shirazi*[1,3], *Behdokht Jamali*[5], *Ali Shirazi*[1,3], *Amir Sadeghi*[6], *Faranak Jamshidian*[1,7], *Neda Zali*[3], *Najma Farahani*[1,*], *Afshin Taheriazam*[1,8,*], *Payman Rahimzadeh*[9,*], *Maliheh Entezari*[1,2,*]

[1]Farhikhtegan Medical Convergent Sciences Research Center, Farhikhtegan Hospital, Faculty of Medicine, TeMs. C., Islamic Azad University, Tehran, Iran

[2]Department of Genetics, Faculty of Advanced Sciences and Technology, TeMs. C, Islamic Azad University, Tehran, Iran

[3]Basic and Molecular Epidemiology of Gastrointestinal Disorders Research Center, Research Institute for Gastroenterology and Liver Diseases, Shahid Beheshti University of Medical Sciences, Tehran, Iran

[4]Department of Immunology, School of Medicine, Shahid Beheshti University of Medical Sciences, Tehran, Iran

[5]Department of Microbiology and Genetics, Kherad Institute of Higher Education, Bushehr, Iran

---

* **Corresponding authors:** Najmafarahani@gmail.com (N.F.); a.taheriazam@iautmu.ac.ir (A.T.); P.rahimzadeh76@gmail.com (P.R.); mentezari@iautmu.ac.ir (M.E.)

[6]Gastroenterology and Liver Diseases Research Center, Research Institute for Gastroenterology and Liver Diseases, Shahid Beheshti University of Medical Sciences, Tehran, Iran
[7]Department of Biology, ET.C., Islamic Azad University, Tehran, Iran
[8]Department of Orthopedics, Faculty of Medicine, TeMs. C, Islamic Azad University, Tehran, Iran
[9]Surgical Research Society (SRS), Students' Scientific Research Center, Tehran University of Medical Sciences, Tehran, Iran

Abstract

Colorectal cancer is the third most prevalent cancer worldwide and the fourth leading cause of cancer-related mortality. Despite advances in surgery, chemotherapy, and targeted therapies, many patients with advanced or metastatic colorectal cancer face poor outcomes due to tumor heterogeneity, therapeutic resistance, and the inability of current treatments to directly address underlying genetic drivers. The advent of CRISPR/Cas9 technology, a highly precise and versatile genome-editing tool, has transformed cancer research by enabling targeted gene modifications, functional genomic screening, and the development of personalized therapeutic strategies. In colorectal cancer, this system has been widely applied to investigate critical oncogenic pathways, including Wnt/β-catenin, MAPK, and PI3K, as well as recurrent mutations in APC, KRAS, and TP53. Emerging applications include the enhancement of immunotherapy, improved tumor modeling, and direct correction of pathogenic mutations. Furthermore, advances in delivery systems, such as nanoparticle-based vectors and engineered CRISPR variants, are addressing challenges related to off-target effects and therapeutic efficacy. This chapter synthesizes current evidence on the use of CRISPR/Cas9 in CRC research and therapy, highlights its potential for overcoming existing clinical limitations, and discusses future directions for integrating CRISPR-based strategies into precision oncology.

Keywords: colorectal cancer; CRISPR/Cas9; genome editing; precision medicine; immunotherapy; tumor modeling; APC; KRAS; TP53; targeted therapy

6.1 Introduction

Colorectal cancer ranks as the third most prevalent cancer worldwide and stands as the fourth major cause of cancer mortality, showing increasing trends especially in Western societies. Individuals face a 4–5% chance of developing colorectal cancer during their lifetime, with various determinants including age, daily habits, and previous health conditions. The development of colorectal cancer has been associated with gut microbiota imbalance (dysbiosis), which triggers persistent inflammation and facilitates tumor development, involving microorganisms like *Escherichia coli*, *Bacteroides fragilis*, and *Fusobacterium* species [1].

The emergence of gene therapy in the late 1980s introduced an innovative approach to gene restoration or modification. While applicable to both flora and fauna, its main application targets human therapeutics. This field has captured significant attention from researchers and pharmaceutical companies due to its potential to address various genetic disorders by targeting their fundamental genetic origins [2, 3]. Through extensive research efforts, CRISPR/Cas9 has emerged as a revolutionary genetic modification technique [4–8].

Despite decades of genetic studies revealing connections between genetic variations and diseases, understanding the exact pathways through which these variations manifest as specific conditions remains challenging. Addressing these genetic disorders requires direct genomic modifications, but achieving precise genetic alterations within the complex human genome poses significant technical challenges. The human genome, containing countless coding and non-coding genes, comprises approximately one meter of DNA within each cell's nucleus [9].

Recent years have witnessed remarkable progress in genetic engineering, particularly in achieving targeted genomic modifications. These breakthrough developments have revolutionized the field, establishing genetic engineering as a crucial component in preclinical studies while offering potential future treatments for previously untreatable conditions. A groundbreaking advancement in genome editing arrived with the development of CRISPR/Cas9.

This revolutionary technology enables precise genome manipulation and regulation with unprecedented versatility. The CRISPR/Cas9 system plays a vital role in advancing our knowledge of genetic functions within the human genome and developing innovative therapeutic approaches [10].

CRISPR/Cas9-based screening libraries have become an invaluable tool in cancer research through bioinformatics-guided screening approaches. These genome-wide studies utilize diverse experimental platforms, including 2D cell cultures, 3D organoid systems, and *in vivo* animal models [11]. The efficacy of CAR-T cell therapy has significantly improved with CRISPR/Cas9 technological advances. A 2021 investigation by Wang and colleagues utilized genome-wide screening in both CAR-T cells and glioma stem cells to identify genetic modifications that could enhance therapeutic efficacy. Their research revealed that eliminating TLE4 and IKZF2 considerably improved the anti-tumor capabilities of CAR-T cells, indicating CRISPR/Cas9's potential to enhance cancer immunotherapy approaches [12].

Colorectal cancer development stems from accumulated genetic and epigenetic modifications affecting crucial signaling pathways, including Wnt/β-catenin, MAPK, and PI3K, alongside frequent alterations in genes such as APC, KRAS, and TP53. These changes influence cancer initiation, development, and treatment resistance. Despite progress in surgical techniques, chemotherapeutic agents, and targeted treatments, patients with advanced or metastatic colorectal cancer face limited therapeutic options and poor survival outcomes. Contemporary treatments often fail to address fundamental genetic factors and tumor heterogeneity. CRISPR/Cas9, with its precision and adaptability in genome editing, presents a novel strategy for directly targeting and correcting colorectal cancer-associated mutations. Its ability to model disease and develop personalized genetic therapies offers a promising direction for overcoming current therapeutic limitations [13, 14].

This research aims to provide a comprehensive analysis of CRISPR/Cas9 applications in colorectal cancer research and treatment, with particular emphasis on its potential in immunotherapy, tumor suppression, and targeted genetic modifications. The investigation encompasses CRISPR/Cas9's effectiveness across different colorectal cancer models, its influence on treatment outcomes, and its role in regulating key cancer-related pathways. The study also examines recent innovations in specialized CRISPR variants and nanoparticle-based delivery systems, while addressing current challenges in CRISPR-based genome editing, such as off-target effects, immune responses, and delivery limitations. Drawing on recent advancements, this research seeks to highlight CRISPR/Cas9's transformative potential in colorectal cancer treatment and its future role in precision oncology.

6.2 Molecular and Genetic Basis of Colorectal Carcinogenesis

The transformation of healthy colon epithelium into colorectal cancer occurs through several distinct mechanisms, with three main pathways identified: chromosomal instability (CIN), microsatellite instability (MSI), and CpG island methylator phenotype (CIMP). Each pathway exhibits unique genetic modifications, tissue characteristics, and clinical progression patterns.

The adenoma-carcinoma progression involves specific genetic and epigenetic changes strongly associated with the CIN pathway [15]. CIN manifests through chromosomal numerical and structural abnormalities, including loss of heterozygosity, chromosomal additions or deletions, and base pair modifications. The conventional adenoma-to-carcinoma transformation typically follows a CIN pathway initiated by APC gene mutations, followed by KRAS activation, alterations in phosphoinositide 3-kinase catalytic subunit alpha and SMAD4 genes, chromosome 18 partial deletion, and TP53 function loss [16].

APC mutations are present in over 80% of non-inherited colorectal tumors, making it one of the most frequently mutated tumor suppressor genes in colorectal cancer [17]. These mutations typically lead to overactivation of the Wnt/β-catenin signaling pathway, which influences cellular growth and differentiation patterns, significantly contributing to colorectal cancer development [18]. KRAS mutations, occurring subsequent to APC alterations, promote carcinogenesis through continuous activation of signaling cascades including Raf-MAPK-ERK and PI3K/AKT/mTOR pathways [19].

The progression from adenomas to malignancy is significantly influenced by TP53 tumor suppressor inactivation [20]. TP53, the most frequently mutated gene across human cancers, regulates cell cycle arrest, cellular aging, and programmed cell death in response to cellular stress. Furthermore, TP53 serves as an indicator of colorectal cancer invasiveness and metastatic potential, with mutations being more prevalent in advanced-stage tumors and correlating with poorer outcomes [21].

MSI represents a defining molecular characteristic of Lynch syndrome, which is the most prevalent inherited form of colorectal cancer, and appears in 15% of non-inherited colorectal cancer cases. The MSI pathway begins when DNA mismatch repair (MMR) genes experience mutations, leading to instability in microsatellite regions. These regions are susceptible to DNA replication errors, which the MMR system normally detects and repairs [22]. When MMR mutations occur, numerous frameshift mutations emerge within repetitive coding sequences of cancer-related genes, closely linked to Lynch syndrome development.

The MSI-driven adenoma-carcinoma pathway differs from the CIN pathway in its mutational profile. MSI tumors show lower mutation frequencies in APC and TP53 genes, while displaying high mutation rates (exceeding 90%) in tumor suppressor genes like transforming growth factor beta receptor 2 [23]. In sporadic colorectal cancer cases, BRAF mutations are commonly observed. A particularly significant mutation is the BRAFV600E variant, where valine is replaced by glutamic acid at position 600 in the v-raf murine sarcoma viral oncogene homolog B1. The high prevalence of this mutation is associated with poor clinical outcomes and reduced survival rates in colorectal cancer patients [24].

MSI's contribution to colorectal cancer development involves disruption of multiple cellular processes, including cell cycle regulation, programmed cell death, DNA repair mechanisms, and proteins controlling cell proliferation [25]. These disruptions collectively promote cancer progression.

The serrated pathway, accounting for 20–30% of colorectal cancer cases, describes the progression from serrated polyps (including sessile serrated adenomas and conventional serrated adenocarcinomas) to colorectal cancer. Unlike traditional adenomatous lesions, this pathway is characterized by widespread DNA methylation. DNA methylation represents a crucial epigenetic modification involving the addition of methyl groups to cytosine bases. CpG islands, predominantly located in gene promoter and exon regions, contain concentrated clusters of cytosine-guanine dinucleotides. Abnormal methylation of these regions can silence cancer-related genes, promoting cancer development through tumor suppressor gene inactivation and MMR system disruption via mutl homolog 1 inactivation [26]. The higher prevalence of methylation in serrated adenomas compared to hyperplastic polyps emphasizes its importance in malignant transformation within the serrated pathway [27].

The pathogenesis of this pathway is closely associated with BRAF mutations and DNA methylation patterns. CIMPhigh tumors typically show BRAF mutations, while CIMPlow tumors are characterized by KRAS mutations [28]. BRAF mutations occur early in the serrated pathway's progression, appearing in serrated proliferative abnormal crypt foci [29]. BRAF activates the MAPK signaling cascade, leading to extracellular signal-regulated kinase activation and subsequent nuclear translocation, where it influences transcription factors controlling cell growth and proliferation genes.

The transformation of normal colorectal epithelial cells into cancerous cells begins with specific genetic mutations, with chronic inflammation potentially accelerating this process under certain conditions. The increased colorectal cancer risk in patients with Crohn's disease and chronic ulcerative colitis demonstrates the crucial role of inflammation in tumor development and progression. Inflammatory pathways encompass cancer-promoting processes triggered by persistent inflammation. Studies consistently demonstrate that inflammatory bowel disease patients, including those with ulcerative colitis and Crohn's disease, have significantly higher colorectal cancer risk compared to individuals with related conditions [27, 30], emphasizing the strong connection between chronic inflammation and cancer development.

The inflammatory pathway differs from the adenoma and serrated pathways in that extensive chronic inflammation typically occurs in multiple areas of flat mucosa, which undergoes abnormal growth and eventual malignant transformation. This pathway progresses through distinct stages: normal cells to atypical hyperplasia, followed by low-grade and high-grade heterogeneous hyperplasia, ultimately leading to cancer formation. While this pathway shares important oncogenic mechanisms with other colorectal cancer types, the sequence and prevalence of molecular events show distinct patterns. In contrast to the adenoma-carcinoma sequence, where APC mutations initiate tumor formation and P53 mutations (influenced by APC and KRAS alterations) drive progression to carcinoma, the inflammatory pathway features early and frequent P53 mutations during atypical hyperplasia, while APC mutations occur less frequently and mainly during the final tumorigenic phase [31, 32].

This pattern suggests that APC mutations are not essential for initiating inflammation-associated cancer. Research has shown that prolonged inflammation can cause DNA damage and intestinal tumor development without external carcinogens [33]. This process may be attributed to excessive production of reactive oxygen species and nitrogen intermediates during chronic inflammation. The inflammatory response activates various signaling pathways including AKT, STAT3, and NF-κB, which promote cell survival and proliferation while enhancing β-catenin activity, thereby facilitating tumor development [34].

Research into the oncogenic mechanisms of colorectal cancer has primarily centered on CIN, MSI, and CIMP. While disease progression patterns vary depending on the specific genomic alterations, these three phenomena often overlap, providing a more comprehensive understanding of colorectal cancer development. Traditional cancer research emphasized the accumulation of oncogene and tumor suppressor gene mutations as primary drivers of cancer progression. However, current genomic analyses indicate that relatively few key genes drive colorectal cancer progression, suggesting the need for deeper investigation into how these crucial mutations influence colorectal cancer cell biology.

6.3 CRISPR/Cas9 as a Therapeutic Strategy in Colorectal Cancer

CRISPR gene knockout technology offers promising strategies for clinical targeting of cancer-related genes, including tumor suppressors and oncogenes. This technology enables identification of novel therapeutic targets associated with cancer stem cells and helps understand metabolic abnormalities in cancer cells, including altered glucose, lipid, and amino acid metabolism, as well as disrupted mitochondrial function and energy metabolism pathways.

Research has demonstrated that nuclear receptor subfamily 1 group H member 4 (NR1H4) is crucial for colon cancer cell survival and proliferation. Studies revealed that NR1H4 knockout enhanced the effectiveness of anticancer drugs like adriamycin and cisplatin. MYC was identified as a key mediator in NR1H4 knockout-induced pathway modifications, suggesting that targeting NR1H4 activity could serve as a therapeutic approach for colon cancer [35].

Studies by Biagioni and colleagues examined how urokinase plasminogen activator receptor (uPAR) gene elimination affects colon cancer cell proliferation. CRISPR-mediated uPAR knockout induced cancer cell death, enhanced chemotherapy drug sensitivity, and reduced EGFR expression, indicating uPAR's potential as a therapeutic target in colon cancer treatment [36].

HNRNPA2B1, an RNA-binding protein that activates the ERK/MAPK pathway, promotes cancer cell growth and regulates cell death. Tang and colleagues used immunohistochemistry and Western blotting to elucidate HNRNPA2B1's mechanism in cancer cells, demonstrating that its knockout inhibited SW480 cell growth [37].

Glycoprotein VI (GPVI), a platelet activation trigger and antithrombotic target, has been implicated in breast and colon cancer metastasis. Mammadova-Bach and colleagues showed reduced tumor metastasis in mice lacking platelet GPVI genes. Gene knockout studies confirmed that platelet GPVI promotes tumor metastasis through interaction with tumor Galectin-3. Additionally, AQ1 F(ab')2-mediated GPVI inhibition was found to reduce tumor metastasis by disrupting tumor-platelet interactions [38].

Research has shown that nuclear receptor binding domain protein 2 (NSD2), a crucial histone methyltransferase, correlates with colorectal cancer progression and metastasis. Zhao and colleagues demonstrated elevated NSD2 mRNA levels in colon cancer tissues. CRISPR/Cas9-mediated NSD2 deletion inhibited colorectal cancer growth and development, identifying NSD2 as a potential therapeutic target [39].

Studies on p38γ, a newly identified CDK-like kinase, revealed its involvement in tumor growth and migration. Su and colleagues investigated tumor cell behavior following p38γ knockout, discovering growth inhibition and noting high p38γ expression in colon cancer tissues. These findings suggest p38γ's potential as a novel therapeutic target for colon cancer treatment [40].

CATSPER1, highly expressed in colon cancer and associated with poor outcomes, appears to promote cancer cell proliferation through PI3K/Akt pathway activation. Huang and colleagues demonstrated that CRISPR-mediated CATSPER1 deletion inhibited colon cancer growth, suggesting its potential as a therapeutic target [41].

Research by Johnson and colleagues revealed that CRISPR/Cas9-mediated NMRAL2P knockdown enhances SFN's therapeutic efficacy in colon cancer. They identified NMRAL2P as an NRF2-regulated functional pseudogene and direct transcriptional target [42].

In metabolic studies, Ždralević and colleagues demonstrated the Warburg effect's crucial role in aggressive tumor growth. Their research showed that simultaneous elimination of LDHA and

LDHB genes disrupts glycolysis, thereby inhibiting aggressive tumor growth. This Warburg effect, characterized by increased glucose consumption in cancer cells, was completely suppressed by LDHA/LDHB double knockout, which eliminated lactate secretion and halted cell growth at ambient temperature, with complete tumor growth inhibition under hypoxic conditions [46].

Research revealed that NAT1 knockout eliminated gain-of-function p53 protein expression in HT-29 cells. During glucose deprivation, NAT1-knockout cells showed increased apoptosis and reduced tumor growth, suggesting HT-29's role in tumor cell growth regulation through p53 protein stabilization [47].

SDHB gene mutations have been correlated with poor tumor outcomes. SDHB knockout resulted in decreased oxygen consumption and enhanced glycolysis. Notably, glycolysis inhibitors effectively suppressed the proliferation of SDHB-knockout cells [48].

Irving and colleagues challenged previous assumptions about vitamin D's role in colon cancer by demonstrating that vitamin D receptor (VDR) knockout neither promoted tumor development nor affected tumor progression and proliferation [49].

Research on cellular signaling molecules revealed that inositol 5-INSP7 and 1,5-Insp8, high-energy signals converted by PPIP5KS, regulate p53 and ATP levels respectively. Gu and colleagues found that CRISPR-mediated PPIP5Ks knockout in colon cancer cells reduced proliferation rates and extended the cell cycle [50].

Studies by Joo and colleagues revealed elevated NoxO1 expression in colon cancer tissues. NoxO1 knockout inhibited tumor growth, while GRB2/CBI-mediated NoxO1 proteolysis regulated NOX1 activity and reactive oxygen species (ROS) production. They found that GRB2's interaction with NOX1 reduced ROS production, with GRB2 overexpression decreasing NOX1 activity [51].

Biagioni and colleagues investigated uPAR, a tumor growth promoter. CRISPR/Cas9-mediated knockout of PLAUR (the uPAR-encoding gene) in colon cancer cells resulted in underdeveloped mitochondria, reduced glycolysis, and enhanced lactate secretion [52].

Further research by Gu and colleagues demonstrated that CRISPR-mediated PPIP5K knockout inhibited colon cancer cell proliferation under glucose-restricted conditions, simulating the tumor microenvironment [53].

Nishi and colleagues elucidated the mechanism of ROS-induced apoptosis, showing that caspase-8 reduces NHLRC2 levels through cleavage, with ROS overproduction triggering this caspase-8-mediated reduction. Their research showed that Caspase-8 knockdown increased NHLRC2 levels and suppressed cell apoptosis [54].

6.4 Targeting Colon Cancer-related Metabolism, Epithelial–Mesenchymal Transition, Aging, and Cachexia Genes by CRISPR/Cas9

Tao et al. demonstrated that hypermethylation of promoters creates aging-like characteristics. Their research using CRISPR to simultaneously deactivate silencing genes showed Wnt pathway activation. These modifications caused aged organs to display increased sensitivity to Braf V600E transformation compared to younger tissues, establishing a connection between aging-related epigenetic changes and colon cancer-driving oncogenes [55].

Kandarian's research revealed LIF as the primary trigger for colon cancer cachexia, a condition linked to poor survival outcomes. Through LIF gene elimination, they observed improvements in various cachexia symptoms, including reduced weight loss, preserved muscle mass, maintained fat tissue, and decreased splenomegaly in experimental mice [56].

Studies by Poghosyan and colleagues explored Nrp2's influence on tumor growth and aggressiveness maintenance. Using CRISPR/Cas9 to eliminate Nrp2 in mesenchymal-type colorectal cancer cells, they observed mesenchymal-to-epithelial conversion with newfound dependence on IR signaling and autophagy. Their findings suggested that combining IR signaling and autophagy inhibition could trigger apoptosis in Nrp2-deficient tumors, offering potential therapeutic strategies [57].

Szeder and team investigated Tks4 scaffold protein's role in colorectal cancer development. Their CRISPR/Cas9-mediated Tks4 elimination resulted in enhanced cell motility, reduced adhesion, and increased fibronectin expression — all characteristic of epithelial-mesenchymal transition (EMT). Their research demonstrated that Tks4 protein absence influences tumor cell EMT [58].

Research conducted by Hosain and colleagues employed CRISPR/Cas9 technology to generate mice with tumor cells containing heterozygous p53 R273H mutations. Their findings revealed enhanced EMT and increased cancer stem cell populations, leading to accelerated tumor development. The study demonstrated that PDMP, through its inhibition of glucosylceramide synthase, could restore p53 expression, reverse the EMT, and decrease cancer stem cell numbers in cells carrying the R273H mutation. This research suggested that targeting ceramide glycosylation to restore p53 function could represent an innovative therapeutic strategy [59].

Li and colleagues investigated the influence of the glycolytic pathway on colorectal cancer progression. Their screening of glycolysis-associated genes identified elevated ALDOB expression in colorectal cancer cells. When ALDOB was eliminated through gene knockout, they observed suppression of EMT and inhibition of cancer cell proliferation and migration. These findings indicated that ALDOB deficiency could restrict colorectal cancer cell growth characteristics by preventing EMT. The study highlighted ALDOB's potential as a novel therapeutic target, offering significant implications for colorectal cancer treatment and outcome prediction [60].

6.5 Restoring Tumor Suppressor Gene Function

Studies by Melo-Hanchuk and colleagues revealed that the 57 kDa regulatory protein HABP4 plays a crucial role in transcriptional regulation and proliferation control of colorectal cancer. Their research demonstrated that HABP4 deletion resulted in increased tumor volume, suggesting its potential as a novel tumor suppressor protein [43].

Cai and team investigated the relationship between zinc finger ZAP antiviral protein expression and colorectal cancer prognosis. They found that ZAP overexpression inhibited tumor development, growth, and invasiveness. Using CRISPR technology, they demonstrated that simultaneous deletion of both ZAP and APC created a synergistic effect that enhanced tumor growth [44].

Research by Liu and colleagues identified PRDM1β as a p53-responsive gene in colorectal cancer cells. Through knockout studies, they discovered that both α and β transcriptional variants of PRDM1 suppress myc response genes and stem cell-associated genes. Their findings showed that PRDM1 gene upregulation could inhibit colorectal cancer growth, suggesting that p53's tumor-suppressing function may operate through PRDM1-mediated silencing of stem cell genes [45].

Taken together, in **Figure 6.1**, the most substantial oncogenes, particularly those involved in colon cancer-related metabolism, EMT, cachexia, and aging and epigenetic changes, as well as key tumor suppressors, which are therapeutically targeted by CRISPR/Cas9 are schematically presented.

6.6 CRISPR/Cas9 in Addressing Drug Resistance

Liu and colleagues investigated colon cancer resistance mechanisms by eliminating PUM1 and DDX5 in trastuzumab-resistant SW480R and Caco-2R cells. Their research revealed reduced proliferation in both cell types and demonstrated PUM1's positive regulation of DDX5 and cell viability. The findings suggested that reducing PUM1 and DDX5 expression could enhance trastuzumab sensitivity in colorectal cancer treatment [61].

Research by Liu et al. explored HMGA2-WHSC1 interactions in cancer cell regulation. They identified WHSC1 as an HMGA2 oncogene target that promotes cancer cell growth and spread. WHSC1 elimination via CRISPR in colorectal cancer cells resulted in decreased proliferation, enhanced drug sensitivity, and reduced metastatic potential [62].

Beck and team studied TFAP2A-encoded AP-2α's tumor-suppressing role in colorectal cancer transcription regulation. Using CRISPR/Cas9 and shRNA to remove TFAP2A expression, they found that AP-2α elimination led to buparlisib BKM120

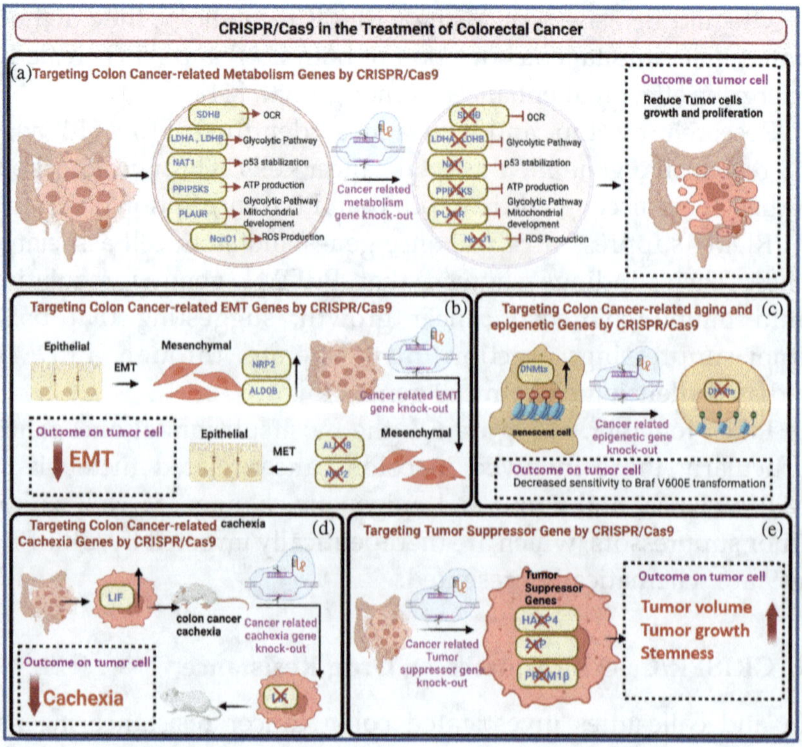

Figure 6.1 CRISPR/Cas9-mediated targeting of key gene networks in the treatment of colorectal cancer. The scheme summarizes the diverse strategies and therapeutic outcomes enabled by CRISPR/Cas9 genome editing in colorectal cancer models through the functional interrogation of crucial genetic pathways. **(a) Targeting metabolism-related genes:** CRISPR/Cas9 knockout of genes involved in cellular metabolism, including SDHB, LDHA, LDHB, NAT1, PPIK5K, PLAUR, and Nox01, disrupts mitochondrial function, glycolytic pathways, ATP and ROS production, and p53 stabilization, cumulatively resulting in reduced tumor cell proliferation and growth. **(b) Disruption of EMT-associated genes:** Knocking out EMT genes such as NRP2 and ALDOB counteracts the mesenchymal phenotype, promoting mesenchymal-to-epithelial transition and attenuating invasive tumor cell behavior. **(c) Targeting aging and epigenetic genes:** CRISPR/Cas9 inactivation of DNA methyltransferases and related epigenetic regulators in senescent tumor cells confers resistance to oncogenic transformation (e.g., BRAF V600E), thus modulating tumorigenesis driven by epigenetic aging signatures. **(d) Cachexia-associated genetic targets:** Disruption of the LIF gene, a key mediator of cancer-associated cachexia, diminishes systemic wasting and tumor-induced cachexia in preclinical models. **(e) Knockout of tumor suppressor genes:** Targeted deletion of tumor suppressors such as HAAI and PKM1B significantly increases tumor volume, growth, and stemness characteristics in colorectal cancer cells, directly implicating them in the suppression of malignancy.

resistance, suggesting that increasing AP-2α levels might enhance BuparlisiB/BKM120 effectiveness [63].

Satapathy and colleagues examined CYSLTR1's role in 5-FU resistance. They observed elevated CYSLTR1 levels in 5-FU resistant cells and demonstrated that CYSLTR1 knockout and Montelukast treatment reduced LTD4/CYSLTR1 signaling, diminishing 5-FU resistance [64].

Tung et al. discovered that oxaliplatin resistance develops through chromatin changes, involving FGFR1 and OXTR genes. CRISPR/Cas9 suppression of these genes helped overcome resistance. Combined treatment with oxaliplatin and either PD166866 or L-368,899 effectively suppressed resistant organoids, offering potential precision treatment approaches [65].

Franke's research connected low SASH1 expression with distant tumor metastasis, noting inverse expression patterns between SASH1 and CRKL in colorectal cancer cells. SASH1 elimination induced EMT, resulting in decreased chemotherapy sensitivity and patient survival [66].

Zhou and colleagues demonstrated through various experimental methods that caspase-3 knockout in HCT116 cells increased sensitivity to chemo- and radiotherapy while reducing tumor invasiveness and metastatic capability, identifying caspase-3 as a potential therapeutic target [67].

Li et al. identified Par3L as a promising therapeutic target, noting lower survival rates in patients with high Par3L expression. Their CRISPR/Cas9 studies showed that Par3L elimination increased cancer cell apoptosis and activated the Lkb1/AMPK signaling cascade, enhancing sensitivity to chemo- and radiotherapy [68].

6.7 CRISPR/Cas9 and Colon Cancer Cell Biology

Zheng and colleagues explored CXCR-4's role in tumor metastasis. Their gene knockout studies revealed decreased tumor cell adhesion without affecting proliferation, operating through AKT and IGF1R signaling pathway modulation [69].

Research by Schwiebs et al. using CRISPR/Cas9 demonstrated that SGPL1 suppression in colonic stem cell niches contributed to cell cycle arrest and cancer progression. They found that SGPL1 influences the cell cycle through Ki-67 and FOXO3 regulation in stem cells [70].

Hu and team investigated DACH1's function in intestinal stem cells and colorectal tumors, noting that elevated DACH1 expression indicated poor prognosis. Their research showed that DACH1 overexpression suppresses cell growth via BMP signal inhibition, while its elimination relieved this growth suppression, suggesting DACH1's potential as a therapeutic target [71].

Gisina and colleagues established a correlation between CEACAM5 expression in colorectal cancer stem cells and CD133 positivity. Their CRISPR/Cas9-mediated CD133 knockout studies demonstrated significant variations in CEACAM5-positive cell populations [72].

Michels et al. studied colon cancer formation through Wnt activation following APC knockout. They distinguished between oncogenic and physiological Wnt-induced transcription, finding that oncogenic Wnt signaling in CMS2 tumors indicated better prognosis, while receptor-mediated signaling in CMS4 tumors suggested poor outcomes [73].

Studies by Eto and colleagues revealed that RNF43 deletion mutations, achieved through CRISPR/Cas9, activated Wnt signaling, enhanced tumor growth, and increased recurrence rates in colorectal cancer patients [74].

Tak and team examined the impact of colorectal cancer risk-associated single nucleotide polymorphisms on gene expression. Their research using CRISPR/Cas9 to eliminate H3K27Ac in the E7 region showed widespread reduction in adjacent gene expression. Notably, similar gene expression decreases occurred in cells lacking H3K27Ac peaks in the E7 region, indicating that the transcriptional effects of enhancer deletion are not solely predicted by H3K27Ac peak characteristics [75].

Rappaport and colleagues investigated GUCY2C's tumor-suppressing role using CRISPR/Cas9 and genome editing. They identified functional enhancers controlling GUCY2C ligand loss and explored the impact of β-catenin/TCF signaling on GUCY2C ligand transcriptional silencing. Their findings established GUCY2C as a primary β-catenin/TCF signaling target, demonstrating transcriptional suppression [76].

Research by Xu et al. demonstrated that METTL3 elimination in SW480 cells led to increased SOCS2 expression and reduced tumor formation capacity. These findings identified METTL3 as a crucial factor in colorectal cancer cell tumorigenicity [77].

Makkar's research explored hyaluronic acid's (HA) role in colorectal cancer progression, noting its correlation with poor outcomes. Their studies showed that HA interaction with CD44 and TLR4 promoted cancer development, while PEP1 blocked these interactions and inhibited growth. CRISPR-mediated CD44 and TLR4 knockout in CT26 cells resulted in slower tumor growth, confirming the significance of HA-receptor interactions in tumor development [78].

Yu and colleagues investigated the interaction between CCAT2 and miR-145 in cancer regulation. They found that nuclear-located CCAT2 prevents pre-miR-145 nuclear-cytoplasmic transport, blocking miR-145 maturation and promoting tumor growth. CRISPR-based CCAT2 elimination increased mature miR-145 levels and inhibited cancer stem cell proliferation [79].

Guo et al. examined the CBS-H2S axis's influence on colorectal cancer liver metastasis. Their CRISPR/Cas9-mediated CBS knockout studies showed reduced VEGF expression, inhibited angiogenesis, and decreased liver metastasis, suggesting CBS as a potential therapeutic target for metastatic colorectal cancer [80].

Malkomes and colleagues explored TGM2's dual functionality in transamidation and GTPase activity. Their research showed that elevated TGM2 expression enhanced colorectal cancer cell activity, while its suppression through gene knockdown reduced tumor proliferation capacity [81].

Research by Xiong et al. investigated STAT3DEL's impact on colorectal cancer development. Their targeted deletion of a short sequence in STAT3's DNA binding domain resulted in decreased cell proliferation and migration. These findings demonstrated that this specific deletion inhibits transcriptional activation and alters DNA motif recognition, influencing cancer progression [82].

Cheng and colleagues demonstrated that mindin deletion promoted cancer cell proliferation through ERK and c-fos pathways. Their CRISPR/Cas9-generated mindin knockout mice showed accelerated tumor growth, while mindin overexpression had the opposite effect, suggesting mindin's potential as a therapeutic target [83].

Studies revealed GSTO1's role in autophagy-related drug resistance development through interaction with TNFαIP3/A20. CRISPR/Cas9-mediated double knockout of both genes showed enhanced chemotherapy sensitivity compared to single gene knockouts, with increased cancer cell apoptosis, highlighting GSTO1's role in drug resistance [84].

Liu et al. identified elevated COMP expression in colorectal cancer tissues, with levels decreasing post-surgery. CRISPR-mediated COMP elimination reduced cancer cell proliferation and chemotherapy resistance. High COMP expression correlated with enhanced proliferation and poor prognosis, establishing COMP as both a prognostic indicator and potential therapeutic target [85].

Yin and colleagues investigated TRIM11, an E3 ubiquitin ligase highly expressed in colorectal cancer tissues correlating with reduced survival. CRISPR-based TRIM11 elimination induced cancer cell apoptosis and inhibited proliferation. Their research revealed miR-24-3P's regulation of TRIM11, where reduced miR-24-3P levels increase TRIM11 expression, identifying TRIM11 as a potential therapeutic target [86].

Hartal-Benishay and colleagues examined MBTPS's role in colorectal cancer proliferation, identifying a positive correlation between MBTPS1 mRNA and SREBPs in tumor tissues. Their research showed that MBTPS1 suppression combined with type 1 interferon pathway inhibition completely halted tumor growth, suggesting MBTPS1's potential as a therapeutic target [87].

Liu et al. investigated RhoB's connection to radiation resistance. CRISPR/Cas9-mediated RhoB elimination reduced Akt phosphorylation and FoxM1 levels, enhancing radiotherapy sensitivity and increasing apoptosis. They found that elevated RhoB expression corresponded with radiotherapy resistance and poor survival outcomes [88].

Research demonstrated that FOLFOX chemotherapy induces CD44v6, MDR1, and YB-1 overexpression, with CD44v6 increasing YB-1 expression. CRISPR/Cas9 elimination of CD44v6 and YB-1 inhibited FOLFOX-resistant CIC growth, indicating CD44v6's role in tumor cell dedifferentiation [89].

Studies revealed CRUMPS3's tumor-suppressing properties and its interaction with FGFR1, which promotes colorectal cancer metastasis and invasion [90].

Dai and colleagues explored PP2A's influence on cancer cell proliferation. Their research showed that LB-100 inhibits PP2A activity and cancer cell survival, while CRISPR-mediated PP2A knockout activated AMPK-induced apoptosis. LB-100 was found to trigger apoptosis and G1-S cell cycle arrest [91].

Huang et al. studied Bid's role in apoptosis, showing its relationship with Caspase8 activation and TRAIL response. Their gene-edited Bid knockout cells demonstrated blocked apoptosis [92].

Chandrasekaran and team investigated USP29's function in colorectal cancer. CRISPR/Cas9-mediated USP29 elimination extended cell cycle duration, increased apoptosis, and reduced proliferation. High USP29 expression was linked to enhanced cancer progression and malignancy [93].

Li and colleagues examined cancer stem cells, finding that CD133 knockout reduced stem cell proliferation and eliminated vimentin expression. While not completely eliminating tumorigenicity, this significantly inhibited tumor characteristics, suggesting CD133 as a potential therapeutic target [94].

6.8 CRISPR in Tumor Microenvironment Modulation and the Immunotherapy

The immunoscore, which measures the density of CD3+ and CD8+ cytotoxic T lymphocytes within and around tumors, serves as a key predictor of colorectal cancer outcomes, including survival rates and recurrence risk. The tumor microenvironment plays an essential role in both promoting cancer growth and facilitating tumor destruction. The complexity of colorectal cancer extends beyond genetic factors, encompassing intricate interactions between malignant cells and various immune system components [95, 96].

Research conducted by the International Society for Immunotherapy of Cancer examined 1,885 stage I-II colon cancer patients, revealing that T cell infiltration in both central tumor regions and peripheral areas correlates with enhanced survival outcomes and longer disease-free intervals, regardless of tumor size [97].

The prognostic value of CD3+ and CD8+ lymphocyte presence extends to patients without detected metastases. Further investigation of 763 stage III colorectal cancer patients demonstrated that higher immunoscores corresponded with improved survival rates and lower recurrence risks, emphasizing significance of T cells in disease prognosis [95, 96].

In colorectal cancer immune responses, CD8+ and CD4+ T lymphocytes play primary roles. These cells typically express T cell receptors consisting of α and β chains. Thymic development includes elimination of self-reactive T cells through programmed cell death, establishing self-tolerance. Following maturation, these T cells circulate to secondary lymphoid tissues for activation by antigen-presenting cells. Within tumor-draining lymph nodes, activated APCs, particularly dendritic cells, present tumor-associated antigens to T cells via distinct MHC molecules: class I for CD8+ cells and class II for CD4+ cells. This specific interaction promotes T cell differentiation into specialized effector cells, generating robust anti-tumor responses [96, 98].

Conventional CD4+ T cells, characterized by their αβ TCR expression, demonstrate multifaceted roles in colorectal cancer. Their diverse helper cell subsets perform distinct functions, with some supporting tumor elimination while others potentially facilitate cancer progression. These cells exhibit remarkable adaptability, modifying their functions based on environmental signals [96, 99, 100].

T helper 17 (Th17) cells demonstrate remarkable plasticity, capable of acquiring characteristics typical of other T helper subtypes [96, 101]. Following activation by antigen-presenting cells,

CD4+ T lymphocytes undergo differentiation into both effector and memory populations [96, 102].

The activation and polarization of naive CD4+ T lymphocytes depend on three critical signals: first, the recognition between T cell receptor and MHC class II complex on antigen-presenting cells; second, antigen-independent co-stimulation through CD28-CD80/CD86 interaction; and third, the presence of antigen-presenting cell-derived cytokines in the surrounding environment.

Colorectal cancer typically maintains an immunosuppressive or "cold" microenvironment that hampers immune system function. One mechanism involves tumor cell expression of PD-L1, which interacts with T-cell PD-1, subsequently suppressing anti-tumor immune responses.

CRISPR-modified T cells, when reinfused, can effectively counter these immunosuppressive mechanisms. PD-1 deletion enables T cells to maintain their anti-tumor activity despite PD-L1 expression. The edited T cells can enhance immune responses through cytokine modulation, such as IL-12 upregulation and TGF-β reduction, counteracting the typical immunosuppressive colorectal cancer environment. These modifications positively influence the immunoscore, a clinical metric of intratumoral immune activity that correlates with improved survival and reduced recurrence in colorectal cancer patients [95, 96, 103].

CD4+ T lymphocytes in colorectal cancer differentiate into multiple distinct subsets, including follicular helper, induced and natural regulatory T cells, and various T helper subtypes (Th1, Th2, Th17, Th22). These subsets are characterized by specific transcription factors (such as T-BET in Th1 and GATA-3 in Th2 cells), distinct cytokine profiles (like IL-4 from Th2 and IL-17 from Th17 cells), and unique combinations of chemokine receptors and STAT proteins [96, 100, 104].

T helper cells, particularly Th17 cells, exhibit significant plasticity. Under conditions like colitis, *in vitro*-generated Th17 cells can transform into IFN-γ-producing Th1 cells after adoptive transfer [96, 105, 106]. Studies have shown that IL-22 contributes to chemotherapy resistance in colorectal cancer patients [107] and enhances tumor development in mouse models [108, 109].

Laboratory studies demonstrate that TGF-β suppresses Th22 cell formation, while in living organisms, it enhances IL-22 production by Th17 cells [110], enabling Th17-to-Th22 cell conversion. Similarly, regulatory T cells can undergo phenotypic shifts, potentially transforming into Th1 or Th17-like ex-regulatory T cells through FOXP3 downregulation [96, 111].

Improved colorectal cancer prognosis correlates with Th1 cells and their cytokine production. These cells impede cancer development through multiple mechanisms: reducing angiogenesis, recruiting cytotoxic CD8+ T cells, and inducing cancer cell senescence [96, 112, 113]. While Th1 cells enhance CD8+ T cell activation supporting anti-tumor responses, they also produce IFN-γ, which increases checkpoint inhibitor expression, including PD-1 on CD8+ T cells [114].

The role of Th2 cells in colorectal cancer remains controversial. Their cytokines (IL-4, IL-5, IL-13) maintain inflammatory conditions that may promote cancer development [115]. However, these cytokines also attract eosinophils, which possess anti-tumor properties and may slow cancer progression by modifying tumor vasculature [96].

CAR-T cell therapy faces significant translational challenges in colorectal cancer despite promising *in vitro* results. While Tauriello et al. reported 90% cytotoxicity in cell cultures, their xenograft models did not account for the immunosuppressive tumor microenvironment, characterized by PD-L1+ myeloid cells and elevated TGF-β levels (2.1–4.8 ng/ml) [116]. The limited focus on colorectal cancer in clinical trials compared to leukemia (two versus 15 Phase I studies) reflects ongoing target validation challenges. Conflicting results regarding EpCAM-targeting CAR-T cells, with one study showing significant toxicity in normal intestinal tissue [117] and another demonstrating effectiveness against peritoneal metastases [118], emphasize the need for consensus molecular subtype (CMS) classification-based subtype-specific approaches (**Table 6.1**) [119].

Table 6.1 T cell immunology in colorectal cancer.

Aspect	Key Finding	Cell Types Involved	Prognostic Significance	Reference
Stage III colorectal cancer prognosis	High immunoscore associated with greater overall survival and decreased recurrence	CD3+, CD8+ cells	Crucial role in colorectal cancer prognosis	[96]
T cell activation	Requires three signals: TCR-MHC interaction, co-stimulation, environmental cytokines	CD8+, CD4+ T cells	Initiates targeted immune response	[96]
CD4+ T cell complexity	Multiple subsets with unique functions, considerable plasticity	Various CD4+ subsets	Complex role in anti-tumor immunity vs. tumor progression	[96]
T cell subsets	Follicular helper cells, regulatory T cells, Th1, Th2, Th17, Th22	Various CD4+ subsets	Defined by specific transcription factors and cytokines	[96]
Th1 cells	Inhibit cancer development, attract cytotoxic CD8+ T cells	Th1 cells	Better prognosis in colorectal cancer	[96]
Th2 cells	May attract eosinophils with anti-tumoral properties	Th2 cells	Controversial role — may help slow cancer progression	[96]

6.9 Risks, Limitations, Ethical Considerations, and Future Directions into Use of CRISPR/Cas System in Colon Cancer

CRISPR/Cas technology represents a groundbreaking advancement in genome editing, offering significant potential for colorectal cancer research and treatment. While its applications span from functional genomics to therapeutic interventions, various obstacles impede its clinical implementation. Artificial intelligence (AI) integration has become crucial in addressing these challenges and enhancing CRISPR-based treatments.

A primary challenge in CRISPR applications involves off-target modifications, where unintended DNA sites undergo editing due to sequence similarities or guide RNA design flaws. In colorectal cancer contexts, such imprecise editing could potentially damage tumor suppressor genes or activate proto-oncogenes, potentially worsening the disease condition or creating new cancer-causing mutations [120]. This concern becomes particularly critical during *in vivo* somatic cell editing, where targeting precision directly impacts treatment safety and effectiveness. Additionally, genetic mosaicism, where both edited and unedited cells coexist, can compromise therapeutic outcomes by reducing the consistency and reproducibility of genetic corrections in colorectal cancer models.

The successful delivery of CRISPR components to colorectal tumors presents significant challenges. While viral vectors provide efficient transduction, they risk immune responses, genetic insertion problems, and face size constraints. Non-viral delivery methods show reduced immunogenicity but struggle with effective delivery to solid tumors [121]. The characteristics of the colorectal cancer tumor microenvironment, including low oxygen levels, tissue scarring, and immune suppression, can hinder CRISPR component distribution and uptake [122].

The diverse tumor characteristics of colorectal cancer, both between and within tumors, lead to variable CRISPR editing results. Different mutation patterns across colorectal cancer subtypes may require individualized guide RNA designs [123]. Tumor evolution during treatment could render initial genetic targets irrelevant. Furthermore, cellular selection following CRISPR-induced DNA alterations might inadvertently promote more aggressive or treatment-resistant cancer cell populations.

The field continues to debate ethical considerations regarding germline editing and potential CRISPR technology misuse in colorectal cancer. Regulatory authorities require thorough preclinical validation, including monitoring of unintended effects, long-term safety, and immune responses. Colorectal cancer patients with inherited genetic instabilities require particularly careful assessment of the broader genomic effects of CRISPR editing [124]. The absence of standardized CRISPR clinical trial protocols in oncology creates implementation challenges, necessitating clear definition of risk-benefit assessments, patient selection methods, and treatment outcomes.

Current CRISPR studies in colorectal cancer primarily utilize cell lines and mouse models, which may inadequately represent human tumor complexity. Model systems differ from human patients in immune responses, tumor microenvironment, and genetic makeup, potentially leading to variations in treatment responses and editing effectiveness. Experimental consistency remains challenging, with CRISPR results varying based on guide RNA sequences, delivery systems, and laboratory conditions [125].

AI is revolutionizing CRISPR applications in colorectal cancer by improving precision, effectiveness, and safety. AI tools can analyze extensive genetic data to enhance guide RNA design, anticipate unintended effects, and predict editing outcomes with remarkable accuracy [126, 127].

Machine learning and deep learning algorithms examine large datasets to identify optimal guide RNA sequences that maximize target specificity while minimizing off-target effects. Advanced tools such as DeepCRISPR, CRISPR-Net, and Elevation employ neural networks trained on experimental data to forecast editing results, reducing trial-and-error approaches. This precision is crucial for colorectal cancer treatment to prevent potential cancer progression [128].

AI enables comprehensive analysis of multiple molecular datasets (genomics, transcriptomics, epigenomics) to identify viable therapeutic targets and pathway relationships in colorectal cancer. AI-driven biomarker discovery helps researchers select editing targets that optimize therapeutic benefits while minimizing systemic effects [129].

The technology facilitates individualized colorectal cancer treatment by analyzing patient-specific mutations and computationally modeling CRISPR editing impacts. AI algorithms can simulate treatments and predict resistance development, enabling proactive strategy adjustments. This personalization is essential given the diverse genetic and epigenetic profiles across colorectal cancer patients.

Machine learning aids in developing more effective tumor-targeting delivery systems. By evaluating physical and chemical properties, cellular uptake, and distribution patterns, AI can guide the development of colorectal cancer-specific nanoparticles and viral vectors.

AI platforms enhance CRISPR clinical trial design through patient stratification, outcome prediction, and early safety assessment. Computer simulations reduce dependence on animal testing and improve translation of research findings to human colorectal cancer treatment.

6.10 Conclusion

Colorectal cancer remains a major global health burden, with limited therapeutic options for patients with advanced disease. The rapid evolution of CRISPR/Cas9 technology offers a unique opportunity to address the genetic and epigenetic complexities of colorectal cancer by enabling direct gene targeting, functional screening, and the development of personalized treatment strategies. Its application spans tumor suppression, immunotherapy enhancement, and the modeling of therapeutic resistance, underscoring its transformative potential in both preclinical and translational research. Nonetheless, significant challenges remain, particularly regarding delivery efficiency, immunogenicity, and off-target effects, which must be resolved for safe clinical implementation. As novel CRISPR variants and improved delivery approaches continue to be developed, CRISPR/Cas9 stands as a powerful tool with the potential to redefine colorectal cancer management and advance the era of precision oncology.

References

1. Mármol I, Sánchez-de-Diego C, Pradilla Dieste A, Cerrada E, Rodriguez Yoldi MJ. Colorectal Carcinoma: A General Overview and Future Perspectives in Colorectal Cancer. Int J Mol Sci. 2017;18(1):197.
2. Ishino Y, Shinagawa H, Makino K, Amemura M, Nakata A. Nucleotide sequence of the iap gene, responsible for alkaline phosphatase isozyme conversion in Escherichia coli, and identification of the gene product. J Bacteriol. 1987;169(12):5429–33.
3. Zhang B. CRISPR/Cas gene therapy. J Cell Physiol. 2021;236(4): 2459–81.
4. Bikard D, Jiang W, Samai P, Hochschild A, Zhang F, Marraffini LA. Programmable repression and activation of bacterial gene expression using an engineered CRISPR-Cas system. Nucleic Acids Res. 2013;41(15):7429–37.
5. Bolotin A, Quinquis B, Sorokin A, Ehrlich SD. Clustered regularly interspaced short palindrome repeats (CRISPRs) have spacers of extrachromosomal origin. Microbiology (Reading). 2005;151(Pt 8): 2551–61.
6. Cyranoski D. CRISPR gene-editing tested in a person for the first time. Nature. 2016;539(7630):479.
7. Garneau JE, Dupuis M, Villion M, Romero DA, Barrangou R, Boyaval P, et al. The CRISPR/Cas bacterial immune system cleaves bacteriophage and plasmid DNA. Nature. 2010;468(7320):67–71.
8. Hu Y, Liu L, Jiang Q, Fang W, Chen Y, Hong Y, Zhai X. CRISPR/Cas9: a powerful tool in colorectal cancer research. J Exp Clin Cancer Res. 2023;42(1):308.
9. Xiong X, Chen M, Lim WA, Zhao D, Qi LS. CRISPR/Cas9 for Human Genome Engineering and Disease Research. Annu Rev Genomics Hum Genet. 2016;17:131–54.

10. Kim H, Kim JS. A guide to genome engineering with programmable nucleases. Nat Rev Genet. 2014;15(5):321–34.
11. Michels BE, Mosa MH, Streibl BI, Zhan T, Menche C, Abou-El-Ardat K, et al. Pooled In Vitro and In Vivo CRISPR-Cas9 Screening Identifies Tumor Suppressors in Human Colon Organoids. Cell Stem Cell. 2020;26(5):782–92.e7.
12. Wang D, Prager BC, Gimple RC, Aguilar B, Alizadeh D, Tang H, et al. CRISPR Screening of CAR T Cells and Cancer Stem Cells Reveals Critical Dependencies for Cell-Based Therapies. Cancer Discov. 2021;11(5):1192–211.
13. Emami A, Mahdavi Sharif P, Rezaei N. KRAS mutations in colorectal cancer: impacts on tumor microenvironment and therapeutic implications. Expert Opin Ther Targets. 2025;29(6):361–83.
14. Takeda M, Yoshida S, Inoue T, Sekido Y, Hata T, Hamabe A, et al. The Role of KRAS Mutations in Colorectal Cancer: Biological Insights, Clinical Implications, and Future Therapeutic Perspectives. Cancers (Basel). 2025;17(3):428.
15. Pino MS, Chung DC. The chromosomal instability pathway in colon cancer. Gastroenterology. 2010;138(6):2059–72.
16. Fearon ER, Vogelstein B. A genetic model for colorectal tumorigenesis. Cell. 1990;61(5):759–67.
17. Comprehensive molecular characterization of human colon and rectal cancer. Nature. 2012;487(7407):330–7.
18. Zhong ZA, Michalski MN, Stevens PD, Sall EA, Williams BO. Regulation of Wnt receptor activity: Implications for therapeutic development in colon cancer. J Biol Chem. 2021;296:100782.
19. Zhu G, Pei L, Xia H, Tang Q, Bi F. Role of oncogenic KRAS in the prognosis, diagnosis and treatment of colorectal cancer. Mol Cancer. 2021;20(1):143.
20. López I, L PO, Tucci P, Alvarez-Valín F, R AC, Marín M. Different mutation profiles associated to P53 accumulation in colorectal cancer. Gene. 2012;499(1):81–7.
21. Iacopetta B, Russo A, Bazan V, Dardanoni G, Gebbia N, Soussi T, et al. Functional categories of TP53 mutation in colorectal cancer: results of an International Collaborative Study. Ann Oncol. 2006; 17(5):842–7.
22. Baretti M, Le DT. DNA mismatch repair in cancer. Pharmacol Ther. 2018;189:45–62.

23. Parsons R, Myeroff LL, Liu B, Willson JK, Markowitz SD, Kinzler KW, Vogelstein B. Microsatellite instability and mutations of the transforming growth factor beta type II receptor gene in colorectal cancer. Cancer Res. 1995;55(23):5548–50.
24. Shimada Y, Tajima Y, Nagahashi M, Ichikawa H, Oyanagi H, Okuda S, et al. Clinical Significance of BRAF Non-V600E Mutations in Colorectal Cancer: A Retrospective Study of Two Institutions. J Surg Res. 2018;232:72–81.
25. Nguyen LH, Goel A, Chung DC. Pathways of Colorectal Carcinogenesis. Gastroenterology. 2020;158(2):291–302.
26. Gallois C, Laurent-Puig P, Taieb J. Methylator phenotype in colorectal cancer: A prognostic factor or not? Crit Rev Oncol Hematol. 2016;99:74–80.
27. Fernando WC, Miranda MS, Worthley DL, Togashi K, Watters DJ, Leggett BA, Spring KJ. The CIMP Phenotype in BRAF Mutant Serrated Polyps from a Prospective Colonoscopy Patient Cohort. Gastroenterol Res Pract. 2014;2014:374926.
28. Shen L, Toyota M, Kondo Y, Lin E, Zhang L, Guo Y, et al. Integrated genetic and epigenetic analysis identifies three different subclasses of colon cancer. Proc Natl Acad Sci U S A. 2007;104(47):18654–9.
29. Rosenberg DW, Yang S, Pleau DC, Greenspan EJ, Stevens RG, Rajan TV, et al. Mutations in BRAF and KRAS differentially distinguish serrated versus non-serrated hyperplastic aberrant crypt foci in humans. Cancer Res. 2007;67(8):3551–4.
30. Jess T, Gamborg M, Matzen P, Munkholm P, Sørensen TI. Increased risk of intestinal cancer in Crohn's disease: a meta-analysis of population-based cohort studies. Am J Gastroenterol. 2005;100(12):2724–9.
31. Itzkowitz SH, Yio X. Inflammation and cancer IV. Colorectal cancer in inflammatory bowel disease: the role of inflammation. Am J Physiol Gastrointest Liver Physiol. 2004;287(1):G7–17.
32. Shah SC, Itzkowitz SH. Colorectal Cancer in Inflammatory Bowel Disease: Mechanisms and Management. Gastroenterology. 2022; 162(3):715–30.e3.
33. Meira LB, Bugni JM, Green SL, Lee CW, Pang B, Borenshtein D, et al. DNA damage induced by chronic inflammation contributes to colon carcinogenesis in mice. J Clin Invest. 2008;118(7):2516–25.
34. Grivennikov SI. Inflammation and colorectal cancer: colitis-associated neoplasia. Semin Immunopathol. 2013;35(2):229–44.

35. Lee YJ, Lee EY, Choi BH, Jang H, Myung JK, You HJ. The Role of Nuclear Receptor Subfamily 1 Group H Member 4 (NR1H4) in Colon Cancer Cell Survival through the Regulation of c-Myc Stability. Mol Cells. 2020;43(5):459–68.
36. Biagioni A, Chillà A, Del Rosso M, Fibbi G, Scavone F, Andreucci E, et al. CRISPR/Cas9 uPAR Gene Knockout Results in Tumor Growth Inhibition, EGFR Downregulation and Induction of Stemness Markers in Melanoma and Colon Carcinoma Cell Lines. Front Oncol. 2021;11:663225.
37. Tang J, Chen Z, Wang Q, Hao W, Gao WQ, Xu H. hnRNPA2B1 Promotes Colon Cancer Progression via the MAPK Pathway. Front Genet. 2021;12:666451.
38. Mammadova-Bach E, Gil-Pulido J, Sarukhanyan E, Burkard P, Shityakov S, Schonhart C, et al. Platelet glycoprotein VI promotes metastasis through interaction with cancer cell-derived galectin-3. Blood. 2020;135(14):1146–60.
39. Zhao LH, Li Q, Huang ZJ, Sun MX, Lu JJ, Zhang XH, et al. Identification of histone methyltransferase NSD2 as an important oncogenic gene in colorectal cancer. Cell Death Dis. 2021;12(11):974.
40. Su C, Sun Q, Liu S, Wang H, Feng L, Cao Y. Targeting p38γ to inhibit human colorectal cancer cell progression. Biochem Biophys Res Commun. 2019;517(1):172–9.
41. Huang Y, Wang Y, Wu Z, Li T, Li S, Wang C, et al. SOX11-dependent CATSPER1 expression controls colon cancer cell growth through regulation the PI3K/AKT signaling pathway. Genes Genomics. 2022;44(11):1415–24.
42. Johnson GS, Li J, Beaver LM, Dashwood WM, Sun D, Rajendran P, et al. A functional pseudogene, NMRAL2P, is regulated by Nrf2 and serves as a coactivator of NQO1 in sulforaphane-treated colon cancer cells. Mol Nutr Food Res. 2017;61(4):1600769.
43. Melo-Hanchuk TD, Colleti C, Saito Â, Mendes MCS, Carvalheira JBC, Vassallo J, Kobarg J. Intracellular hyaluronic acid-binding protein 4 (HABP4): a candidate tumor suppressor in colorectal cancer. Oncotarget. 2020;11(46):4325–37.
44. Cai J, Liu W, Wong CW, Zhu W, Lin Y, Hu J, et al. Zinc-finger antiviral protein acts as a tumor suppressor in colorectal cancer. Oncogene. 2020;39(37):5995–6008.
45. Liu C, Banister CE, Weige CC, Altomare D, Richardson JH, Contreras CM, Buckhaults PJ. PRDM1 silences stem cell-related genes and

inhibits proliferation of human colon tumor organoids. Proc Natl Acad Sci U S A. 2018;115(22):E5066-e75.

46. Ždralević M, Brand A, Di Ianni L, Dettmer K, Reinders J, Singer K, et al. Double genetic disruption of lactate dehydrogenases A and B is required to ablate the "Warburg effect" restricting tumor growth to oxidative metabolism. J Biol Chem. 2018;293(41):15947–61.
47. Wang L, Minchin RF, Butcher NJ. Arylamine N-acetyltransferase 1 protects against reactive oxygen species during glucose starvation: Role in the regulation of p53 stability. PLoS One. 2018;13(3): e0193560.
48. Kitazawa S, Ebara S, Ando A, Baba Y, Satomi Y, Soga T, Hara T. Succinate dehydrogenase B-deficient cancer cells are highly sensitive to bromodomain and extra-terminal inhibitors. Oncotarget. 2017;8(17):28922–38.
49. Irving AA, Waters BJ, Seeman JR, Plum LA, DeLuca HF. Vitamin D receptor absence does not enhance intestinal tumorigenesis in ApcPirc/+rats. Biol Open. 2022;11(7):bio059290.
50. Gu C, Nguyen HN, Ganini D, Chen Z, Jessen HJ, Gu Z, et al. KO of 5-InsP(7) kinase activity transforms the HCT116 colon cancer cell line into a hypermetabolic, growth-inhibited phenotype. Proc Natl Acad Sci U S A. 2017;114(45):11968–73.
51. Joo JH, Oh H, Kim M, An EJ, Kim RK, Lee SY, et al. NADPH Oxidase 1 Activity and ROS Generation Are Regulated by Grb2/Cbl-Mediated Proteasomal Degradation of NoxO1 in Colon Cancer Cells. Cancer Res. 2016;76(4):855–65.
52. Biagioni A, Laurenzana A, Chillà A, Del Rosso M, Andreucci E, Poteti M, et al. uPAR Knockout Results in a Deep Glycolytic and OXPHOS Reprogramming in Melanoma and Colon Carcinoma Cell Lines. Cells. 2020;9(2):308.
53. Gu C, Liu J, Liu X, Zhang H, Luo J, Wang H, et al. Metabolic supervision by PPIP5K, an inositol pyrophosphate kinase/phosphatase, controls proliferation of the HCT116 tumor cell line. Proc Natl Acad Sci U S A. 2021;118(10):e2020187118.
54. Nishi K, Iwaihara Y, Tsunoda T, Doi K, Sakata T, Shirasawa S, Ishikura S. ROS-induced cleavage of NHLRC2 by caspase-8 leads to apoptotic cell death in the HCT116 human colon cancer cell line. Cell Death Dis. 2017;8(12):3218.
55. Tao Y, Kang B, Petkovich DA, Bhandari YR, In J, Stein-O'Brien G, et al. Aging-like Spontaneous Epigenetic Silencing Facilitates Wnt

Activation, Stemness, and Braf(V600E)-Induced Tumorigenesis. Cancer Cell. 2019;35(2):315–28.e6.

56. Kandarian SC, Nosacka RL, Delitto AE, Judge AR, Judge SM, Ganey JD, et al. Tumour-derived leukaemia inhibitory factor is a major driver of cancer cachexia and morbidity in C26 tumour-bearing mice. J Cachexia Sarcopenia Muscle. 2018;9(6):1109–20.
57. Poghosyan S, Frenkel N, Lentzas A, Laoukili J, Rinkes IB, Kranenburg O, Hagendoorn J. Loss of Neuropilin-2 in Murine Mesenchymal-like Colon Cancer Organoids Causes Mesenchymal-to-Epithelial Transition and an Acquired Dependency on Insulin-Receptor Signaling and Autophagy. Cancers (Basel). 2022;14(3):671.
58. Szeder B, Tárnoki-Zách J, Lakatos D, Vas V, Kudlik G, Merő B, et al. Absence of the Tks4 Scaffold Protein Induces Epithelial-Mesenchymal Transition-Like Changes in Human Colon Cancer Cells. Cells. 2019;8(11):1343.
59. Hosain SB, Khiste SK, Uddin MB, Vorubindi V, Ingram C, Zhang S, et al. Inhibition of glucosylceramide synthase eliminates the oncogenic function of p53 R273H mutant in the epithelial-mesenchymal transition and induced pluripotency of colon cancer cells. Oncotarget. 2016;7(37):60575–92.
60. Li Q, Li Y, Xu J, Wang S, Xu Y, Li X, Cai S. Aldolase B Overexpression is Associated with Poor Prognosis and Promotes Tumor Progression by Epithelial-Mesenchymal Transition in Colorectal Adenocarcinoma. Cell Physiol Biochem. 2017;42(1):397–406.
61. Liu Q, Xin C, Chen Y, Yang J, Chen Y, Zhang W, Ye L. PUM1 Is Overexpressed in Colon Cancer Cells With Acquired Resistance to Cetuximab. Front Cell Dev Biol. 2021;9:696558.
62. Liu HH, Lee CH, Hsieh YC, Hsu DW, Cho EC. Multiple myeloma driving factor WHSC1 is a transcription target of oncogene HMGA2 that facilitates colon cancer proliferation and metastasis. Biochem Biophys Res Commun. 2021;567:183–9.
63. Beck AC, Cho E, White JR, Paemka L, Li T, Gu VW, et al. AP-2α Regulates S-Phase and Is a Marker for Sensitivity to PI3K Inhibitor Buparlisib in Colon Cancer. Mol Cancer Res. 2021;19(7):1156–67.
64. Satapathy SR, Sjölander A. Cysteinyl leukotriene receptor 1 promotes 5-fluorouracil resistance and resistance-derived stemness in colon cancer cells. Cancer Lett. 2020;488:50–62.
65. Tung KL, Chen KY, Negrete M, Chen T, Safi A, Aljamal AA, et al. Integrated chromatin and transcriptomic profiling of

patient-derived colon cancer organoids identifies personalized drug targets to overcome oxaliplatin resistance. Genes Dis. 2021;8(2): 203–14.
66. Franke FC, Müller J, Abal M, Medina ED, Nitsche U, Weidmann H, et al. The Tumor Suppressor SASH1 Interacts With the Signal Adaptor CRKL to Inhibit Epithelial-Mesenchymal Transition and Metastasis in Colorectal Cancer. Cell Mol Gastroenterol Hepatol. 2019;7(1):33–53.
67. Zhou M, Liu X, Li Z, Huang Q, Li F, Li CY. Caspase-3 regulates the migration, invasion and metastasis of colon cancer cells. Int J Cancer. 2018;143(4):921–30.
68. Li T, Liu D, Lei X, Jiang Q. Par3L enhances colorectal cancer cell survival by inhibiting Lkb1/AMPK signaling pathway. Biochem Biophys Res Commun. 2017;482(4):1037–41.
69. Zheng F, Zhang Z, Flamini V, Jiang WG, Cui Y. The Axis of CXCR4/ SDF-1 Plays a Role in Colon Cancer Cell Adhesion Through Regulation of the AKT and IGF1R Signalling Pathways. Anticancer Res. 2017;37(8):4361–9.
70. Schwiebs A, Faqar-Uz-Zaman F, Herrero San Juan M, Radeke HH. S1P Lyase Regulates Intestinal Stem Cell Quiescence via Ki-67 and FOXO3. Int J Mol Sci. 2021;22(11):5682.
71. Hu X, Zhang L, Li Y, Ma X, Dai W, Gao X, et al. Organoid modelling identifies that DACH1 functions as a tumour promoter in colorectal cancer by modulating BMP signalling. EBioMedicine. 2020;56:102800.
72. Gisina A, Novikova S, Kim Y, Sidorov D, Bykasov S, Volchenko N, et al. CEACAM5 overexpression is a reliable characteristic of CD133-positive colorectal cancer stem cells. Cancer Biomark. 2021; 32(1):85–98.
73. Michels BE, Mosa MH, Grebbin BM, Yepes D, Darvishi T, Hausmann J, et al. Human colon organoids reveal distinct physiologic and oncogenic Wnt responses. J Exp Med. 2019;216(3):704–20.
74. Eto T, Miyake K, Nosho K, Ohmuraya M, Imamura Y, Arima K, et al. Impact of loss-of-function mutations at the RNF43 locus on colorectal cancer development and progression. J Pathol. 2018; 245(4):445–55.
75. Tak YG, Hung Y, Yao L, Grimmer MR, Do A, Bhakta MS, et al. Effects on the transcriptome upon deletion of a distal element cannot be predicted by the size of the H3K27Ac peak in human cells. Nucleic Acids Res. 2016;44(9):4123–33.

76. Rappaport JA, Entezari AA, Caspi A, Caksa S, Jhaveri AV, Stanek TJ, et al. A β-Catenin-TCF-Sensitive Locus Control Region Mediates GUCY2C Ligand Loss in Colorectal Cancer. Cell Mol Gastroenterol Hepatol. 2022;13(4):1276–96.
77. Xu J, Chen Q, Tian K, Liang R, Chen T, Gong A, et al. m6A methyltransferase METTL3 maintains colon cancer tumorigenicity by suppressing SOCS2 to promote cell proliferation. Oncol Rep. 2020;44(3): 973–86.
78. Makkar S, Riehl TE, Chen B, Yan Y, Alvarado DM, Ciorba MA, Stenson WF. Hyaluronic Acid Binding to TLR4 Promotes Proliferation and Blocks Apoptosis in Colon Cancer. Mol Cancer Ther. 2019; 18(12):2446–56.
79. Yu Y, Nangia-Makker P, Farhana L, Majumdar APN. A novel mechanism of lncRNA and miRNA interaction: CCAT2 regulates miR-145 expression by suppressing its maturation process in colon cancer cells. Mol Cancer. 2017;16(1):155.
80. Guo S, Li J, Huang Z, Yue T, Zhu J, Wang X, et al. The CBS-H(2)S axis promotes liver metastasis of colon cancer by upregulating VEGF through AP-1 activation. Br J Cancer. 2022;126(7):1055–66.
81. Malkomes P, Lunger I, Oppermann E, Abou-El-Ardat K, Oellerich T, Günther S, et al. Transglutaminase 2 promotes tumorigenicity of colon cancer cells by inactivation of the tumor suppressor p53. Oncogene. 2021;40(25):4352–67.
82. Xiong YJ, Liu DY, Shen RR, Xiong Y. A short deletion in the DNA-binding domain of STAT3 suppresses growth and progression of colon cancer cells. Aging (Albany NY). 2021;13(4):5185–96.
83. Cheng XS, Huo YN, Fan YY, Xiao CX, Ouyang XM, Liang LY, et al. Mindin serves as a tumour suppressor gene during colon cancer progression through MAPK/ERK signalling pathway in mice. J Cell Mol Med. 2020;24(15):8391–404.
84. Paul S, Bhardwaj M, Kang SC. GSTO1 confers drug resistance in HCT-116 colon cancer cells through an interaction with TNFαIP3/A20. Int J Oncol. 2022;61(5):136.
85. Liu TT, Liu XS, Zhang M, Liu XN, Zhu FX, Zhu FM, et al. Cartilage oligomeric matrix protein is a prognostic factor and biomarker of colon cancer and promotes cell proliferation by activating the Akt pathway. J Cancer Res Clin Oncol. 2018;144(6):1049–63.

86. Yin Y, Zhong J, Li SW, Li JZ, Zhou M, Chen Y, et al. TRIM11, a direct target of miR-24–3p, promotes cell proliferation and inhibits apoptosis in colon cancer. Oncotarget. 2016;7(52):86755–65.
87. Hartal-Benishay LH, Saadi E, Toubiana S, Shaked L, Lalzar M, Abu Hatoum O, et al. MBTPS1 regulates proliferation of colorectal cancer primarily through its action on sterol regulatory element-binding proteins. Front Oncol. 2022;12:1004014.
88. Liu N, Cui W, Jiang X, Zhang Z, Gnosa S, Ali Z, et al. The Critical Role of Dysregulated RhoB Signaling Pathway in Radioresistance of Colorectal Cancer. Int J Radiat Oncol Biol Phys. 2019;104(5): 1153–64.
89. Ghatak S, Hascall VC, Markwald RR, Misra S. FOLFOX Therapy Induces Feedback Upregulation of CD44v6 through YB-1 to Maintain Stemness in Colon Initiating Cells. Int J Mol Sci. 2021;22(2):753.
90. Iioka H, Saito K, Sakaguchi M, Tachibana T, Homma K, Kondo E. Crumbs3 is a critical factor that regulates invasion and metastasis of colon adenocarcinoma via the specific interaction with FGFR1. Int J Cancer. 2019;145(10):2740–53.
91. Dai C, Zhang X, Xie D, Tang P, Li C, Zuo Y, et al. Targeting PP2A activates AMPK signaling to inhibit colorectal cancer cells. Oncotarget. 2017;8(56):95810–23.
92. Huang K, Zhang J, O'Neill KL, Gurumurthy CB, Quadros RM, Tu Y, Luo X. Cleavage by Caspase 8 and Mitochondrial Membrane Association Activate the BH3-only Protein Bid during TRAIL-induced Apoptosis. J Biol Chem. 2016;291(22):11843–51.
93. Chandrasekaran AP, Suresh B, Sarodaya N, Ko NR, Oh SJ, Kim KS, Ramakrishna S. Ubiquitin Specific Protease 29 Functions as an Oncogene Promoting Tumorigenesis in Colorectal Carcinoma. Cancers (Basel). 2021;13(11):2706.
94. Li W, Cho MY, Lee S, Jang M, Park J, Park R. CRISPR-Cas9 mediated CD133 knockout inhibits colon cancer invasion through reduced epithelial-mesenchymal transition. PLoS One. 2019;14(8):e0220860.
95. Mlecnik B, Bifulco C, Bindea G, Marliot F, Lugli A, Lee JJ, et al. Multicenter International Society for Immunotherapy of Cancer Study of the Consensus Immunoscore for the Prediction of Survival and Response to Chemotherapy in Stage III Colon Cancer. J Clin Oncol. 2020;38(31):3638–51.

96. Zheng Z, Wieder T, Mauerer B, Schäfer L, Kesselring R, Braumüller H. T Cells in Colorectal Cancer: Unravelling the Function of Different T Cell Subsets in the Tumor Microenvironment. Int J Mol Sci. 2023;24(14):11673.
97. Mlecnik B, Lugli A, Bindea G, Marliot F, Bifulco C, Lee JJ, et al. Multicenter International Study of the Consensus Immunoscore for the Prediction of Relapse and Survival in Early-Stage Colon Cancer. Cancers (Basel). 2023;15(2):418.
98. Oliveira G, Wu CJ. Dynamics and specificities of T cells in cancer immunotherapy. Nat Rev Cancer. 2023;23(5):295–316.
99. Bell HN, Huber AK, Singhal R, Korimerla N, Rebernick RJ, Kumar R, et al. Microenvironmental ammonia enhances T cell exhaustion in colorectal cancer. Cell Metab. 2023;35(1):134–49.e6.
100. Geginat J, Paroni M, Maglie S, Alfen JS, Kastirr I, Gruarin P, et al. Plasticity of human CD4 T cell subsets. Front Immunol. 2014;5:630.
101. Bhaumik S, Basu R. Cellular and Molecular Dynamics of Th17 Differentiation and its Developmental Plasticity in the Intestinal Immune Response. Front Immunol. 2017;8:254.
102. Kruse B, Buzzai AC, Shridhar N, Braun AD, Gellert S, Knauth K, et al. CD4(+) T cell-induced inflammatory cell death controls immune-evasive tumours. Nature. 2023;618(7967):1033–40.
103. Marin-Acevedo JA, Kimbrough EO, Lou Y. Next generation of immune checkpoint inhibitors and beyond. J Hematol Oncol. 2021; 14(1):45.
104. Takeuchi A, Saito T. CD4 CTL, a Cytotoxic Subset of CD4(+) T Cells, Their Differentiation and Function. Front Immunol. 2017;8:194.
105. Harbour SN, Maynard CL, Zindl CL, Schoeb TR, Weaver CT. Th17 cells give rise to Th1 cells that are required for the pathogenesis of colitis. Proc Natl Acad Sci U S A. 2015;112(22):7061–6.
106. Hirota K, Duarte JH, Veldhoen M, Hornsby E, Li Y, Cua DJ, et al. Fate mapping of IL-17-producing T cells in inflammatory responses. Nat Immunol. 2011;12(3):255–63.
107. Wu T, Cui L, Liang Z, Liu C, Liu Y, Li J. Elevated serum IL-22 levels correlate with chemoresistant condition of colorectal cancer. Clin Immunol. 2013;147(1):38–9.
108. Huber S, Gagliani N, Zenewicz LA, Huber FJ, Bosurgi L, Hu B, et al. IL-22BP is regulated by the inflammasome and modulates tumorigenesis in the intestine. Nature. 2012;491(7423):259–63.

109. Kirchberger S, Royston DJ, Boulard O, Thornton E, Franchini F, Szabady RL, et al. Innate lymphoid cells sustain colon cancer through production of interleukin-22 in a mouse model. J Exp Med. 2013;210(5):917–31.
110. Perez LG, Kempski J, McGee HM, Pelzcar P, Agalioti T, Giannou A, et al. TGF-β signaling in Th17 cells promotes IL-22 production and colitis-associated colon cancer. Nat Commun. 2020;11(1):2608.
111. Sawant DV, Vignali DA. Once a Treg, always a Treg? Immunol Rev. 2014;259(1):173–91.
112. Brenner E, Schörg BF, Ahmetlić F, Wieder T, Hilke FJ, Simon N, et al. Cancer immune control needs senescence induction by interferon-dependent cell cycle regulator pathways in tumours. Nat Commun. 2020;11(1):1335.
113. Rentschler M, Braumüller H, Briquez PS, Wieder T. Cytokine-Induced Senescence in the Tumor Microenvironment and Its Effects on Anti-Tumor Immune Responses. Cancers (Basel). 2022;14(6):1364.
114. Wozniakova M, Skarda J, Raska M. The Role of Tumor Microenvironment and Immune Response in Colorectal Cancer Development and Prognosis. Pathol Oncol Res. 2022;28:1610502.
115. Braumüller H, Mauerer B, Andris J, Berlin C, Wieder T, Kesselring R. The Cytokine Network in Colorectal Cancer: Implications for New Treatment Strategies. Cells. 2022;12(1):138.
116. Tauriello DVF, Palomo-Ponce S, Stork D, Berenguer-Llergo A, Badia-Ramentol J, Iglesias M, et al. TGFβ drives immune evasion in genetically reconstituted colon cancer metastasis. Nature. 2018; 554(7693):538–43.
117. Gires O, Pan M, Schinke H, Canis M, Baeuerle PA. Expression and function of epithelial cell adhesion molecule EpCAM: where are we after 40 years? Cancer Metastasis Rev. 2020;39(3):969–87.
118. Katz SC, Moody AE, Guha P, Hardaway JC, Prince E, LaPorte J, et al. HITM-SURE: Hepatic immunotherapy for metastases phase Ib anti-CEA CAR-T study utilizing pressure enabled drug delivery. J Immunother Cancer. 2020;8(2):e001097.
119. Guinney J, Dienstmann R, Wang X, de Reyniès A, Schlicker A, Soneson C, et al. The consensus molecular subtypes of colorectal cancer. Nat Med. 2015;21(11):1350–6.
120. Le QA, Wittayarat M, Namula Z, Lin Q, Takebayashi K, Hirata M, et al. Multiple gene editing in porcine embryos using a combination

of microinjection, electroporation, and transfection methods. Vet World. 2022;15(9):2210–6.

121. Xu X, Wan T, Xin H, Li D, Pan H, Wu J, Ping Y. Delivery of CRISPR/Cas9 for therapeutic genome editing. J Gene Med. 2019;21(7):e3107.
122. Horii T, Hatada I. Generation of Genome-Edited Mice by Cytoplasmic Injection of CRISPR-Cas9 RNA. Methods Mol Biol. 2023;2637:75–86.
123. Hu W, Yang Y, Qi L, Chen J, Ge W, Zheng S. Subtyping of microsatellite instability-high colorectal cancer. Cell Commun Signal. 2019;17(1):79.
124. Kleiderman E, Ogbogu U. Realigning gene editing with clinical research ethics: What the "CRISPR Twins" debacle means for Chinese and international research ethics governance. Account Res. 2019;26(4):257–64.
125. Li C, Du X, Zhang H, Liu S. Knockdown of ribosomal protein L22-like 1 arrests the cell cycle and promotes apoptosis in colorectal cancer. Cytojournal. 2024;21:45.
126. Muhammad Rafid AH, Toufikuzzaman M, Rahman MS, Rahman MS. CRISPRpred(SEQ): a sequence-based method for sgRNA on target activity prediction using traditional machine learning. BMC Bioinformatics. 2020;21(1):223.
127. Qian FC, Zhou LW, Li YY, Yu ZM, Li LD, Wang YZ, et al. SEanalysis 2.0: a comprehensive super-enhancer regulatory network analysis tool for human and mouse. Nucleic Acids Res. 2023;51(W1):W520-w7.
128. Abbasi AF, Asim MN, Dengel A. Transitioning from wet lab to artificial intelligence: a systematic review of AI predictors in CRISPR. J Transl Med. 2025;23(1):153.
129. Liang L, Liang X, Yu X, Xiang W. Bioinformatic Analyses and Integrated Machine Learning to Predict prognosis and therapeutic response Based on E3 Ligase-Related Genes in colon cancer. J Cancer. 2024;15(16):5376–95.

https://doi.org/10.1142/9789819826759_0007

CHAPTER 7

CRISPR/Cas9 in the Treatment of Hepatocellular Carcinoma

Mehrdad Hashemi[1,2], *Alireza Khosravinejad*[1,3], *Mina Alimohammadi*[4], *Reza Mohajer Shirazi*[1,3], *Ali Shirazi*[1,3], *Kimia Sadat Esfahani*[1,3], *Behdokht Jamali*[5], *Amir Sadeghi*[6], *Faranak Jamshidian*[1,7], *Neda Zali*[3], *Najma Farahani*[1,*], *Afshin Taheriazam*[1,8,*], *Payman Rahimzadeh*[9,*], *Maliheh Entezari*[1,2,*]

[1]Farhikhtegan Medical Convergent Sciences Research Center, Farhikhtegan Hospital, Faculty of Medicine, TeMs. C., Islamic Azad University, Tehran, Iran

[2]Department of Genetics, Faculty of Advanced Sciences and Technology, TeMs. C, Islamic Azad University, Tehran, Iran

[3]Basic and Molecular Epidemiology of Gastrointestinal Disorders Research Center, Research Institute for Gastroenterology and Liver Diseases, Shahid Beheshti University of Medical Sciences, Tehran, Iran

[4]Department of Immunology, School of Medicine, Shahid Beheshti University of Medical Sciences, Tehran, Iran

[5]Department of Microbiology and Genetics, Kherad Institute of Higher Education, Bushehr, Iran

---

* **Corresponding authors:** Najmafarahani@gmail.com (N.F.); a.taheriazam@iautmu.ac.ir (A.T.); P.rahimzadeh76@gmail.com (P.R.); mentezari@iautmu.ac.ir (M.E.)

[6]Gastroenterology and Liver Diseases Research Center, Research Institute for Gastroenterology and Liver Diseases, Shahid Beheshti University of Medical Sciences, Tehran, Iran
[7]Department of Biology, ET.C., Islamic Azad University, Tehran, Iran
[8]Department of Orthopedics, Faculty of Medicine, TeMs. C, Islamic Azad University, Tehran, Iran
[9]Surgical Research Society (SRS), Students' Scientific Research Center, Tehran University of Medical Sciences, Tehran, Iran

Abstract

Liver cancer is a leading global health burden, ranking as the seventh most commonly diagnosed malignancy and the second most lethal cancer worldwide. Hepatocellular carcinoma, which constitutes more than 90% of primary liver cancer cases, is strongly associated with chronic hepatitis B and C infections, alcoholic cirrhosis, and non-alcoholic fatty liver disease. Despite a variety of therapeutic strategies, including surgical resection, liver transplantation, transcatheter arterial chemoembolization, and molecular targeted drugs such as sorafenib and lenvatinib, hepatocellular carcinoma continues to demonstrate poor prognosis due to high recurrence rates and late-stage diagnosis. Advances in genomics have identified numerous oncogenes, tumor suppressors, and novel biomarkers that are reshaping the landscape of hepatocellular carcinoma diagnosis and treatment. Among emerging therapeutic approaches, the CRISPR/Cas9 genome-editing system has gained attention as a powerful and versatile technology capable of modifying specific oncogenic and tumor suppressor pathways with high efficiency and relative ease. CRISPR/Cas9 has demonstrated significant promise in both basic research and preclinical models of hepatocellular carcinoma, enabling functional genomic studies, the development of novel therapeutic targets, and the potential for precision medicine applications. This chapter summarizes the mechanisms, advantages, and current limitations of CRISPR/Cas9, explores its applications in hepatocellular carcinoma research and therapy, and highlights future perspectives for integrating genome-editing strategies into liver cancer treatment.

Keywords: liver cancer; hepatocellular carcinoma; CRISPR/Cas9; genome editing; gene therapy; targeted therapy; biomarkers; precision oncology

7.1 Introduction

Among global malignancies, liver cancer ranks as the seventh most prevalent cancer worldwide [1]. Hepatocellular carcinoma, representing over 90% of cases, and intrahepatic cholangiocarcinoma constitute the primary histological variants of liver cancer [2, 3]. Research has demonstrated strong associations between hepatocellular carcinoma development and various risk factors, including hepatitis B virus (HBV) and hepatitis C virus (HCV) infections, as well as both alcoholic and non-alcoholic liver diseases [4, 5].

Current therapeutic approaches remain limited in their effectiveness. Treatment options, selected based on disease staging and individual patient conditions, encompass surgical interventions like hepatic resection and transplantation, alongside procedures such as radiofrequency ablation, transarterial chemoembolization, and targeted therapies including sorafenib and levabinib [6, 7]. Despite these diverse treatment modalities, liver cancer maintains its position as the second leading cause of cancer-related deaths, primarily due to frequent recurrence and challenges in early detection [1]. The current medical landscape demands enhanced diagnostic and therapeutic strategies for hepatocellular carcinoma management.

Recent advances in genetic research have yielded promising developments. Scientists have successfully identified additional oncogenes and tumor suppressor genes implicated in hepatocellular carcinoma progression. The discovery of novel biomarkers showing superior specificity compared to the traditional AFP marker suggests potential improvements in diagnostic capabilities [8]. Contemporary genetic studies have produced significant findings through both laboratory and animal model investigations [9]. These developments indicate that genetic therapeutic approaches may offer promising alternatives to conventional treatment methods.

The advancement of cancer research, particularly in hepatocellular carcinoma, has been significantly enhanced by gene editing technologies, which enable detailed studies through gene knockout and knockin techniques. The CRISPR/Cas9 system, which evolved from a microbial immune defense mechanism known as the CRISPR family, has emerged as a revolutionary tool [10]. This refined technology has largely superseded traditional gene editing methods, gaining prominence due to its user-friendly nature, cost-effectiveness, and versatile applications [11].

This section examines the evolutionary development of CRISPR/Cas9 technology through a comprehensive analysis of its operational principles, highlighting both its strengths and limitations. Additionally, we provide an overview of its current applications in hepatocellular carcinoma research by evaluating relevant scientific studies. Drawing insights from breakthrough discoveries in various cancer fields, we explore the expanding potential of CRISPR/Cas9 in developing novel therapeutic strategies for hepatocellular carcinoma.

7.2 Molecular and Genetic Alterations in Hepatocellular Carcinoma

Hepatocellular carcinoma, the predominant form of liver cancer, presents significant therapeutic challenges, with global statistics placing it as the sixth most common cancer and the third leading cause of cancer mortality [12]. While HBV infection remains the primary risk factor, responsible for roughly 50% of hepatocellular carcinoma cases, the landscape is shifting. The prevalence of viral hepatitis-induced hepatocellular carcinoma (both HBV and HCV) continues to decrease, thanks to improved antiviral medications and vaccination programs. Conversely, non-alcoholic steatohepatitis (NASH)-related hepatocellular carcinoma, associated with metabolic disorders and diabetes, is becoming increasingly prevalent [13].

The molecular pathogenesis varies significantly based on underlying causes and genetic damage patterns. For instance, HBV-related hepatocellular carcinoma exhibits distinct molecular profiles and immune responses compared to NASH-induced cases. Understanding these etiology-specific molecular mechanisms is crucial for developing targeted therapeutic approaches.

Complicating this effort is the fact that only about 25% of hepatocellular carcinoma cases possess actionable mutations. Although approximately half of the patients harbor recurring oncogenic mutations in genes such as TP53, CTNNB1, or TERT, conventional pharmaceutical interventions rarely effectively target these alterations. Despite the development of inhibitors targeting TERT promoter mutations and WNT/β-catenin pathway components, achieving optimal therapeutic outcomes remains challenging [14, 15]. Research into downstream signaling pathways affected by these mutations may provide insights for developing treatments targeting currently undruggable mutations.

For early-stage hepatocellular carcinoma, surgical interventions — specifically hepatic resection and transplantation — remain the primary treatment options. Radiofrequency ablation serves as the main non-surgical approach for early-stage cases [16], while transarterial chemoembolization has been the standard treatment for intermediate-stage hepatocellular carcinoma over the past 20 years [17]. Traditional treatment paradigms are now being complemented by targeted therapies and immunotherapy. Sorafenib, the first 'targeted' therapy approved for advanced hepatocellular carcinoma, acts on multiple kinases including RAF, MEK, VEGFR, and PDGFR, improving median overall survival from 7.9 to 10.7 months. Subsequently, lenvatinib emerged as another first-line treatment option [18], showing particular efficacy in cases with portal vein involvement.

The 2020 IMbrave150 trial marked a revolutionary advancement in hepatocellular carcinoma treatment by demonstrating the effectiveness of combining anti-PD-L1 immunotherapy (atezolizumab) with anti-angiogenic therapy (bevacizumab). This therapeutic approach demonstrated better outcomes than sorafenib across multiple metrics, including overall survival, progression-free survival, and objective response rate. Recent studies have also shown improved recurrence-free survival in early-stage hepatocellular carcinoma patients [19]. Another significant milestone occurred in November 2022 with the U.S. Food and Drug Administration (FDA)'s approval of combined durvalumab (anti-PD-L1) and tremelimumab (anti-CTLA-4) therapy. The HIMALAYA trial revealed impressive results, with advanced hepatocellular carcinoma patients achieving a 25.2% 4-year overall survival rate. However, the limited number of advanced-stage patients experiencing sustained clinical benefits underscores the persistent therapeutic challenges [20].

The landscape of clinical trials in hepatocellular carcinoma has evolved significantly over the past five years, with phase II trials comprising more than 50% of all studies. Phase III trials have primarily shifted their focus toward investigating second-line treatments and combination therapies. Current research priorities include developing more effective and safer agents targeting immune checkpoint pathways and angiogenesis-related mechanisms, such as VEGFR and TGF-β signaling. Additional areas of investigation include epigenetic modifications and dysregulated pathways, encompassing MAPK, PI3K-AKT, and JAKs/STATs signaling systems.

7.3 Mechanistic Insights: CRISPR/Cas9 Gene Editing Platform in Hepatocellular Carcinoma Therapy

Through genome-wide CRISPR/Cas9 knockdown screening, Yang and colleagues identified the significance of PDHB, PC, and PDHA in hepatocellular carcinoma metabolism. Their research demonstrated that disrupting these genes impairs tricarboxylic acid (TCA) cycling and mitochondrial function, thereby inhibiting hepatocellular carcinoma cell proliferation. They observed that hepatocellular carcinoma cells efficiently process pyruvate into acetyl-CoA and oxaloacetate via pyruvate dehydrogenase (PDH) and pyruvate carboxylase (PC) for TCA cycle initiation. Furthermore, they showed that PDH and PC inhibitors could compensate for pyruvate metabolism during glutamine deficiency [21].

The pyruvate dehydrogenase complex, comprised of PDHA and PDHB, forms a crucial metabolic bridge between glycolysis and the Krebs cycle by converting pyruvate to acetyl-CoA [22]. Hepatocellular carcinoma cells, like many cancer cells, exhibit the

Warburg effect — preferentially utilizing aerobic glycolysis for energy production. CRISPR/Cas9-mediated disruption of PDHA and PDHB leads to pyruvate accumulation and acetyl-CoA reduction, ultimately disrupting the Warburg effect and triggering hepatocellular carcinoma cell apoptosis through energy depletion.

PC enzyme's conversion of pyruvate to oxaloacetate is essential for both gluconeogenesis and the citric acid cycle. Similar to PDH, PC maintains metabolic homeostasis through anaplerotic reactions. PC inhibition reduces oxaloacetate availability, compromising both the citric acid cycle and gluconeogenesis. This metabolic disruption impairs cancer cell growth by limiting energy and biosynthetic precursors, while potentially inducing oxidative stress-mediated cell death [22, 23].

Research by Hu et al. revealed that CRISPR/Cas9-mediated Traf3 deletion enhanced HepG2 cell proliferation, migration, and invasion, providing crucial insights into Traf3's regulatory role [24].

Studies showed that PTEN knockout combined with NRAS overexpression promoted the formation of stress-resistant lipid droplets in hepatocytes, preventing metabolic stress, senescence, and immune clearance. This mechanism facilitates cell survival and proliferation, potentially driving cancer development. These findings emphasize the critical role of hepatocellular lipid droplets in liver cancer progression, particularly in contexts of somatic PTEN loss and NRAS overexpression [25].

Research has demonstrated that CRISPR/Cas9-guided targeting of Ctnnb1's exon 3 generates an exon-skipping variant *in vivo*. When combined with YAPS127A, this CRISPR/Cas9-mediated Ctnnb1 modification successfully induced liver tumor formation in mice, highlighting the utility of this system for studying β-catenin-dependent oncogenesis through gain-of-function mutations [26].

TRAF3, PTEN, and CTNNB1 represent crucial regulatory elements in cancer pathogenesis, with their manipulation via CRISPR/Cas9 showing significant therapeutic potential [27–29]. TRAF3, a multifunctional signaling adapter, influences both innate immunity and cellular survival through negative regulation of NF-κB signaling. TRAF3 deficiency can lead to NF-κB pathway hyperactivation, promoting inflammatory responses that support tumor development [30–33]. However, TRAF3's role exhibits context-dependent complexity, sometimes functioning as a tumor promoter where its deletion may actually enhance apoptosis and reduce tumor progression.

PTEN, a key tumor suppressor, regulates the tumor microenvironment by inhibiting PI3K/AKT signaling, which controls cell proliferation and survival. PTEN dysfunction in hepatocellular carcinoma results in unrestricted cellular growth. Therapeutic strategies often focus on restoring PTEN function through CRISPR/Cas9-mediated gene correction, which can suppress PI3K/AKT signaling, induce cell cycle arrest, promote apoptosis, and inhibit tumor growth [34].

CTNNB1, encoding β-catenin, plays a central role in Wnt signaling. When inactive, β-catenin accumulates and translocates to the nucleus, activating genes that promote hepatocellular carcinoma progression [35, 36]. CRISPR/Cas9-mediated CTNNB1 knockout had been found to disrupt aberrant Wnt/β-catenin signaling in other cancers [37], reducing cell proliferation and survival while potentially inhibiting tumor invasion, metastasis, and modifying the tumor microenvironment.

Research has shown that inhibiting the Wnt/β-catenin pathway effectively reduces cancer cell proliferation, migration, and invasion. These findings were validated both *in vitro* and through nude mouse xenograft models. The knockout of NSD1, H3, and Wnt10b in hepatocellular carcinoma cells suggests their potential as therapeutic targets [38].

LBP4-delivered pCas9 has demonstrated effective oncogene editing capabilities, enhancing cancer inhibition and drug sensitivity *in vivo*. Studies showed that LBP/pCas9 complexes, through Survivin knockout, improved drug antineoplastic effects and inhibited hepatocellular carcinoma cell proliferation *in vitro* [39].

Liu and colleagues demonstrated that CRISPR/Cas9-mediated HIF-1α knockout enhanced the effectiveness of transarterial embolization in hepatocellular carcinoma. The HIF-1α knockout increased apoptosis and reduced cancer cell invasion, suggesting its potential as a therapeutic target when combined with transarterial embolization/chemoembolization procedures [40].

Studies identified DOCK1 as a synthetic lethal target for metformin, with DOCK1 levels influencing metformin's antitumor efficacy. Metformin resistance develops through RAC1 activation via DOCK1 phosphorylation, promoting cell survival. This suggests that combining DOCK1 inhibition with metformin could benefit patients with metformin-resistant hepatocellular carcinoma [41].

PTPMT1 knockout under hypoxic conditions prevents cardiolipin formation, leading to electron transport chain complex dysfunction and subsequent reactive oxygen species (ROS) accumulation. Alexidine dihydrochloride, a PTPMT1 inhibitor, shows particular effectiveness against hepatocellular carcinoma cells in hypoxic environments, indicating PTPMT1's protective role in hypoxia-related cancer development [42].

Wang and colleagues revealed CXCR4's role in modulating cisplatin sensitivity through MDR1. CXCR4 downregulation in HepG2 cells increased cisplatin tolerance. CRISPR/Cas9-mediated intervention reversed epithelial-mesenchymal transition, enhanced chemosensitivity, and reduced cancer malignancy [43].

Lu and colleagues demonstrated that CRISPR/Cas9-mediated SQSTM1/p62 knockout influenced hepatocellular carcinoma invasion and migration through the Keap1/Rhf2/MMP2 pathway, both *in vitro* and *in vivo*. While SQSTM1/p62 shows promise as a therapeutic target for controlling progression, additional research is needed to fully understand its potential [44].

A groundbreaking mouse model of liver cancer was developed using single oncogenic modifications, marking the first instance of somatic liver cancer generation without carcinogens or toxins. The model accurately replicates human fibrolamellar hepatocellular carcinoma's hepatocytic and cholangiocytic markers [45]. The discovery of DNAJB1-PRKACA fusion's role in the oncogenesis presents a promising therapeutic target, with these mouse models serving as valuable tools for studying disease progression and therapeutic development [46].

Researchers achieved precise NFE2L2 gene knockdown using ultrasound-controlled CRISPR/Cas9, enhancing sonodynamic therapy effectiveness through increased oxidative stress. This approach offers advantages for treating deep-seated tumors like hepatocellular carcinoma compared to light-controlled techniques. The technology shows potential for treating various conditions, including degenerative brain diseases, genetic disorders, and inflammatory conditions, with possible applications in immunotherapy for preventing metastasis and recurrence [47].

CRISPR/Cas9 screening identified XAGE1B and MYADML2 as genes associated with liver tumor invasion and metastasis in mouse models. MYADML2 expression showed correlation with reduced chemotherapy sensitivity and increased prevalence in patients over 60, suggesting new therapeutic targets for improved treatment outcomes [48].

Studies of CRISPR-hepatocyte growth factor (HGF) transfection in hepatocellular carcinoma cell lines revealed its role in suppressing natural apoptotic responses and reducing HGF production. Transfected cells showed decreased colony formation compared to controls. These findings suggest that CRISPR/Cas9-mediated HGF regulation could be crucial for understanding and controlling cell apoptosis, though further research is needed for specific targeting of cancer cells [49].

Research has identified PSTK as a novel mediator of ferroptosis resistance in cancer cells. PSTK depletion increased vulnerability of hepatocellular carcinoma cells to ferroptosis-inducing targeted therapies by inhibiting GPX4 activation, GSH metabolism, and folate synthesis. Studies showed punicalin's synergistic effects with sorafenib in hepatocellular carcinoma treatment both *in vitro* and *in vivo*, suggesting PSTK inhibition as a potential strategy to overcome therapy resistance in patients [50].

Porcine models have proven valuable for studying human diseases due to their similarities in anatomy, physiology, genetics, and drug metabolism. Researchers used CRISPR/Cas9 to generate genetically modified porcine hepatocellular carcinoma cells for studying TP53R167H- and KRASG12D-driven hepatocellular carcinoma through autologous liver transplantation. This approach, combined with next-generation sequencing analysis, enabled investigation of the effects of clinically relevant mutations on cancer development and treatment response [51].

CRISPR/Cas9-mediated exon skipping has been shown to activate β-catenin signaling while suppressing immunoactivating cytokines like CCL20 and CXCL2, affecting immune evasion. This finding is particularly relevant for CTNNB1-mutated hepatocellular carcinoma (approximately 30% of cases), which typically responds poorly to immune checkpoint inhibitor therapy. Research continues on recombinant cytokines as immunostimulants and trans-arterial cytokine delivery [52].

GeCKO library screening identified ADAMTSL3 and PTEN as key genes in hepatocellular carcinoma proliferation and metastasis. The study revealed ADAMTSL3's novel role in proliferation, while confirming PTEN's function in tumor invasion, validating CRISPR-based *in vivo* screening methodology [53].

Song and colleagues pioneered the use of CRISPR/Cas9 to generate HBsAg-knockout hepatocellular carcinoma cells, demonstrating HBsAg's role in enhancing HBV-hepatocellular carcinoma malignancy through IL-6/STAT3 signaling pathways. This approach of targeting the open reading frame of HBsAg presents a promising therapeutic strategy for HBV-related hepatocellular carcinoma [54].

Saputra et al.'s research suggests that non-synergistic (anti-synergistic or additive) drug combinations may be more effective than synergistic ones in preventing resistance subclone proliferation and providing sustained resistance protection [55].

CRISPR knockout studies of AXIN1 and ARID1A in porcine hepatocellular carcinoma cells demonstrated reduced sensitivity to sorafenib and doxorubicin. The research proposes using autologous cell injection to create genetically customized tumors in pigs, with intrahepatic injection of CRISPR-edited cells enabling development of tailored models. This approach, including *in vivo* editing of hepatocellular carcinoma driver genes in porcine hepatocytes, offers promising tools for testing precision medicine approaches and identifying effective treatments for common genetic mutations [56].

Genome-wide CRISPR screening identified NCAPG as a significant predictor of tumor recurrence in non-structural maintenance of chromosomes. The study demonstrated NCAPG transcript levels and liver cirrhosis could distinguish early recurrent from non-recurrent tumors with 0.80 area-under-curve across two datasets. NCAPG protein levels accurately identified seven of eight early recurrent tumors, with high NCAPG levels correlating with reduced disease-free survival [57].

Research using CRISPR/Cas9 to knockout Axl receptor in HLF and SNU449 hepatoma cell lines revealed incomplete editing effects. While SNU449-Axl-1 cells showed detectable total and soluble Axl in supernatant, Axl protein expression was absent in immunoblotting, suggesting the role of genomic heterogeneity in incomplete CRISPR/Cas9 editing in cancer cells [58].

Studies on Huh-7 and HepG2 cell lines using CRISPR/Cas9 to eliminate MT family binding sites showed increased MT transcription compared to normal liver cells. Analysis of CTCF binding domain destruction revealed changes in H3K4me3 and H3K9me3 levels, suggesting potential therapeutic approaches through manipulation of local genomic organization [59].

The collective research findings demonstrate CRISPR/Cas9's effectiveness as a gene editing tool in experimental hepatocellular carcinoma models, revealing specific and quantifiable impacts on cancer development and progression. These studies emphasize the crucial role of molecular characteristics in determining cancer behavior and treatment approaches, showcasing the potential of precision genetic interventions as therapeutic strategies.

While CRISPR/Cas9 has shown promise in both *in vitro* and *in vivo* hepatocellular carcinoma studies, successful clinical implementation requires deeper understanding of mechanisms and potential therapeutic targets. Translation of laboratory findings into clinical applications necessitates extensive human trials. **Table 7.1** summarizes key applications of CRISPR/Cas9 in hepatocellular carcinoma research.

Table 7.1 CRISPR/Cas9 applications in hepatocellular carcinoma research.

Target	Primary Function or Pathway	CRISPR/Cas9 Effect and Consequence in Hepatocellular Carcinoma	References
PDHA/PDHB	Pyruvate dehydrogenase complex (glycolysis to TCA cycle)	Knockout disrupts TCA cycle, inhibits mitochondrial function, and induces apoptosis by disrupting the Warburg effect.	[21]
PC	Anaplerosis, gluconeogenesis	Knockout reduces oxaloacetate, disrupting the TCA cycle and gluconeogenesis, leading to energy starvation and oxidative stress.	[21]
TRAF3	NF-κB signaling regulation	Knockout increases proliferation, migration, and invasion of HepG2 cells (context-dependent tumor promoter/suppressor role).	[24, 30]
PTEN	PI3K/AKT pathway suppression	Knockout (with NRAS overexpression) promotes cell survival, proliferation, and resistance to metabolic stress and immune clearance.	[25]
CTNNB1 (β-catenin)	Wnt/β-catenin signaling	Exon-skipping mutation leads to β-catenin accumulation, activating pro-survival/proliferation genes and driving tumorigenesis.	[26, 35, 36]
HIF-1α	Hypoxia response	Knockout enhances the efficacy of transarterial embolization/chemoembolization by increasing apoptosis and suppressing invasion.	[40]

(*Continued*)

Table 7.1 (*Continued*)

Target	Primary Function or Pathway	CRISPR/Cas9 Effect and Consequence in Hepatocellular Carcinoma	References
DOCK1	RAC1 activation, cell survival	Knockout reveals that metformin's antitumor activity depends on DOCK1 levels, suggesting a combo therapy to overcome resistance.	[41]
PTPMT1	Cardiolipin biosynthesis	Knockout causes defective electron transport chain assembly, ROS buildup, and increased sensitivity to inhibitors, especially in hypoxia.	[42]
CXCR4	Chemokine receptor	Knockdown reverses epithelial-mesenchymal transition, increases cisplatin sensitivity, and decreases cancer malignancy.	[43]
SQSTM1/ p62	Keap1/Nrf2/ MMP2 pathway	Knockout slows hepatocellular carcinoma invasion and migration *in vitro* and *in vivo*, identifying it as a potential target.	[44]
DNAJB1-PRKACA	Fusion gene (driver of fibrolamellar hepatocellular carcinoma)	Somatic editing in mice replicates human fibrolamellar hepatocellular carcinoma phenotypes and genotypes without toxins.	[45, 46]
NFE2L2	Oxidative stress response	Ultrasound-controlled knockdown synergizes with sonodynamic therapy to increase oxidative stress for treating deep tumors.	[47]
Survivin	Apoptosis inhibition	Knockout via LBP/pCas9 delivery inhibits proliferation *in vitro* and enhances drug sensitivity *in vivo*.	[39]

Table 7.1 (*Continued*)

Target	Primary Function or Pathway	CRISPR/Cas9 Effect and Consequence in Hepatocellular Carcinoma	References
HGF	Apoptosis regulation	CRISPR-mediated regulation suppresses the natural apoptotic response and reduces colony formation in hepatocellular carcinoma cells.	[49]
PSTK	Ferroptosis resistance	Depletion increases susceptibility to ferroptosis by suppressing GPX4, GSH metabolism, and folate synthesis.	[50]
AXIN1 / ARID1A	Tumor suppressors	Knockout in porcine cells reduces susceptibility to sorafenib and doxorubicin, creating tailored models for drug testing.	[56]
NCAPG	Chromosome condensation	Identified via screening; high expression predicts tumor recurrence and reduced disease-free survival.	[57]
GeCKO Library	Genome-wide screening	Screening identified novel genes like ADAMTSL3 (promotes proliferation/ metastasis) and validated PTEN (inhibits invasion).	[53]
HBsAg	Viral antigen	Knockout of HBsAg open reading frame reduces malignant potential of HBV-hepatocellular carcinoma by disrupting IL-6/STAT3 signaling, suggesting a novel therapy.	[54]

7.4 CRISPR/Cas9 System and Hepatitis B Virus Infection as a Predominant Cause of Hepatocellular Carcinoma

HBV persistent infection significantly contributes to the development of liver cancer, with research indicating that 30–40% of individuals carrying HBV eventually develop hepatocellular carcinoma [60]. Currently available antiviral medications cannot completely eradicate HBV [61], prompting researchers to look toward gene therapy as an alternative for reducing liver cancer incidence.

The virus's life cycle centers around covalently closed circular DNA (cccDNA). Following hepatocyte entry, viral double-stranded DNA either incorporates into the host's chromosomes or forms cccDNA, which serves as a template for transcription. This process generates vital viral proteins including core (HBcAg), polymerase, surface (HBsAg), and X (HBxAg) proteins, enabling viral replication while maintaining cccDNA levels [62, 63]. Building on earlier successes with transcription activator-like effector nuclease and zinc finger nuclease technologies, CRISPR/Cas9 has emerged as a superior tool for HBV suppression or elimination [64, 65].

The pioneering work by Lin et al. in 2014 demonstrated CRISPR/Cas9's capability to target specific HBV sequences and lower surface antigen levels [66]. Their findings revealed reduced HBcAg and HBsAg expression both *in vitro* and *in vivo*, with enhanced effectiveness using multiple single-guide RNAs (sgRNAs). Subsequent studies have validated these results [67–70]. Additionally, targeting conserved genetic sequences across HBV genotypes effectively decreased viral replication [71].

Studies show that disrupting the HBsAg gene sequence leads to reduced cccDNA copies, decreased HBsAg secretion, and diminished tumorigenic potential in HBV-related liver cancer [54, 72]. Conversely, HBsAg accumulation has been linked to increased invasiveness in HBV-associated hepatocellular carcinoma [73].

A breakthrough 2019 study by Dash et al. successfully eliminated HIV in experimental mouse models [74] using a combined approach of LASER ART and CRISPR/Cas9 gene editing. Given the similarities between HIV and HBV treatment approaches, this strategy could potentially be adapted for HBV elimination.

As research progresses, additional genetic targets for HBV therapy and liver cancer treatment continue to emerge. CRISPR/Cas9 technology shows promise in vaccine development against HBV infection [75]. However, challenges remain in efficiently delivering Cas9 plasmids *in vivo*. Future research must focus on improving delivery methods for Cas9 and sgRNA to target cells while ensuring biological safety.

7.5 CRISPR/Cas9 in Overcoming Drug Resistance in Hepatocellular Carcinoma

Through comprehensive screening using CRISPR/Cas9 libraries with multiple sgRNAs, Wei and colleagues identified PHGDH as a key contributor to sorafenib resistance, along with other genes including AKT1S1, TBL1Y, SKAP2, and AMPD2. This finding complemented earlier research using pooled short hairpin RNA knockdown libraries in mouse models, which had previously implicated MAPK in resistance to sorafenib. Studies demonstrated that when PHGDH is inactivated in sorafenib-treated hepatocellular carcinoma cells, there is an increase in apoptotic activity and cell death [76].

A fundamental challenge in hepatocellular carcinoma research involves developing models of sorafenib resistance. PHGDH, which catalyzes the initial step in serine biosynthesis, is crucial for both nucleotide and protein synthesis. Cancer cells typically exhibit altered metabolism, requiring increased serine levels to support rapid cell division. PHGDH not only controls serine synthesis flux but also supports DNA and RNA replication through nucleotide synthesis, making it essential for cell proliferation. When PHGDH is eliminated using CRISPR technology, the disruption of the serine synthesis pathway leads to multiple cellular effects: decreased nucleotide availability, increased oxidative stress, DNA damage, and compromised antioxidant defenses. These changes enhance sensitivity of the cells to sorafenib. Understanding PHGDH's role in cell survival, proliferation, and stress response mechanisms explains why its knockout increases vulnerability of hepatocellular carcinoma cells to sorafenib-induced cell death [76].

Research utilizing CRISPR in hepatoma cells has revealed that certain gene overexpression patterns contribute to regorafenib resistance. Specifically, mutations in the HK1 gene render hepatoma cells resistant to regorafenib treatment. While glycolysis inhibitors like lonidamine can potentially restore regorafenib sensitivity, these inhibitors await FDA approval. Given HK1's universal expression pattern, targeting alternative identified genes may prove more practical for treating tyrosine kinase inhibitor-resistant patients, pending further validation. Additionally, monitoring expression levels of HK1 or other target genes could serve as predictive markers for tyrosine kinase inhibitor therapy outcomes, potentially preventing unnecessary treatment-related complications and expenses [77].

Drug resistance to lenvatinib presents a significant challenge in advanced liver cancer treatment. Through comprehensive CRISPR/Cas9 genome library screening, researchers identified DUSP4 as a crucial gene associated with lenvatinib resistance. In hepatocellular carcinoma patients lacking DUSP4, lenvatinib treatment leads to ERK and MEK reactivation. This finding, validated through *in vivo* xenograft mouse models, suggests DUSP4 could be a valuable target for developing strategies to overcome tyrosine kinase inhibitor resistance [78].

DUSP4's normal expression serves as a tumor suppressor by deactivating the MAPK pathway, particularly ERK1/2. When DUSP4 levels decrease, reduced dephosphorylation leads to increased ERK1/2 activation, promoting the transcription of genes associated with cell survival, growth, and proliferation. This activation mechanism enables cells to resist lenvatinib's growth-inhibiting effects. While lenvatinib functions by inhibiting multiple tyrosine kinase receptors that are commonly overexpressed in cancers, DUSP4 deficiency allows sustained ERK pathway activation, circumventing the drug's anti-tumor effects despite upstream receptor inhibition. Understanding this DUSP4-ERK signaling relationship suggests potential therapeutic strategies, such as combining lenvatinib with MEK inhibitors to directly target ERK1/2 signaling, potentially overcoming resistance by blocking these DUSP4-loss-induced survival signals [79].

Chen and colleagues demonstrated that KEAP1 gene suppression prevented sorafenib resistance through NRF2 regulation. Their research revealed FGF21's critical role in NRF2 downstream regulation, where FGF21 binds to NRF2's C-terminus, creating a positive feedback loop that reduces NRF2 ubiquitination and enhances protein stability. These findings suggest that targeting FGF21 could provide a novel approach for addressing sorafenib resistance in hepatocellular carcinoma [80].

The first application of genome-wide CRISPR transcriptional activation libraries (SAM) to study sorafenib resistance yielded distinct findings compared to previous GeCKO v.2 screening studies [81]. By integrating gene expression profiling data from Huh7 cells with SAM library analysis, researchers identified LRP8 as a key contributor to sorafenib resistance in hepatocellular carcinoma cells. The study found high copy numbers of all three LRP8-targeting sgRNAs in Huh7 cells, along with significantly elevated LRP8 expression in sorafenib-treated hepatocellular carcinoma cells. LRP8 overexpression was linked to reduced apoptosis and enhanced β-catenin activity in hepatocellular carcinoma cells [82].

Research has revealed that LAPTM5 upregulation in hepatocellular carcinoma occurs through hypomethylation and TP53 driver mutations. The combination of lenvatinib and hydroxychloroquine effectively inhibits autolysosome formation and tumor growth. Either LAPTM5 knockdown or hydroxychloroquine administration, when combined with lenvatinib, shows promise in overcoming resistance through autophagy inhibition, potentially improving patient outcomes [83].

Using CRISPR kinome libraries in Cas9-expressing hepatocellular carcinoma cells for xenograft studies, researchers compared regorafenib and vehicle treatments. Sequence analysis identified 31 genes, including LATS2 paralogs of the Hippo pathway, that were more abundant in regorafenib-treated tumors. Notably, inhibiting YAP or Bcl-xL restored regorafenib sensitivity in previously resistant cells, supporting the efficacy of regorafenib against hepatocellular carcinoma based on CRISPR loss-of-function screening [84].

CRISPR/Cas9 screening has identified the potential of combining ifenprodil with sorafenib for hepatocellular carcinoma treatment. While this combination shows promise for treating sorafenib-resistant cancer cells, its effectiveness may be limited in highly resistant cases [85].

CRISPR screens combined with next-generation sequencing have identified SGOL1 as a prognostic marker for sorafenib treatment response. High SGOL1 expression in hepatocellular carcinoma cells correlates with poor prognosis, suggesting that targeting SGOL1 alongside sorafenib could significantly extend patient survival [81].

Research showed enhanced HUH-7 cell viability under moderate doses of sorafenib or lenvatinib compared to controls. MAGeCK analysis identified KEAP1 as a prime candidate gene, with KEAP1-disrupted hepatocellular carcinoma cells showing reduced sensitivity to sorafenib in both short- and long-term treatments. These cells demonstrated lower sorafenib-induced ROS levels and exhibited resistance to other treatments, including regorafenib [86].

Recent findings indicate that downregulating IQGAP1 and FOXM1 enhances the therapeutic effect of sorafenib by inhibiting PI3K/AKT and MAPK/ERK pathways. This combination also impairs CD133+ cancer stem cells, which contribute to sorafenib resistance. The potential combination of sorafenib with extracellular vesicles may offer improved treatment outcomes compared to sorafenib monotherapy [87].

All the reviewed findings on CRISPR/Cas9 roles in overcoming hepatocellular carcinoma drug resistance are summarily illustrated in **Figure 7.1**.

7.6 CRISPR/Cas9 to Promote Immunotherapy

Recent advances in cancer immunotherapy have highlighted gene editing of PD-L1 or PD-1 and CAR-T cell modifications as

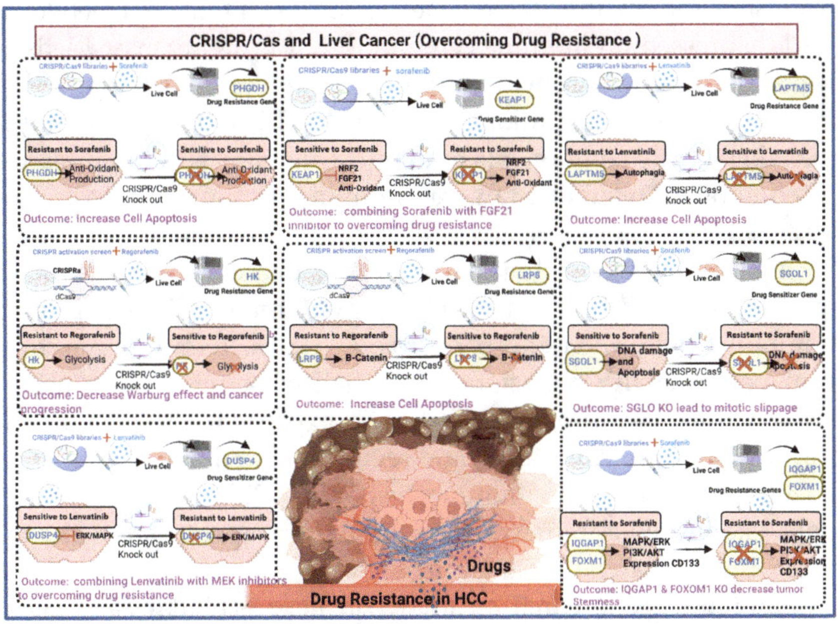

Figure 7.1 CRISPR/Cas9-mediated functional genomics for overcoming drug resistance in liver cancer, particularly hepatocellular carcinoma. CRISPR/Cas9 genome editing platforms are leveraged to dissect and counteract the molecular mechanisms underlying drug resistance in hepatocellular carcinoma, highlighting a range of gene targets and combination therapies. **Overcoming sorafenib resistance:** *PHGDH and PHX knockout:* Disruption of these genes elevates cell apoptosis and restores sensitivity to sorafenib by attenuating antioxidant production; *KEAP1 knockout and FGF21 combination:* Loss of KEAP1, a drug sensitizer gene, combined with FGF21 inhibitors disrupts NRF2-mediated antioxidant responses, enhancing sorafenib efficacy; *SGOL1 knockout:* Enhances DNA damage and apoptosis upon sorafenib treatment, where its deletion causes mitotic slippage and increases drug response. **Overcoming lenvatinib resistance:** *LAPTM5 knockout:* Promotes tumor cell apoptosis via impaired autophagic flux, sensitizing cells to lenvatinib; *DUSP4 knockout and MEK inhibitor combination:* Dual targeting with lenvatinib and MEK inhibitors inhibits ERK/MAPK signaling, overcoming resistance. **Overcoming regorafenib resistance:** *HK (hexokinase) knockout:* Suppresses glycolysis and the Warburg effect, hampering tumor progression and restoring drug sensitivity; *LRP8 knockout:* Blocks β-catenin signaling, induces apoptosis, and overcomes resistance to regorafenib. **Multi-drug resistance pathways:** *IQGAP1 and FOXM1 knockout:* Combined loss reduces MAPK/ERK and PI3K/AKT signaling, diminishes the expression of cancer stem cell marker CD133, and curtails tumor stemness and drug resistance.

promising therapeutic approaches [88]. The interaction between PD-1, expressed on immune cells, and PD-L1, highly expressed in tumor tissues, compromises immune regulation and reduces the body's ability to fight tumors [89, 90]. CAR-T cell therapy employs specialized ScFv components to identify and attach to tumor-associated antigens, enabling targeted immune responses against cancer cells [91].

A groundbreaking clinical trial in 2016 marked the first human application of CRISPR/Cas9 technology to modify the PD-1 gene in immune cells. Their approach involved extracting immune cells from patients with metastatic non-small cell lung cancer, using CRISPR/Cas9 to disable the PD-1 gene, expanding these modified cells in laboratory conditions, and reintroducing them into patients to enhance anti-cancer immune responses [92]. This pioneering work established a framework for similar therapeutic strategies in hepatocellular carcinoma treatment.

Fundamental research on PD-L1 in hepatocellular carcinoma has yielded significant insights. Guo and colleagues' investigation into effects of CAR-T cells on hepatocellular carcinoma growth revealed that CAR-T cells with modified PD-1 expression demonstrated substantially prolonged anti-tumor activity. Their findings confirmed that PD-1 modification could enhance CAR-T cell therapy effectiveness against hepatocellular carcinoma [93], underscoring the crucial role of PD-L1 and PD-1 pathways in treatment strategies.

CRISPR/Cas9 technology enhances CAR-T therapy for hepatocellular carcinoma through two main approaches: by eliminating genes that code for signal molecules or immune response inhibitors to boost anti-tumor immune responses, and by removing HLA I gene fragments from T cells to prevent xenograft rejection. This latter modification opens the possibility of developing universal CAR-T cells suitable for multiple patients, significantly improving treatment accessibility and efficiency [94].

The versatility of CRISPR/Cas9 extends to genetic engineering of both human stem cells and induced pluripotent stem cells. Research has demonstrated that CRISPR/Cas9-modified pluripotent stem cells maintain their ability to form organ-like structures in culture [91]. This capability has been successfully demonstrated in treating β-thalassemia and duchenne muscular dystrophypatients using their own modified induced pluripotent stem cells [95, 96]. In hepatocellular carcinoma treatment applications, CRISPR/Cas9 enables genetic modification of pluripotent stem cells and their directed differentiation into immune cells, particularly natural killer cells. When combined with CAR-T gene therapy, this approach enhances immune-mediated tumor cell destruction following autologous transplantation. Furthermore, Yin and colleagues' discovery of cancer stem cell characteristics in CD133-positive cells [97] has opened new avenues for using CRISPR/Cas9 to study gene function in liver cancer stem cells and develop strategies to reduce their activity.

7.7 Preclinical Studies in CRISPR/Cas-Based Manipulation of Cancer Genome

CRISPR/Cas9 has emerged as a powerful tool for genetic manipulation across various cancer types. Studies have shown that CRISPR/Cas9-mediated elimination of HIF-1α enhances the effectiveness of transarterial embolization in cell cultures and extends survival in hepatocellular carcinoma-bearing mice [40]. Similarly, research investigating the role of NSD1 demonstrated that its deletion through CRISPR/Cas9 suppresses cancer cell proliferation, migration, and invasion by deactivating the Wnt/β-catenin signaling pathway [38].

CRISPR/Cas9 technology also enables the strategic insertion of drug-target sequences into cells to enhance treatment effectiveness. Chen and colleagues demonstrated this by using CRISPR/Cas9 to integrate HSV1-tk into hepatocellular carcinoma cell genomes. This modification enables cells to convert ganciclovir into its active form (ganciclovir triphosphate), which interferes with DNA replication. When treated with ganciclovir, the modified cells underwent extensive necrosis *in vitro*. In mouse xenograft models, this approach resulted in reduced tumor size and mortality rates [98].

Looking ahead, as more oncogenes are discovered in hepatocellular carcinoma, research priorities should focus on identifying the most suitable targets for gene therapy and developing strategies to prevent cancer cell resistance and escape mechanisms.

7.8 Challenges and Future Perspectives

The development of biomedical modeling has been revolutionized by the ability to create genetically customized tumors through *in vitro* cell editing and orthotopic implantation. This approach has been extended to porcine models and can be adapted for various cancer types using immunocompromised animals implanted with human gene-edited cells. Optimizing CRISPR delivery components for *in vivo* porcine gene editing models will significantly advance the development and testing of precision medicine strategies.

Due to their anatomical and physiological similarities to humans, pigs serve as ideal test subjects for evaluating novel CRISPR-based therapies prior to human clinical trials. Although CRISPR/Cas systems show great promise for treating genetic disorders, their clinical application remains limited during the model evaluation phase. Testing in porcine models provides a valuable platform for assessing both the safety and efficacy of CRISPR/Cas9 interventions.

Current research on CRISPR/Cas9-based hepatocellular carcinoma treatment is evolving toward more precise and targeted approaches. Future developments are expected to focus on enhanced genetic modifications targeting multiple genes such as SNHG9 and CASC11 to more effectively inhibit hepatocellular carcinoma growth and metastasis, combining CRISPR/Cas9 with existing therapies to overcome the limitations of current treatments like sorafenib, and improving delivery systems through advanced nanoparticle technologies that offer greater specificity, stability, and safety. Additionally, personalized gene therapy approaches that account for genetic heterogeneity among hepatocellular carcinoma patients are being explored, alongside comprehensive clinical trials aimed at evaluating long-term outcomes and safety.

However, several key limitations must be addressed to ensure successful clinical translation. These include target specificity and off-target effects, delivery efficiency, immunogenicity, *in vivo* editing efficiency, gene editing control, and scale-up and manufacturing challenges. Overcoming these obstacles will require the integration of advances in materials science, immunology, genomic analysis, and cellular biology to ensure precision, safety, and control in therapeutic applications.

Scientific collaboration is essential for overcoming technical challenges and establishing robust ethical and regulatory frameworks that will enable CRISPR to become a mainstream therapeutic tool. Key development priorities span several critical domains.

In preclinical modeling, the use of patient-derived xenografts and organoids offers improved prediction of clinical outcomes, while diverse animal models help elucidate CRISPR system behavior and reduce off-target effects. For safety optimization, high-resolution genome-wide techniques are being employed to map potential off-target sites. Safe delivery methods and transient expression strategies are under development, alongside engineering of higher-fidelity Cas enzymes. Comprehensive toxicological assessments particularly those focused on liver-specific effects are vital to ensure therapeutic safety.

Target validation efforts focus on confirming the roles of identified long non-coding RNAs and genetic elements in hepatocellular carcinoma through independent studies. Establishing clear mechanistic links between therapeutic targets and hepatocellular carcinoma pathogenesis, as well as determining optimal dosing strategies, are crucial for maximizing efficacy while minimizing risk.

In the realm of clinical translation, optimizing delivery vectors for hepatocyte targeting and investigating the long-term effects of gene editing are key priorities. Ensuring full compliance with legal and ethical requirements for gene therapy, and meeting all regulatory standards for human trials, are foundational to advancing CRISPR-based treatments.

The future of CRISPR/Cas9 in hepatocellular carcinoma therapy holds significant promise. However, its success will depend on rigorous scientific research, unwavering adherence to ethical standards, patient-centered approaches, and careful navigation of the scientific, ethical, and clinical pathways. These elements are indispensable for translating CRISPR/Cas9 technology into effective clinical treatments that genuinely improve patient outcomes.

7.9 Conclusion

Hepatocellular carcinoma remains a pressing global health challenge, with limited advances in survival outcomes despite the availability of diverse treatment modalities. The integration of genetic insights has revealed key molecular drivers and potential biomarkers for improving diagnosis and prognosis, yet therapeutic breakthroughs remain urgently needed. CRISPR/Cas9 has emerged as a transformative tool in this context, offering a precise and robust method for interrogating gene function, correcting pathogenic mutations, and developing novel therapeutic strategies. Preliminary studies in hepatocellular carcinoma models underscore its potential in tumor suppression, immunotherapy enhancement, and biomarker discovery. However, challenges such as off-target effects, delivery efficiency, and safety in clinical applications must be addressed before its full therapeutic value can be realized. With ongoing refinements in delivery technologies and engineered Cas variants, CRISPR/Cas9 is poised to contribute significantly to the future of hepatocellular carcinoma management, advancing the field toward more effective and personalized therapeutic interventions.

References

1. Bray F, Ferlay J, Soerjomataram I, Siegel RL, Torre LA, Jemal A. Global cancer statistics 2018: GLOBOCAN estimates of incidence and mortality worldwide for 36 cancers in 185 countries. CA Cancer J Clin. 2018;68(6):394–424.
2. Role of endoscopy in primary sclerosing cholangitis: European Society of Gastrointestinal Endoscopy (ESGE) and European

Association for the Study of the Liver (EASL) Clinical Guideline. J Hepatol. 2017;66(6):1265–81.
3. Sia D, Villanueva A, Friedman SL, Llovet JM. Liver Cancer Cell of Origin, Molecular Class, and Effects on Patient Prognosis. Gastroenterology. 2017;152(4):745–61.
4. de Martel C, Maucort-Boulch D, Plummer M, Franceschi S. World-wide relative contribution of hepatitis B and C viruses in hepatocellular carcinoma. Hepatology. 2015;62(4):1190–200.
5. Massarweh NN, El-Serag HB. Epidemiology of Hepatocellular Carcinoma and Intrahepatic Cholangiocarcinoma. Cancer Control. 2017;24(3):1073274817729245.
6. 2018 Korean Liver Cancer Association-National Cancer Center Korea Practice Guidelines for the Management of Hepatocellular Carcinoma. Korean J Radiol. 2019;20(7):1042–113.
7. Kudo M, Finn RS, Qin S, Han KH, Ikeda K, Piscaglia F, et al. Lenvatinib versus sorafenib in first-line treatment of patients with unresectable hepatocellular carcinoma: a randomised phase 3 non-inferiority trial. Lancet. 2018;391(10126):1163–73.
8. Zhang B, Yang B. Combined alpha fetoprotein testing and ultrasonography as a screening test for primary liver cancer. J Med Screen. 1999;6(2):108–10.
9. Wang C, Vegna S, Jin H, Benedict B, Lieftink C, Ramirez C, et al. Inducing and exploiting vulnerabilities for the treatment of liver cancer. Nature. 2019;574(7777):268–72.
10. Barrangou R, Fremaux C, Deveau H, Richards M, Boyaval P, Moineau S, et al. CRISPR provides acquired resistance against viruses in prokaryotes. Science. 2007;315(5819):1709–12.
11. Jinek M, Chylinski K, Fonfara I, Hauer M, Doudna JA, Charpentier E. A programmable dual-RNA-guided DNA endonuclease in adaptive bacterial immunity. Science. 2012;337(6096):816–21.
12. Llovet JM, Kelley RK, Villanueva A, Singal AG, Pikarsky E, Roayaie S, et al. Hepatocellular carcinoma. Nat Rev Dis Primers. 2021;7(1):6.
13. Anstee QM, Reeves HL, Kotsiliti E, Govaere O, Heikenwalder M. From NASH to HCC: current concepts and future challenges. Nat Rev Gastroenterol Hepatol. 2019;16(7):411–28.
14. Goswami VG, Patel BD. Recent updates on Wnt signaling modulators: a patent review (2014–2020). Expert Opin Ther Pat. 2021; 31(11):1009–43.

15. Tornesello ML, Tornesello AL, Starita N, Cerasuolo A, Izzo F, Buonaguro L, Buonaguro FM. Telomerase: a good target in hepatocellular carcinoma? An overview of relevant preclinical data. Expert Opin Ther Targets. 2022;26(9):767–80.
16. Nevola R, Ruocco R, Criscuolo L, Villani A, Alfano M, Beccia D, et al. Predictors of early and late hepatocellular carcinoma recurrence. World J Gastroenterol. 2023;29(8):1243–60.
17. Raoul JL, Forner A, Bolondi L, Cheung TT, Kloeckner R, de Baere T. Updated use of TACE for hepatocellular carcinoma treatment: How and when to use it based on clinical evidence. Cancer Treat Rev. 2019;72:28–36.
18. Sperandio RC, Pestana RC, Miyamura BV, Kaseb AO. Hepatocellular Carcinoma Immunotherapy. Annu Rev Med. 2022;73:267–78.
19. Qin S, Chen M, Cheng AL, Kaseb AO, Kudo M, Lee HC, et al. Atezolizumab plus bevacizumab versus active surveillance in patients with resected or ablated high-risk hepatocellular carcinoma (IMbrave050): a randomised, open-label, multicentre, phase 3 trial. Lancet. 2023;402(10415):1835–47.
20. Llovet JM, Castet F, Heikenwalder M, Maini MK, Mazzaferro V, Pinato DJ, et al. Immunotherapies for hepatocellular carcinoma. Nat Rev Clin Oncol. 2022;19(3):151–72.
21. Yang C, Lee D, Zhang MS, Tse AP, Wei L, Bao MH, et al. Genome-Wide CRISPR/Cas9 Library Screening Revealed Dietary Restriction of Glutamine in Combination with Inhibition of Pyruvate Metabolism as Effective Liver Cancer Treatment. Adv Sci (Weinh). 2022;9(34):e2202104.
22. Vernieri C, Casola S, Foiani M, Pietrantonio F, de Braud F, Longo V. Targeting Cancer Metabolism: Dietary and Pharmacologic Interventions. Cancer Discov. 2016;6(12):1315–33.
23. Daye D, Wellen KE. Metabolic reprogramming in cancer: unraveling the role of glutamine in tumorigenesis. Semin Cell Dev Biol. 2012;23(4):362–9.
24. Hu W, Guo G, Chi Y, Li F. Construction of Traf3 knockout liver cancer cell line using CRISPR/Cas9 system. J Cell Biochem. 2019;120(9):14908–15.
25. Gao M, Liu D. CRISPR/Cas9-based Pten knock-out and Sleeping Beauty Transposon-mediated Nras knock-in induces hepatocellular carcinoma and hepatic lipid accumulation in mice. Cancer Biol Ther. 2017;18(7):505–12.

26. Mou H, Eskiocak O, Özler KA, Gorman M, Yue J, Jin Y, et al. CRISPR-induced exon skipping of β-catenin reveals tumorigenic mutants driving distinct subtypes of liver cancer. J Pathol. 2023;259(4):415–27.
27. Chen Z, Krinsky A, Woolaver RA, Wang X, Chen SMY, Popolizio V, et al. TRAF3 Acts as a Checkpoint of B Cell Receptor Signaling to Control Antibody Class Switch Recombination and Anergy. J Immunol. 2020;205(3):830–41.
28. He JQ, Zarnegar B, Oganesyan G, Saha SK, Yamazaki S, Doyle SE, et al. Rescue of TRAF3-null mice by p100 NF-kappa B deficiency. J Exp Med. 2006;203(11):2413–8.
29. Liao G, Zhang M, Harhaj EW, Sun SC. Regulation of the NF-kappaB-inducing kinase by tumor necrosis factor receptor-associated factor 3-induced degradation. J Biol Chem. 2004;279(25):26243–50.
30. Shi JH, Sun SC. Tumor Necrosis Factor Receptor-Associated Factor Regulation of Nuclear Factor κB and Mitogen-Activated Protein Kinase Pathways. Front Immunol. 2018;9:1849.
31. Vallabhapurapu S, Matsuzawa A, Zhang W, Tseng PH, Keats JJ, Wang H, et al. Nonredundant and complementary functions of TRAF2 and TRAF3 in a ubiquitination cascade that activates NIK-dependent alternative NF-kappaB signaling. Nat Immunol. 2008;9(12):1364–70.
32. Xie P, Kraus ZJ, Stunz LL, Liu Y, Bishop GA. TNF receptor-associated factor 3 is required for T cell-mediated immunity and TCR/CD28 signaling. J Immunol. 2011;186(1):143–55.
33. Yang XD, Sun SC. Targeting signaling factors for degradation, an emerging mechanism for TRAF functions. Immunol Rev. 2015;266(1):56–71.
34. Amjad E, Pezzani R, Sokouti B. A review of the literature on the use of CRISPR/Cas9 gene therapy to treat hepatocellular carcinoma. Oncol Res. 2024;32(3):439–61.
35. Huang Y, Zeng J, Liu T, Xu Q, Song X, Zeng J. Deubiquitinating enzyme JOSD2 promotes hepatocellular carcinoma progression through interacting with and inhibiting CTNNB1 degradation. Cell Biol Int. 2022;46(7):1089–97.
36. Rebouissou S, Franconi A, Calderaro J, Letouzé E, Imbeaud S, Pilati C, et al. Genotype-phenotype correlation of CTNNB1 mutations reveals different ß-catenin activity associated with liver tumor progression. Hepatology. 2016;64(6):2047–61.
37. Guan L, Zhu S, Han Y, Yang C, Liu Y, Qiao L, et al. Knockout of CTNNB1 by CRISPR-Cas9 technology inhibits cell proliferation

through the Wnt/β-catenin signaling pathway. Biotechnol Lett. 2018;40(3):501–8.
38. Zhang S, Zhang F, Chen Q, Wan C, Xiong J, Xu J. CRISPR/Cas9-mediated knockout of NSD1 suppresses the hepatocellular carcinoma development via the NSD1/H3/Wnt10b signaling pathway. J Exp Clin Cancer Res. 2019;38(1):467.
39. Qi Y, Liu Y, Yu B, Hu Y, Zhang N, Zheng Y, et al. A Lactose-Derived CRISPR/Cas9 Delivery System for Efficient Genome Editing In Vivo to Treat Orthotopic Hepatocellular Carcinoma. Adv Sci (Weinh). 2020;7(17):2001424.
40. Liu Q, Fan D, Adah D, Wu Z, Liu R, Yan QT, et al. CRISPR/Cas9-mediated hypoxia inducible factor-1α knockout enhances the antitumor effect of transarterial embolization in hepatocellular carcinoma. Oncol Rep. 2018;40(5):2547–57.
41. Feng J, Lu H, Ma W, Tian W, Lu Z, Yang H, et al. Genome-wide CRISPR screen identifies synthetic lethality between DOCK1 inhibition and metformin in liver cancer. Protein Cell. 2022;13(11):825–41.
42. Bao MH, Yang C, Tse AP, Wei L, Lee D, Zhang MS, et al. Genome-wide CRISPR-Cas9 knockout library screening identified PTPMT1 in cardiolipin synthesis is crucial to survival in hypoxia in liver cancer. Cell Rep. 2021;34(4):108676.
43. Wang X, Zhang W, Ding Y, Guo X, Yuan Y, Li D. CRISPR/Cas9-mediated genome engineering of CXCR4 decreases the malignancy of hepatocellular carcinoma cells in vitro and in vivo. Oncol Rep. 2017;37(6):3565–71.
44. Lu J, Ding Y, Zhang W, Qi Y, Zhou J, Xu N, et al. SQSTM1/p62 Knockout by Using the CRISPR/Cas9 System Inhibits Migration and Invasion of Hepatocellular Carcinoma. Cells. 2023;12(9):1238.
45. Riggle KM, Turnham R, Scott JD, Yeung RS, Riehle KJ. Fibrolamellar Hepatocellular Carcinoma: Mechanistic Distinction From Adult Hepatocellular Carcinoma. Pediatr Blood Cancer. 2016;63(7):1163–7.
46. Engelholm LH, Riaz A, Serra D, Dagnæs-Hansen F, Johansen JV, Santoni-Rugiu E, et al. CRISPR/Cas9 Engineering of Adult Mouse Liver Demonstrates That the Dnajb1-Prkaca Gene Fusion Is Sufficient to Induce Tumors Resembling Fibrolamellar Hepatocellular Carcinoma. Gastroenterology. 2017;153(6):1662–73.e10.
47. Yin H, Sun L, Pu Y, Yu J, Feng W, Dong C, et al. Ultrasound-Controlled CRISPR/Cas9 System Augments Sonodynamic Therapy of Hepatocellular Carcinoma. ACS Cent Sci. 2021;7(12):2049–62.

48. Zhang B, Ren Z, Zheng H, Lin M, Chen G, Luo OJ, Zhu G. CRISPR activation screening in a mouse model for drivers of hepatocellular carcinoma growth and metastasis. iScience. 2023;26(3):106099.
49. Lee HK, Lim HM, Park SH, Nam MJ. Knockout of Hepatocyte Growth Factor by CRISPR/Cas9 System Induces Apoptosis in Hepatocellular Carcinoma Cells. J Pers Med. 2021;11(10):983.
50. Chen Y, Li L, Lan J, Cui Y, Rao X, Zhao J, et al. CRISPR screens uncover protective effect of PSTK as a regulator of chemotherapy-induced ferroptosis in hepatocellular carcinoma. Mol Cancer. 2022;21(1):11.
51. Elkhadragy L, Regan MR, W MT, Goli KD, Patel S, Garcia K, et al. Generation of genetically tailored porcine liver cancer cells by CRISPR/Cas9 editing. Biotechniques. 2021;70(1):37–48.
52. Akasu M, Shimada S, Kabashima A, Akiyama Y, Shimokawa M, Akahoshi K, et al. Intrinsic activation of β-catenin signaling by CRISPR/Cas9-mediated exon skipping contributes to immune evasion in hepatocellular carcinoma. Sci Rep. 2021;11(1):16732.
53. Zhou X, Li R, Jing R, Zuo B, Zheng Q. Genome-wide CRISPR knockout screens identify ADAMTSL3 and PTEN genes as suppressors of HCC proliferation and metastasis, respectively. J Cancer Res Clin Oncol. 2020;146(6):1509–21.
54. Song J, Zhang X, Ge Q, Yuan C, Chu L, Liang HF, et al. CRISPR/Cas9-mediated knockout of HBsAg inhibits proliferation and tumorigenicity of HBV-positive hepatocellular carcinoma cells. J Cell Biochem. 2018;119(10):8419–31.
55. Saputra EC, Huang L, Chen Y, Tucker-Kellogg L. Combination Therapy and the Evolution of Resistance: The Theoretical Merits of Synergism and Antagonism in Cancer. Cancer Res. 2018;78(9):2419–31.
56. Elkhadragy L, Dasteh Goli K, Totura WM, Carlino MJ, Regan MR, Guzman G, et al. Effect of CRISPR Knockout of AXIN1 or ARID1A on Proliferation and Migration of Porcine Hepatocellular Carcinoma. Front Oncol. 2022;12:904031.
57. Wang Y, Gao B, Tan PY, Handoko YA, Sekar K, Deivasigamani A, et al. Genome-wide CRISPR knockout screens identify NCAPG as an essential oncogene for hepatocellular carcinoma tumor growth. Faseb j. 2019;33(8):8759–70.
58. Scharf I, Bierbaumer L, Huber H, Wittmann P, Haider C, Pirker C, et al. Dynamics of CRISPR/Cas9-mediated genomic editing of the

AXL locus in hepatocellular carcinoma cells. Oncol Lett. 2018;15(2): 2441–50.

59. Gong W, Liu Y, Qu H, Liu A, Sun P, Wang X. The effect of CTCF binding sites destruction by CRISPR/Cas9 on transcription of metallothionein gene family in liver hepatocellular carcinoma. Biochem Biophys Res Commun. 2019;510(4):530–8.
60. Lok AS. Prevention of hepatitis B virus-related hepatocellular carcinoma. Gastroenterology. 2004;127(5 Suppl 1):S303–9.
61. Trépo C, Chan HL, Lok A. Hepatitis B virus infection. Lancet. 2014;384(9959):2053–63.
62. Guo JT, Guo H. Metabolism and function of hepatitis B virus cccDNA: Implications for the development of cccDNA-targeting antiviral therapeutics. Antiviral Res. 2015;122:91–100.
63. Lin G, Zhang K, Li J. Application of CRISPR/Cas9 Technology to HBV. Int J Mol Sci. 2015;16(11):26077–86.
64. Bloom K, Ely A, Mussolino C, Cathomen T, Arbuthnot P. Inactivation of hepatitis B virus replication in cultured cells and in vivo with engineered transcription activator-like effector nucleases. Mol Ther. 2013;21(10):1889–97.
65. Weber ND, Stone D, Sedlak RH, De Silva Feelixge HS, Roychoudhury P, Schiffer JT, et al. AAV-mediated delivery of zinc finger nucleases targeting hepatitis B virus inhibits active replication. PLoS One. 2014;9(5):e97579.
66. Lin SR, Yang HC, Kuo YT, Liu CJ, Yang TY, Sung KC, et al. The CRISPR/Cas9 System Facilitates Clearance of the Intrahepatic HBV Templates In Vivo. Mol Ther Nucleic Acids. 2014;3(8):e186.
67. Dong C, Qu L, Wang H, Wei L, Dong Y, Xiong S. Targeting hepatitis B virus cccDNA by CRISPR/Cas9 nuclease efficiently inhibits viral replication. Antiviral Res. 2015;118:110–7.
68. Kennedy EM, Kornepati AV, Cullen BR. Targeting hepatitis B virus cccDNA using CRISPR/Cas9. Antiviral Res. 2015;123:188–92.
69. Ramanan V, Shlomai A, Cox DB, Schwartz RE, Michailidis E, Bhatta A, et al. CRISPR/Cas9 cleavage of viral DNA efficiently suppresses hepatitis B virus. Sci Rep. 2015;5:10833.
70. Seeger C, Sohn JA. Complete Spectrum of CRISPR/Cas9-induced Mutations on HBV cccDNA. Mol Ther. 2016;24(7):1258–66.
71. Liu X, Hao R, Chen S, Guo D, Chen Y. Inhibition of hepatitis B virus by the CRISPR/Cas9 system via targeting the conserved regions of the viral genome. J Gen Virol. 2015;96(8):2252–61.

72. Zhen S, Hua L, Liu YH, Gao LC, Fu J, Wan DY, et al. Harnessing the clustered regularly interspaced short palindromic repeat (CRISPR)/CRISPR-associated Cas9 system to disrupt the hepatitis B virus. Gene Ther. 2015;22(5):404–12.
73. Cheng S, Zhang B, Du JY, Jin YH, Lang HY, Zeng LH. Hepatitis B Surface Antigen Promotes the Invasion of Hepatitis B Virus-Related Hepatocellular Carcinoma Cells by Upregulation of Toll-Like Receptor 2. Viral Immunol. 2017;30(3):232–9.
74. Dash PK, Kaminski R, Bella R, Su H, Mathews S, Ahooyi TM, et al. Sequential LASER ART and CRISPR Treatments Eliminate HIV-1 in a Subset of Infected Humanized Mice. Nat Commun. 2019;10(1):2753.
75. Okoli A, Okeke MI, Tryland M, Moens U. CRISPR/Cas9-Advancing Orthopoxvirus Genome Editing for Vaccine and Vector Development. Viruses. 2018;10(1):50.
76. Wei L, Lee D, Law CT, Zhang MS, Shen J, Chin DW, et al. Genome-wide CRISPR/Cas9 library screening identified PHGDH as a critical driver for Sorafenib resistance in HCC. Nat Commun. 2019;10(1):4681.
77. Sofer S, Lamkiewicz K, Armoza Eilat S, Partouche S, Marz M, Moskovits N, et al. A genome-wide CRISPR activation screen reveals Hexokinase 1 as a critical factor in promoting resistance to multi-kinase inhibitors in hepatocellular carcinoma cells. Faseb J. 2022;36(3):e22191.
78. Huang S, Ma Z, Zhou Q, Wang A, Gong Y, Li Z, et al. Genome-Wide CRISPR/Cas9 Library Screening Identified that DUSP4 Deficiency Induces Lenvatinib Resistance in Hepatocellular Carcinoma. Int J Biol Sci. 2022;18(11):4357–71.
79. Mebratu Y, Tesfaigzi Y. How ERK1/2 activation controls cell proliferation and cell death: Is subcellular localization the answer? Cell Cycle. 2009;8(8):1168–75.
80. Chen J, Jiang S, Shao H, Li B, Ji T, Staiculescu D, et al. CRISPR-Cas9-based genome-wide screening identified novel targets for treating sorafenib-resistant hepatocellular carcinoma: a cross-talk between FGF21 and the NRF2 pathway. Sci China Life Sci. 2022;65(10):1998–2016.
81. Sun W, He B, Yang B, Hu W, Cheng S, Xiao H, et al. Genome-wide CRISPR screen reveals SGOL1 as a druggable target of sorafenib-treated hepatocellular carcinoma. Lab Invest. 2018;98(6):734–44.
82. Cai J, Chen J, Wu T, Cheng Z, Tian Y, Pu C, et al. Genome-scale CRISPR activation screening identifies a role of LRP8 in Sorafenib

resistance in Hepatocellular carcinoma. Biochem Biophys Res Commun. 2020;526(4):1170–6.

83. Pan J, Zhang M, Dong L, Ji S, Zhang J, Zhang S, et al. Genome-Scale CRISPR screen identifies LAPTM5 driving lenvatinib resistance in hepatocellular carcinoma. Autophagy. 2023;19(4):1184–98.
84. Suemura S, Kodama T, Myojin Y, Yamada R, Shigekawa M, Hikita H, et al. CRISPR Loss-of-Function Screen Identifies the Hippo Signaling Pathway as the Mediator of Regorafenib Efficacy in Hepatocellular Carcinoma. Cancers (Basel). 2019;11(9):1362.
85. Xu F, Tong M, Tong CSW, Chan BKC, Chu HY, Wong TL, et al. A Combinatorial CRISPR-Cas9 Screen Identifies Ifenprodil as an Adjunct to Sorafenib for Liver Cancer Treatment. Cancer Res. 2021;81(24):6219–32.
86. Zheng A, Chevalier N, Calderoni M, Dubuis G, Dormond O, Ziros PG, et al. CRISPR/Cas9 genome-wide screening identifies KEAP1 as a sorafenib, lenvatinib, and regorafenib sensitivity gene in hepatocellular carcinoma. Oncotarget. 2019;10(66):7058–70.
87. He C, Jaffar Ali D, Qi Y, Li Y, Sun B, Liu R, et al. Engineered extracellular vesicles mediated CRISPR-induced deficiency of IQGAP1/FOXM1 reverses sorafenib resistance in HCC by suppressing cancer stem cells. J Nanobiotechnology. 2023;21(1):154.
88. Iwai Y, Hamanishi J, Chamoto K, Honjo T. Cancer immunotherapies targeting the PD-1 signaling pathway. J Biomed Sci. 2017;24(1):26.
89. Iwai Y, Ishida M, Tanaka Y, Okazaki T, Honjo T, Minato N. Involvement of PD-L1 on tumor cells in the escape from host immune system and tumor immunotherapy by PD-L1 blockade. Proc Natl Acad Sci U S A. 2002;99(19):12293–7.
90. Okazaki T, Honjo T. The PD-1-PD-L pathway in immunological tolerance. Trends Immunol. 2006;27(4):195–201.
91. Wang Z, Wu Z, Liu Y, Han W. New development in CAR-T cell therapy. J Hematol Oncol. 2017;10(1):53.
92. Cyranoski D. CRISPR gene-editing tested in a person for the first time. Nature. 2016;539(7630):479.
93. Guo X, Jiang H, Shi B, Zhou M, Zhang H, Shi Z, et al. Disruption of PD-1 Enhanced the Anti-tumor Activity of Chimeric Antigen Receptor T Cells Against Hepatocellular Carcinoma. Front Pharmacol. 2018;9:1118.

94. Liu X, Zhang Y, Cheng C, Cheng AW, Zhang X, Li N, et al. CRISPR-Cas9-mediated multiplex gene editing in CAR-T cells. Cell Res. 2017;27(1):154–7.
95. Li HL, Fujimoto N, Sasakawa N, Shirai S, Ohkame T, Sakuma T, et al. Precise correction of the dystrophin gene in duchenne muscular dystrophy patient induced pluripotent stem cells by TALEN and CRISPR-Cas9. Stem Cell Reports. 2015;4(1):143–54.
96. Xie F, Ye L, Chang JC, Beyer AI, Wang J, Muench MO, Kan YW. Seamless gene correction of β-thalassemia mutations in patient-specific iPSCs using CRISPR/Cas9 and piggyBac. Genome Res. 2014;24(9):1526–33.
97. Yin S, Li J, Hu C, Chen X, Yao M, Yan M, et al. CD133 positive hepatocellular carcinoma cells possess high capacity for tumorigenicity. Int J Cancer. 2007;120(7):1444–50.
98. Chen ZH, Yu YP, Zuo ZH, Nelson JB, Michalopoulos GK, Monga S, et al. Targeting genomic rearrangements in tumor cells through Cas9-mediated insertion of a suicide gene. Nat Biotechnol. 2017;35(6):543–50.

https://doi.org/10.1142/9789819826759_0008

CHAPTER 8

CRISPR/Cas9 in the Treatment of Prostate Cancer

Mehrdad Hashemi[1,2], *Alireza Khosravinejad*[1,3], *Mina Alimohammadi*[4], *Faranak Jamshidian*[1,5], *Reza Mohajer Shirazi*[1,3], *Rojin Ghannad Zadeh*[1,6], *Behdokht Jamali*[7], *Kimia Sadat Esfahani*[1,3], *Ali Shirazi*[1,3], *Neda Zali*[3], *Najma Farahani*[1,*], *Afshin Taheriazam*[1,8,*], *Payman Rahimzadeh*[9,*], *Maliheh Entezari*[1,2,*]

[1]Farhikhtegan Medical Convergent Sciences Research Center, Farhikhtegan Hospital, Faculty of Medicine, TeMs. C., Islamic Azad University, Tehran, Iran
[2]Department of Genetics, Faculty of Advanced Sciences and Technology, TeMs. C, Islamic Azad University, Tehran, Iran
[3]Basic and Molecular Epidemiology of Gastrointestinal Disorders Research Center, Research Institute for Gastroenterology and Liver Diseases, Shahid Beheshti University of Medical Sciences, Tehran, Iran
[4]Department of Immunology, School of Medicine, Shahid Beheshti University of Medical Sciences, Tehran, Iran
[5]Department of Biology, ET.C., Islamic Azad University, Tehran, Iran

* **Corresponding authors:** Najmafarahani@gmail.com (N.F.); a.taheriazam@iautmu.ac.ir (A.T.); P.rahimzadeh76@gmail.com (P.R.); mentezari@iautmu.ac.ir (M.E.)

[6]Department of Art & Sciences, Faculty of Biology, University of North Florida, Jacksonville, Florida, USA
[7]Department of Microbiology and Genetics, Kherad Institute of Higher Education, Bushehr, Iran
[8]Department of Orthopedics, Faculty of Medicine, TeMs. C, Islamic Azad University, Tehran, Iran
[9]Surgical Research Society (SRS), Students' Scientific Research Center, Tehran University of Medical Sciences, Tehran, Iran

Abstract

Prostate cancer is the second most frequently diagnosed solid-organ malignancy in men and remains a major contributor to global cancer-related mortality. While most cases are adenocarcinomas originating from luminal epithelial cells, disease progression varies markedly, ranging from indolent localized tumors with excellent long-term survival to aggressive metastatic prostate cancer associated with poor prognosis. Despite advances in early detection and diverse therapeutic approaches, including androgen deprivation therapy, chemotherapy, immunotherapy, and next-generation targeted agents, treatment outcomes remain suboptimal, particularly in metastatic castration-resistant prostate cancer, which is frequently characterized by therapeutic resistance. Given this challenge, understanding the genetic underpinnings of prostate cancer progression has become a central priority. The CRISPR/Cas9 system, a versatile and efficient genome-editing technology, has emerged as a powerful tool for functional genomic studies, identification of metastasis-driving mutations, validation of therapeutic targets, and development of innovative precision medicine strategies. In preclinical prostate cancer models, CRISPR/Cas9 has been employed to dissect key signaling pathways, investigate drug resistance mechanisms, and design novel therapeutic interventions. Here, we highlight the latest insights into the role of CRISPR/Cas9 in prostate cancer research and therapy, highlighting its potential to reshape current treatment paradigms through gene-based precision oncology.

Keywords: prostate cancer; metastatic castration-resistant prostate cancer; CRISPR/Cas9; genome editing; metastasis; gene therapy; personalized medicine; drug resistance; precision oncology

8.1 Introduction

Representing the second most prevalent solid-organ malignancy in males [1], prostate cancer affected 1,414,259 new patients and claimed 375,304 lives [2]. While prostate cancer incidence has maintained stability between 2014–2018, it constitutes 29% of all cancer cases. Since 2011, advanced prostate cancer cases in the United States have shown an annual increase of 4–6%. The disease predominantly affects older men, with approximately 60% of cases occurring in those above 65 years. Current projections indicate 35,250 deaths in the USA by 2024, with a mortality rate of 18.8% observed from 2017–2021 [3].

Adenocarcinomas comprise over 95% of prostate cancer instances, predominantly originating from acinar rather than ductal tissue. The majority of cases (approximately 80%) emerge from luminal or basal epithelial cells within the peripheral zones, which make up more than 70% of prostatic tissue.

Localized disease characterizes roughly 80% of prostate cancer diagnoses [4]. Early detection significantly improves outcomes, with survival rates reaching 99% beyond 10 years [5]. The Cancer of the Prostate Strategic Urological Research Endeavor database indicates that despite prostate-specific antigen (PSA) testing, about 40% of new diagnoses present as intermediate-risk localized disease [6].

Metastatic spread varies, with 8% of patients showing distant metastases across multiple sites and 13% exhibiting locoregional spread. The five-year survival rate drops dramatically to 34% when distant metastases are present [7]. Metastatic prostate cancer (mPCa) causes over 400,000 annual deaths globally, with projections suggesting a doubling of this figure by 2040 [8].

Despite early diagnosis being common, treatment decisions remain complex due to significant therapy-related morbidity [9, 10]. Given that 20–30% of patients develop metastases and the emergence of metastatic castration-resistant prostate cancer (mCRPC) leads to treatment resistance, understanding metastatic mechanisms is crucial. The high mutation rate in mPCa necessitates identifying key metastasis-driving genes for personalized treatment approaches. CRISPR/Cas9 technology provides promising opportunities for identifying metastasis drivers and developing gene therapy-based treatments. This discussion examines the underlying causes of mPCa and explores recent therapeutic advances, including ongoing experimental studies.

8.2 Molecular and Genetic Landscape of Prostate Cancer

While metabolic changes are not primary cancer triggers, they enhance cancer cell growth and survival. Unlike normal cells that predominantly use aerobic metabolism, cancer cells favor anaerobic pathways. Though this glycolytic process yields less efficient ATP production, it generates energy more rapidly. Cancer cells exhibit unusual metabolic patterns, including increased fatty acid synthesis from elevated glucose intake. These malignant cells typically show heightened expression of lipogenic enzymes, including acetyl-CoA carboxylase and fatty acid synthase (FASN). Elevated FASN levels correlate with worse outcomes. Research has shown that FASN inhibition using cerulenin effectively reduces cell proliferation and triggers cell death [11].

The androgen receptor (AR) pathway plays a central role in prostate cancer development and progression. Both testosterone and 5α-dihydrotestosterone are key drivers in this process. These sex hormones influence cell growth and anti-apoptotic mechanisms by binding to gene promoter regions within the nucleus. They also affect cell cycle regulation and migration through extranuclear interactions. AKT serine/threonine kinase facilitates AR dimerization and nuclear membrane translocation. Since 80–90% of prostate malignancies depend on androgens for growth, antiandrogen therapy remains fundamental in treatment. However, some cases evolve into CRPC, which maintains growth through autonomous androgen production [12].

The AR splice variant 7 (AR-V7) involves genetic modifications of the X chromosome-located AR gene. Recent studies suggest that AR-V7 mutations correlate with more aggressive disease progression and reduced survival, though findings remain controversial. These mutations also show links to resistance against abiraterone and enzalutamide, making AR-V7 status a potential prognostic indicator for mCRPC [13]. Non-coding RNAs serve crucial regulatory functions across multiple molecular processes, including transcription and translation. They influence cancer cell proliferation, apoptosis resistance, metastasis, and treatment resistance, while also modulating AR activity. Their stability in biological fluids makes them promising biomarker candidates for liquid biopsies. Therapeutic approaches targeting these RNAs could potentially suppress AR expression and disease advancement [14].

The phosphatidylinositol 3-kinase (PI3K) signaling pathway frequently underlies castration resistance in prostate cancer, correlating with heightened tumor aggressiveness and unfavorable outcomes. This pathway mediates phosphatidylinositol-3,4,5-triphosphate (PIP3) production and AKT activation, with PTEN (phosphatase and tensin homolog) serving as a PIP3 inhibitor through plasma membrane binding. Between 70–100% of advanced prostate cancer cases exhibit PI3K/AKT/mTOR pathway irregularities. When membrane-bound PTEN is lost, PI3K pathway overactivation triggers prostatic tumorigenesis. AKT signaling inhibition shows promise in halting tumor development and reducing tumor size. The PI3K pathway's extensive involvement in castration-resistant disease includes interactions with androgen signaling mechanisms [15, 16].

Autophagy exhibits dual roles in cancer progression, initially promoting cell death in early tumor development before supporting cancer cell proliferation in established tumors. Three primary forms exist: chaperone-mediated autophagy, microautophagy, and the predominant form, macroautophagy, which maintains cellular homeostasis [17]. The process involves multiple phases from initiation through elongation to lysosomal fusion, regulated by various molecular pathways. Key regulators include AMPK (5′AMP adenosine monophosphate-activated protein kinase), mTOR (mechanistic target of rapamycin), and ATGs [18]. The PI3K/AKT/mTOR pathway plays a crucial role, with PTEN and AMPK acting as down regulators that promote autophagy. Evidence suggests the involvement of autophagy in chemotherapy resistance, warranting further investigation into autophagy modulators as potential therapeutic targets [19].

TMPRSS2 (transmembrane serine protease 2) appears predominantly in prostatic secretory epithelium, prostate cancer cells, and certain pancreatic and colon cancers. TMPRSS2-ERG gene fusions serve as molecular diagnostic markers for prostate cancer, defining fusion-positive cases. These tumors display characteristic genetic alterations, including oncogene overexpression and tumor suppressor inactivation. ERG protein influences AR pathway regulation, with stronger expression in the prostate's peripheral zone. TMPRSS2-ERG fusions disrupt cell cycle checkpoints, enhance tumor proliferation, and increase invasiveness through MMP9 and plexin A2 overexpression. This chromosome 21-affecting fusion occurs most frequently in Indian and Caucasian populations [20, 21].

A distinctive biochemical marker of prostate malignancies is the significant reduction in both citrate and zinc concentrations compared to healthy prostatic tissue. This biochemical alteration stems from the compromised ability of cancer cells to accumulate zinc, attributed to the complete or partial deletion of genes encoding zinc uptake transporters. The restoration of normal zinc levels could potentially serve as a preventive or therapeutic strategy in prostate cancer management. While healthy prostate tissue, particularly in the peripheral zone, typically maintains high zinc concentrations, this characteristic is lost in cancer cells. Given zinc's essential role in citrate synthesis, the reduction in zinc levels consequently leads to decreased citrate production. These biochemical changes often manifest during pre-malignant stages, preceding the development of frank malignancy. However, research has not demonstrated any preventive benefits from zinc dietary supplementation in prostate cancer [22].

8.3 Mechanistic Insights: CRISPR/Cas9 in Prostate Cancer-related Genes

The central role of AR in prostate cancer development has prompted various therapeutic approaches targeting this pathway. Initial successes were achieved using small interference RNA [23, 24], followed by the development of next-generation AR signaling inhibitors, bone-targeting agents, and poly(ADP-ribose) polymerase inhibitors [25]. CRISPR technology has emerged as a promising tool in this field. Wei et al. demonstrated successful AR gene elimination in androgen-positive prostate cancer cells using CRISPR/Cas methodology. Their research identified the most effective single-guide RNA (sgRNA) among three candidates targeting different AR gene regions. This approach induced targeted AR gene disruption, promoting cellular apoptosis and inhibiting proliferation, suggesting CRISPR/Cas as a viable therapeutic strategy [26].

AR signaling regulates various genes including PSA, an androgen-responsive gene [27] expressed in embryonic and cancerous prostate cells but absent in normal tissue. Researchers developed a CRISPR/dCas9-KRAB system targeting the PSA promoter to suppress PSA gene transcription. This intervention successfully inhibited tumor growth and migration while inducing apoptosis, demonstrating the potential of CRISPR-dCas9-KRAB in controlling PSA expression as a therapeutic approach [28].

The steroid type II 5-alpha-reductase (SRD5α2) enzyme, which converts testosterone to dihydrotestosterone, represents another therapeutic target in prostate cancer and benign prostatic hyperplasia. Akbaba et al. developed an innovative cationic liposome system incorporating Cas9 protein with surface-bound sgRNA. This formulation demonstrated favorable properties including stability, low toxicity, efficient cellular uptake, and effective gene knockout capability. The system achieved a 29.7% reduction in SRD5α2 mRNA expression, offering a promising alternative to conventional treatments with fewer side effects [29].

Survivin influences both AR-dependent and AR-independent drug resistance mechanisms in prostate cancer, showing increased expression in response to androgens in both AR-positive LNCaP and AR-negative cancer cells [30]. CRISPR-based Survivin suppression successfully triggered apoptosis in prostate cancer cells [31].

NANOG affects AR signaling by facilitating castration resistance through AR/FOXA1 signaling pathway suppression [32]. Kaneda et al.'s research using CRISPR/Cas9 to create NANOG- and NANOGP8-knockout DU145 cells revealed significant reductions in cancer cell characteristics including sphere formation, anchorage-independent growth, migration, and chemoresistance. While cell proliferation *in vitro* remained unchanged, tumorigenic potential decreased markedly. Their findings demonstrated equivalent roles for NANOG and NANOGP8 in cancer aggressiveness, suggesting CRISPR-based targeting of these genes as a potential therapeutic approach [33].

Researchers successfully developed mouse prostate models featuring the TMPRSS2-ERG gene fusion using CRISPR/Cas9 technology. This fusion led to ERG overexpression in cancer cells, with nilutamide (an AR antagonist) treatment normalizing fusion transcript expression. This model provides valuable insights into TMPRSS2-ERG fusion mechanisms and potential treatments [34].

The homeodomain transcription factor NKX3.1 contains androgen-responsive regions in its 3′ untranslated region [35] and functions as a crucial gatekeeper in prostate cancer. Its haplo-insufficient nature means pathogenic protein reduction can result from genetic loss, reduced transcription, or increased protein degradation due to inflammation or PTEN loss. Using CRISPR/Cas9, researchers introduced a specific missense mutation (alanine to serine at position 186) in murine Nkx3.1, affecting Dyrk1b phosphorylation. The resulting Nkx3.1S186A/– mice showed increased Nkx3.1 protein levels, reduced prostate size, normal histology, decreased cell growth, and enhanced DNA labeling. These results demonstrated

Table 8.1 CRISPR/Cas9 approaches for targeting androgen receptor signaling pathway in prostate cancer.

Target Gene or Pathway	CRISPR/Cas9-based Approach	Purpose/Effect	Cancer Type or Model	Reference
Androgen receptor	CRISPR/Cas9 with sgRNAs targeting different AR gene regions	Gene knockout, inhibition of cell proliferation, induction of apoptosis	Androgen-positive prostate cancer cells	[26]
Prostate-specific antigen	CRISPR/dCas9-KRAB system using PSA promoter	Transcriptional repression of PSA gene, inhibition of tumor growth and migration	Prostate cancer	[28]
SRD5α2 (5-alpha-reductase)	Cationic liposome encapsulated Cas9 with surface sgRNA	29.7% reduction in SRD5α2 mRNA expression	Prostate cancer/BPH	[29]
Survivin	CRISPR-mediated silencing	Induction of apoptosis in prostate cancer cells	AR-positive and AR-negative prostate cancer cells	[31]
NANOG and NANOGP8	CRISPR/Cas9 knockout	Inhibition of malignant characteristics (sphere formation, migration, chemoresistance)	DU145 prostate cancer cells	[33]
TMPRSS2-ERG fusion	CRISPR/Cas9-based technique	Creation of prostate cancer model with gene fusion, ERG overexpression	Mouse prostate models	[34]
NKX3.1	CRISPR/Cas9 missense mutation (S186A)]	Increased protein levels, reduced prostate size, decreased cell growth	Mouse prostate model	[36]

that targeted Nkx3.1 modification could provide long-term control over DNA damage-related precancerous changes, highlighting the potential of CRISPR-mediated NKX3.1 modulation as a therapeutic strategy (**Table 8.1**) [36].

8.4 CRISPR/Cas9 and PI3K/AKT/mTOR Signaling in Prostate Cancer

The PI3K/AKT/mTOR pathway, crucial in prostate cancer development, has been extensively studied using CRISPR-mediated knockout approaches. This pathway shows hyperactivation in most advanced prostate cancers, primarily through PTEN loss [37, 38]. The mTOR protein kinase, a key component of this pathway, regulates various cellular processes including growth, survival, autophagy, and metabolism [39]. mTOR forms two distinct complexes (mTORC1 and mTORC2), with DEPTOR serving as a common inhibitory component. Studies revealed decreased DEPTOR expression in prostate cancer correlating with disease progression. CRISPR-based DEPTOR elimination enhanced cellular proliferation, survival, and invasiveness, triggering AKT-dependent EMT and β-catenin nuclear translocation. Animal models demonstrated accelerated tumor growth following DEPTOR knockout, suggesting DEPTOR reactivation as a potential therapeutic strategy [40].

A novel approach utilizing aptamer-liposome CRISPR/Cas9 chimeras achieved targeted delivery to prostate cancer cells. This system incorporated RNA aptamers specifically binding to prostate-specific membrane antigen-expressing cells. The aptamer-conjugated cationic liposomes effectively delivered CRISPR/Cas9 components, achieving significant gene silencing *in vitro* and tumor regression *in vivo*. This innovation presents a versatile solution for cell-specific CRISPR/Cas9 delivery, addressing a major challenge in therapeutic applications [41].

CRISPR/Cas9 technology enabled simultaneous multi-gene modification in mouse prostate cells, focusing on the activating protein-1 (AP-1) transcription factor's role. Research showed that combined loss of either JunB or Fos with Pten deletion promoted invasive cancer progression. Fos deletion increased Jun expression, while Jun knockout reduced cell proliferation. This revealed dual roles for AP-1 factors: JunB and Fos as tumor suppressors preventing invasive disease, and Jun as an oncogene promoting cell proliferation. These findings demonstrated complex involvement of AP-1 factors in different stages of cancer progression [42, 43].

Research examining GPRC6A's role in prostate cancer focused on the "Y.K" polymorphism in its third intracellular loop, which replaced the ancestral RKLP sequence and appears in all human prostate cancer cell lines. Using CRISPR/Cas9 technology, researchers generated GPRC6A-deficient PC-3 cells to study its effects on cellular behavior. The results showed inhibition of cell proliferation and migration *in vitro*. Furthermore, xenograft studies demonstrated that GPRC6A-deficient PC-3 cells exhibited reduced proliferation and diminished response to osteocalcin-mediated cancer progression compared to GPRC6A-expressing controls. These findings suggest GPRC6A as a potential therapeutic target, particularly relevant to addressing racial disparities in prostate cancer treatment [44].

The androgen-responsive NKX3.1 gene also influences PI3K/AKT pathway activity. CRISPR-based deletion of its first exon resulted in increased prostate weight. The modified tissue showed enhanced Ki67 staining in epithelial cells alongside reduced p53 levels. Additionally, NKX3.1 deletion led to suppression of the PI3K/AKT/mTOR pathway in the affected cells [45].

8.5 CRISPR/Cas9 in Metastatic Prostate Cancer

Many mCRPC patients exhibit mutations in DNA damage response pathway genes, with a significant portion of these alterations being inherited. Gene therapy has evolved significantly through genome editing advances, with CRISPR/Cas9 emerging as a promising precision medicine tool for cancer treatment due to its exceptional accuracy and efficiency in genetic modification (**Figure 8.1**).

The CRISPR/Cas9 system consists of two key components: the Cas9 enzyme and gRNA. The Doudna laboratory pioneered the development of sgRNA capable of targeting specific DNA sequences, along with purified Cas9 enzyme that precisely cuts DNA at predetermined locations [46]. The process involves sgRNA-directed target binding, where the gRNA/Cas9 RNP complex hybridizes with specific DNA regions containing complementary protospacer sequences and protospacer-adjacent motif. This technique enables precise DNA modifications, including insertions, deletions, and single-base pair alterations [47, 48], revolutionizing multiple fields including medicine and agriculture.

Current CRISPR applications in cancer research focus on three main areas: drug resistance mechanisms, metastasis, and treatment development. Key strategies include: (i) oncogene suppression or repair of genetic mutations, such as BRCA1 and BRCA2 alterations [49], and (ii) enhancement of anti-cancer immune responses through CRISPR-engineered T cells.

8.5.1 *CRISPR/Cas9 and Drug Resistance*

Despite the survival benefits provided by AR signaling and PARP inhibitors in mPCa, the emergence of drug resistance poses a significant challenge. CRISPR/Cas9 technology offers potential solutions by identifying novel targets that could enhance the effectiveness of conventional monotherapy approaches.

Certain germline mutations, particularly those affecting homologous recombination, can predict PARP inhibitor treatment outcomes. Tsujino et al. discovered that checkpoint kinase 2 (CHEK2) deficiency leads to PARP inhibitor resistance by increasing BRCA2 expression [50]. Their comprehensive CRISPR knockout screening across four BRCA1/2-deficient prostate cancer cell lines (LNCaP, C4-2B, 22Rv1, and DU145) with and without olaparib targeted over

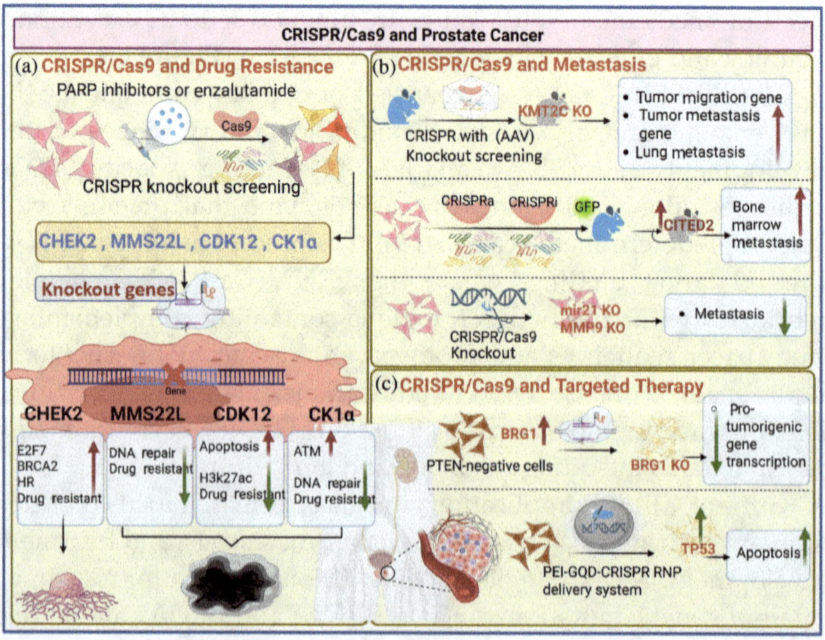

Figure 8.1 CRISPR/Cas9 applications in prostate cancer therapeutics: drug resistance, metastasis, and targeted therapy. (a) Drug resistance: CRISPR/Cas9 knockout screening identifies key genes conferring resistance to PARP inhibitors and enzalutamide in prostate cancer. Genome-wide screens revealed four critical genes: CHEK2, MMS22L, CDK12, and CK1α. Loss of CHEK2 unexpectedly confers resistance to PARP inhibition through enhanced homologous recombination via E2F7-BRCA2 upregulation, contradicting its traditional role as a BRCAness biomarker. MMS22L depletion sensitizes cells to PARP inhibitors and represents a novel predictive biomarker frequently deleted in prostate cancer. CDK12 inhibition combined with AR antagonists induces apoptosis through attenuated H3K27ac signaling on AR targets and enhanced super-enhancer-associated apoptotic pathways. CK1α knockout stabilizes ATM protein through phosphorylation, activating downstream DNA damage response signaling and sensitizing cells to enzalutamide. **(b) Metastasis:** CRISPR/Cas9 screens identify genetic drivers of prostate cancer metastasis using *in vivo* knockout models with AAV delivery. KMT2C knockout promotes tumor migration genes, tumor metastasis genes, and lung metastasis through dysregulation of a conserved genomic region on chromosome 5 (mouse) or chromosome 4 (human), particularly upregulating Odam and Cabs1 genes. Depletion of these downstream targets prevents metastasis, confirming their critical role in metastatic progression. The CRISPRa (activation) and CRISPRi (inhibition) screening approaches identified CITED2 as

Figure 8.1 (*Continued on facing page*) a novel driver of bone marrow metastasis, the most common site of prostate cancer dissemination. Combined knockout of miR-21 and MMP9 using CRISPR/Cas9 reduces metastatic potential by decreasing cell proliferation, increasing apoptosis through upregulated BAX expression, and reducing invasion capacity. **(c) Targeted therapy:** CRISPR/Cas9 enables targeted therapeutic interventions in prostate cancer through gene editing of oncogenic drivers. BRG1 upregulation occurs in PTEN-negative cells, and BRG1 knockout in PTEN-deficient models inhibits pro-tumorigenic gene transcription, establishing a synthetic lethal relationship between these genes. This approach demonstrates therapeutic potential for PTEN-deficient prostate cancers through BRG1 inhibition. The PEI-GQD CRISPR RNP delivery system enables non-viral delivery of CRISPR/Cas9 complexes to restore TP53 function in prostate cancer cells. This nanotechnology-based approach achieves 40% apoptotic cancer cell death specifically in PC-3 prostate cancer cells while sparing non-cancerous HeK293 cells, with GQD intrinsic fluorescence enabling tracking of gene editing tool delivery and nuclear localization.

18,000 protein-coding genes. Gene ontology analysis of the results revealed 67 negatively selected genes common to at least two cell lines, primarily involved in DNA repair and replication. Additionally, 103 positively selected genes shared across multiple cell lines showed enrichment in cell cycle phase transition and gene expression regulation. Notably, MMS22L loss, a component of TONSL involved in double-strand break repair at compromised replication forks [51], enhanced PARP inhibitor response through homologous recombination function impairment, with effects dependent on TP53 status.

The research also revealed an unexpected mechanism where CHEK2 loss promotes homologous recombination function through E2F7-mediated BRCA2 expression, resulting in olaparib resistance. This finding was particularly surprising given CHEK2's traditional classification as a BRCAness gene due to its role in BRCA1 phosphorylation and homologous recombination promotion, and its use as an olaparib treatment biomarker in clinical trials [52, 53]. This discovery highlights the value of CRISPR/Cas9 screening in challenging conventional understanding and revealing novel mechanisms.

Studies on AR signaling inhibition revealed significant findings. Through CRISPR/Cas9 screening combined with enzalutamide treatment, Lei and colleagues demonstrated that CDK12 plays an essential role in prostate cancer cell viability [54]. Their research showed that blocking CDK12 reduces cell growth and triggers cell death in prostate cancer cells. While these results differ from earlier studies on CDK12 loss-of-function mutations, they observed clear enhanced anti-cancer effects when combining CDK12 inhibitors with AR antagonists. These outcomes may be attributed to reduced H3K27ac signaling on AR targets and enhanced super-enhancer-related apoptotic pathways. This groundbreaking study was the first to identify CDK12 as a conserved prostate cancer target using CRISPR/Cas9 screening, suggesting its potential as a therapeutic target [54].

In a separate investigation, Liu and collaborators employed CRISPR knockout screening to identify casein kinase 1α (CK1α) as a potential target for addressing enzalutamide resistance in mPCa [55]. They found that when CK1α was either eliminated or inhibited, it led to ATM protein stabilization through phosphorylation and activated downstream DNA damage response signaling, which enhanced the effectiveness of enzalutamide treatment.

8.5.2 *CRISPR/Cas9 and Metastasis*

CRISPR technology has been instrumental in identifying crucial metastasis drivers in prostate cancer. In one breakthrough study, researchers engineered a mouse model enabling concurrent multiple gene mutations in prostate epithelial cells. This approach significantly improved upon previous methods that required time-consuming crossbreeding of multiple mouse strains. By combining CRISPR with an adeno-associated virus (AAV) delivery mechanism, scientists successfully created a mouse model exhibiting simultaneous mutations in five tumor suppressor genes (TP53, PTEN, Rb1, Stk11, and RnaseL). This innovation produced a quick-developing, invasive, androgen-independent tumor model. Further investigation of three additional gene deletions (Zbtb16, KMT2C, and Kmt2d) demonstrated that KMT2C loss was crucial for lung metastasis development, though not for tumor progression. KMT2C, a histone methyltransferase frequently mutated in various cancers [56], had previously unknown functions in prostate cancer. This research contributed both a novel CRPC mouse model and insights into metastasis mechanisms.

Research using CRISPR also uncovered mechanisms driving bone metastasis in prostate cancer [57]. Investigators developed comprehensive genome-wide CRISPRa (activation) and CRISPRi (inhibition) libraries, each containing five sgRNAs targeting 18,915 genes plus 1,895 non-targeting control sgRNAs in the non-metastatic prostate cancer cell line 22Rv1. They modified dCas9 by linking it to either a transcriptional activator (sunCas9) or repressor (dCas9-KRAB) and incorporated it into GFP-luciferase-labeled 22Rv1 cells [58]. The research identified CITED2, a transcriptional co-activator known to promote metastasis in other cancers [59], as a key bone metastasis driver in prostate cancer.

Scientists have also investigated the role of non-coding RNA in metastatic prostate cancer using CRISPR. Previous studies highlighted miR-34a's anti-cancer stem cell properties and its ability to target invasiveness and metastasis [60], leading to the development of various delivery methods [61, 62]. Additional research by Camargo et al. examined metalloproteinase 9 (MMP9) and miR-21's influence on prostate cancer metastasis [63]. MMP9, an extracellular matrix-degrading enzyme, facilitates tumor cell infiltration into other organs [64]. miR-21, which enhances MMP9 expression, shows elevated levels in prostate cancer. Its suppression reduced metastasis in xenograft models by downregulating RECK signaling [65]. miR-21 also influences BTG2, associated with prostate cancer progression [66], and MARCKS, which regulates cellular invasion [67]. When researchers introduced sgRNAs targeting MMP9 and miR-21 sequences via PX-330 plasmid into DU145 and PC-3 cells, they observed decreased cell proliferation and invasion, along with increased apoptosis through enhanced RECK expression.

8.5.3 *CRISPR/Cas9 and Targeted Therapy*

In the realm of targeted therapy, researchers have utilized CRISPR/Cas9 screening to discover novel synthetic lethal targets in mPCa. A significant study by Ding and colleagues conducted CRISPR knockout screening, both with and without PTEN suppression, to identify epigenetic regulators that create synthetic lethality in PTEN-deficient mPCa [68]. Their findings demonstrated that suppressing the SWI/SNF subunit BRG1 (SMARCA4) reduced cell proliferation specifically in PTEN-negative cells (LNCaP, C4-2, and PC3), while PTEN-competent cells (22Rv1, BPH-1, and LAPC4) remained unaffected. Testing in a PTEN-null pre-clinical model showed that BRG1 inhibition effectively slowed the progression of PTEN-deficient prostate cancer. The research revealed that increased BRG1 expression in PTEN-deficient cells triggers chromatin restructuring, leading to enhanced pro-tumorigenic gene transcription.

The effective delivery of CRISPR systems into human subjects remains a significant challenge for treatment efficacy. While AAV viral delivery systems show promise due to their reduced genomic integration risk, natural tissue specificity, and manageable immune response, they face limitations including potential carcinogenesis, restricted cargo capacity, and scaling challenges for human application. This has led to extensive research into non-viral delivery alternatives. A notable advancement came from Lee and colleagues, who developed an innovative polyethyleneimine-graphene quantum dot (PEI-GQD) CRISPR ribonucleoprotein delivery system designed to overcome physiological barriers while enabling visual gene tracking [69]. GQD technology offers significant advantages in scalability, thanks to straightforward synthesis processes and readily available source materials. This delivery method successfully restored wild-type TP53 gene function in PC-3 cells, resulting in a 40% reduction in cancer cell viability. The system induced apoptosis levels comparable to staurosporine treatment (a known apoptosis inducer), while showing minimal impact on healthy HEK293T cells. These outcomes suggest promising potential for GQD-based delivery of CRISPR-Cas9 therapeutics in clinical applications.

8.6 CRISPR/Cas9 in Regulation of Immune-related Genes and the Immune Function

CRISPR-mediated gene editing has been applied to investigate immune-related genes in prostate cancer, particularly those associated with the NF-κB signaling pathway. Research has shown that TUBB4A, which is overexpressed in prostate cancer and correlates with aggressive disease characteristics and poor survival outcomes, can be effectively targeted using CRISPR technology [70]. When TUBB4A was knocked out using CRISPR, researchers observed decreased cell growth and migration, alongside increased DNA damage markers (elevated γH2AX and 53BP1 levels). The knockout resulted in extensive DNA damage, suppressed NF-κB signaling, and inhibited both tumor growth and metastatic spread. The underlying mechanism involved reduced MYH9-dependent GSK3β ubiquitination and degradation, which subsequently led to β-catenin signaling inactivation and disrupted EMT processes.

In a separate investigation, Wang and colleagues explored the relationship between FGFR isoform conversion and prostate cancer progression [71]. Their findings demonstrated that FGF enhanced NF-κB signaling in prostate cancer cells, particularly in conjunction with FGFR1 expression. When FGFR1 was disrupted using CRISPR/Cas, both FGF activity and NF-κB signaling were suppressed. Additional research revealed that FGFR1's influence on NF-κB signaling was mediated through TGF β-activating kinase 1 (TAK1). Specifically, FGFR1 sustained NF-κB activation by reducing TAK1 degradation. This research established that FGFR1 contributes to prostate cancer progression by triggering inflammatory responses within the tumor microenvironment.

8.7 Preclinical and Clinical Insights into Therapeutic Potentials of CRISPR/Cas9

CRISPR technology has opened new avenues in prostate cancer research, particularly through its RNA-targeting capabilities, offering innovative diagnostic approaches. However, the predominant use of mouse models in these studies presents challenges for clinical translation.

Research has demonstrated that CRISPR/Cas9-based gene suppression can potentiate the effects of traditional chemotherapy, suggesting promising combination treatment strategies [72]. The technology has helped map molecular pathways involved in various stages of prostate cancer development. Through genome-wide CRISPR activation and inhibition screening, researchers have identified key regulators of metastatic processes. *In vivo* applications have clarified the roles of frequently mutated genes in tumor growth, cell fate determination, and cancer spread.

CAR-T cell therapy has shown safety and efficacy in prostate cancer patients, with evidence of T cell receptor repertoire diversification and immune microenvironment modulation [73]. CRISPR/Cas9 technology has enhanced CAR-T cell performance by improving their proliferation and persistence [74]. The system has been used to generate memory phenotypes, reduce exhaustion, and identify novel targets for improved anti-tumor activity.

The primary challenge in clinical implementation remains effective delivery of CRISPR/Cas to prostate tumors. An ideal delivery system requires a protective vehicle for RNA stability in circulation and specific targeting mechanisms [41]. This approach needs highly selective ligands with strong affinity for cellular receptors [75]. Aptamer-liposome-CRISPR/Cas9 chimeras have demonstrated promising results, showing specific cell-type binding and significant anti-tumor effects both *in vitro* and *in vivo* [41].

CRISPR therapy has achieved remarkable progress, advancing to clinical applications within just 11 years [76]. Current clinical trials are recruiting patients with both hematological malignancies (NCT05885464) and solid tumors (NCT05795595). The technology's future success in prostate cancer treatment depends on identifying optimal targets that play fundamental roles in carcinogenesis and are consistently dysregulated across diverse patient populations with varying pathological characteristics.

8.8 Future Perspectives

While CRISPR technology has not yet entered clinical trials for prostate cancer, its successful applications in other cancers, particularly in immunotherapy, suggest promising potential for prostate cancer treatment.

The success of CAR-T cell therapy in blood cancers has driven its development for mCRPC treatment. Given that solid tumors present an immunosuppressive microenvironment, enhancing T cell function is crucial for effective immunotherapy. Current clinical trials are evaluating CAR-T cells against various solid tumors, including prostate cancer, with several studies demonstrating feasibility through T cell engineering [73, 77].

CRISPR technology offers ways to enhance CAR-T cell persistence and cancer-killing capability [74]. A major advancement in cancer immunotherapy involves blocking PD-1/PD-L1 interaction between T cells and tumor cells [78]. Research by Dötsch and colleagues showed that CRISPR/Cas9-modified PD-1 knockout CD19-CAR-T cells-maintained antigen exposure sensitivity for over 390 days in immunocompetent mouse models [79]. Similarly, CRISPR-mediated LAG-3 knockout in CAR-T cells demonstrated strong antitumor activity both *in vitro* and in mouse xenografts [80].

Despite challenges like off-target effects and potential DNA cleavage-related cytotoxicity in human applications, newer techniques such as base editing and prime editing offer solutions by avoiding double-strand breaks [81].

CRISPR/Cas9 technology shows promise for both targeted gene therapy and immunotherapy advancement. It can help identify new genetic targets in mPCa to improve CAR-T cell therapy effectiveness through genetic modification. The technology's precision and efficiency make it particularly suitable for personalized medicine approaches. CRISPR/Cas9 represents a potential breakthrough in providing prostate cancer patients with effective, personalized treatment options at manageable costs.

8.9 Conclusion

Prostate cancer represents a heterogeneous malignancy in which clinical outcomes are highly dependent on the stage at diagnosis and the molecular complexity of the tumor. Although localized prostate cancer is often manageable with current therapies, a significant proportion of patients progress to advanced or metastatic disease, where therapeutic resistance and limited treatment efficacy remain critical challenges. CRISPR/Cas9 technology provides a unique opportunity to address these obstacles by enabling precise dissection of metastatic drivers, modeling of treatment resistance, and the development of novel gene editing-based therapies. Its capacity to accelerate target discovery, augment therapeutic strategies, and personalize medicine places CRISPR/Cas9 at the forefront of next-generation prostate cancer management. Nevertheless, significant barriers — including delivery systems, safety concerns, and off-target events — must be resolved before clinical translation. With continued advancements in CRISPR engineering and delivery methods, this technology holds the promise of transforming prostate cancer therapy, particularly for patients with metastatic and drug-resistant disease.

References

1. Bray F, Ferlay J, Soerjomataram I, Siegel RL, Torre LA, Jemal A. Global cancer statistics 2018: GLOBOCAN estimates of incidence and mortality worldwide for 36 cancers in 185 countries. CA Cancer J Clin. 2018;68(6):394–424.
2. Wani M, Madaan S. What Is New in the Management of High-Risk Localized Prostate Cancer? J Clin Med. 2023;12(2):455.
3. Siegel RL, Miller KD, Jemal A. Cancer statistics, 2018. CA Cancer J Clin. 2018;68(1):7–30.
4. Wasim S, Lee SY, Kim J. Complexities of Prostate Cancer. Int J Mol Sci. 2022;23(22).
5. Rebello RJ, Oing C, Knudsen KE, Loeb S, Johnson DC, Reiter RE, et al. Prostate cancer. Nat Rev Dis Primers. 2021;7(1):9.

6. Kinsella N, Helleman J, Bruinsma S, Carlsson S, Cahill D, Brown C, Van Hemelrijck M. Active surveillance for prostate cancer: a systematic review of contemporary worldwide practices. Transl Androl Urol. 2018;7(1):83–97.
7. Posdzich P, Darr C, Hilser T, Wahl M, Herrmann K, Hadaschik B, Gruenwald V. Metastatic prostate cancer — a review of current treatment options and promising new approaches. Cancers. 2023;15(2):461.
8. Sandhu S, Moore CM, Chiong E, Beltran H, Bristow RG, Williams SG. Prostate cancer. Lancet. 2021;398(10305):1075–90.
9. Cuzick J, Thorat MA, Andriole G, Brawley OW, Brown PH, Culig Z, et al. Prevention and early detection of prostate cancer. Lancet Oncol. 2014;15(11):e484–92.
10. Desai MM, Cacciamani GE, Gill K, Zhang J, Liu L, Abreu A, Gill IS. Trends in incidence of metastatic prostate cancer in the US. JAMA Network Open. 2022;5(3):e222246-e.
11. Benedettini E, Nguyen P, Loda M. The pathogenesis of prostate cancer: from molecular to metabolic alterations. Diagn Histopathol (Oxf). 2008;14(5):195–201.
12. Aurilio G, Cimadamore A, Mazzucchelli R, Lopez-Beltran A, Verri E, Scarpelli M, et al. Androgen Receptor Signaling Pathway in Prostate Cancer: From Genetics to Clinical Applications. Cells. 2020;9(12):2653.
13. Sobhani N, Neeli PK, D'Angelo A, Pittacolo M, Sirico M, Galli IC, et al. AR-V7 in Metastatic Prostate Cancer: A Strategy beyond Redemption. Int J Mol Sci. 2021;22(11):5515.
14. Yang Y, Liu KY, Liu Q, Cao Q. Androgen Receptor-Related Noncoding RNAs in Prostate Cancer. Front Cell Dev Biol. 2021;9:660853.
15. Caforio M, de Billy E, De Angelis B, Iacovelli S, Quintarelli C, Paganelli V, Folgiero V. PI3K/Akt Pathway: The Indestructible Role of a Vintage Target as a Support to the Most Recent Immunotherapeutic Approaches. Cancers (Basel). 2021;13(16):4040.
16. Crumbaker M, Khoja L, Joshua AM. AR Signaling and the PI3K Pathway in Prostate Cancer. Cancers (Basel). 2017;9(4):34.
17. Mizushima N, Ohsumi Y, Yoshimori T. Autophagosome formation in mammalian cells. Cell Struct Funct. 2002;27(6):421–9.
18. Ashrafizadeh M, Paskeh MDA, Mirzaei S, Gholami MH, Zarrabi A, Hashemi F, et al. Targeting autophagy in prostate cancer: preclinical and clinical evidence for therapeutic response. J Exp Clin Cancer Res. 2022;41(1):105.

19. Loizzo D, Pandolfo SD, Rogers D, Cerrato C, di Meo NA, Autorino R, et al. Novel Insights into Autophagy and Prostate Cancer: A Comprehensive Review. Int J Mol Sci. 2022;23(7):3826.
20. Afshari A, Janfeshan S, Yaghobi R, Roozbeh J, Azarpira N. Covid-19 pathogenesis in prostatic cancer and TMPRSS2-ERG regulatory genetic pathway. Infect Genet Evol. 2021;88:104669.
21. Khosh Kish E, Choudhry M, Gamallat Y, Buharideen SM, D D, Bismar TA. The Expression of Proto-Oncogene ETS-Related Gene (ERG) Plays a Central Role in the Oncogenic Mechanism Involved in the Development and Progression of Prostate Cancer. Int J Mol Sci. 2022;23(9):4772.
22. Costello LC, Feng P, Milon B, Tan M, Franklin RB. Role of zinc in the pathogenesis and treatment of prostate cancer: critical issues to resolve. Prostate Cancer Prostatic Dis. 2004;7(2):111–7.
23. Hååg P, Bektic J, Bartsch G, Klocker H, Eder IE. Androgen receptor down regulation by small interference RNA induces cell growth inhibition in androgen sensitive as well as in androgen independent prostate cancer cells. J Steroid Biochem Mol Biol. 2005;96(3–4):251–8.
24. Yu Y, Papukashvili D, Ren R, Rcheulishvili N, Feng S, Bai W, et al. siRNA-based approaches for castration-resistant prostate cancer therapy targeting the androgen receptor signaling pathway. Future Oncol. 2023;19(30):2055–73.
25. He Y, Xu W, Xiao YT, Huang H, Gu D, Ren S. Targeting signaling pathways in prostate cancer: mechanisms and clinical trials. Signal Transduct Target Ther. 2022;7(1):198.
26. Wei C, Wang F, Liu W, Zhao W, Yang Y, Li K, et al. CRISPR/Cas9 targeting of the androgen receptor suppresses the growth of LNCaP human prostate cancer cells. Mol Med Rep. 2018;17(2):2901–6.
27. Obinata D, Takayama K, Inoue S, Takahashi S. Exploring androgen receptor signaling pathway in prostate cancer: A path to new discoveries. Int J Urol. 2024;31(6):590–7.
28. Yang Y, Mei H, Han X, Zhang X, Cheng J, Zhang Z, et al. Synthetic CRISPR/dCas9-KRAB system driven by specific PSA promoter suppresses malignant biological behavior of prostate cancer cells through negative feedback inhibition of PSA expression. Cell Mol Biol Lett. 2023;28(1):96.
29. Akbaba H, Erel-Akbaba G, Başpınar Y, Şentürk Ş. Design of Liposome Formulations for CRISPR/Cas9 Enzyme Immobilization: Evaluation

of 5-Alpha-Reductase Enzyme Knockout for Androgenic Disorders. ACS Omega. 2023;8(48):46101–12.
30. Zhang M, Yang J, Li F. Transcriptional and post-transcriptional controls of survivin in cancer cells: novel approaches for cancer treatment. J Exp Clin Cancer Res. 2006;25(3):391–402.
31. Farhadi L, Fakhari S, Soleimani F, Jalili A. Survivin Gene Disruption via CRISPR/Cas9 Induces Apoptosis Through Down-regulation of FBXO5 and RRM2 in Prostate Cancer Cell Line PC3. Cres J Med Biol Sci. 2021;8(3):191–7.
32. Jeter CR, Liu B, Lu Y, Chao HP, Zhang D, Liu X, et al. NANOG reprograms prostate cancer cells to castration resistance via dynamically repressing and engaging the AR/FOXA1 signaling axis. Cell Discov. 2016;2:16041.
33. Kawamura N, Nimura K, Nagano H, Yamaguchi S, Nonomura N, Kaneda Y. CRISPR/Cas9-mediated gene knockout of NANOG and NANOGP8 decreases the malignant potential of prostate cancer cells. Oncotarget. 2015;6(26):22361–74.
34. Driehuis E, Clevers H. CRISPR-Induced TMPRSS2-ERG Gene Fusions in Mouse Prostate Organoids. JSM Biotechnol Biomed Eng. 2017;4(1):1076.
35. Thomas MA, Preece DM, Bentel JM. Androgen regulation of the prostatic tumour suppressor NKX3.1 is mediated by its 3′ untranslated region. Biochem J. 2010;425(3):575–83.
36. Bowen C, Shibata M, Zhang H, Bergren SK, Shen MM, Gelmann EP. CRISPR/Cas9-Mediated Point Mutation in Nkx3.1 Prolongs Protein Half-Life and Reverses Effects Nkx3.1 Allelic Loss. Cancer Res. 2020;80(21):4805–14.
37. Lee YR, Chen M, Pandolfi PP. The functions and regulation of the PTEN tumour suppressor: new modes and prospects. Nat Rev Mol Cell Biol. 2018;19(9):547–62.
38. Taylor BS, Schultz N, Hieronymus H, Gopalan A, Xiao Y, Carver BS, et al. Integrative genomic profiling of human prostate cancer. Cancer Cell. 2010;18(1):11–22.
39. Laplante M, Sabatini DM. mTOR signaling in growth control and disease. Cell. 2012;149(2):274–93.
40. Chen X, Xiong X, Cui D, Yang F, Wei D, Li H, et al. DEPTOR is an in vivo tumor suppressor that inhibits prostate tumorigenesis via the inactivation of mTORC1/2 signals. Oncogene. 2020;39(7):1557–71.

41. Zhen S, Takahashi Y, Narita S, Yang YC, Li X. Targeted delivery of CRISPR/Cas9 to prostate cancer by modified gRNA using a flexible aptamer-cationic liposome. Oncotarget. 2017;8(6):9375–87.
42. Riedel M, Berthelsen MF, Cai H, Haldrup J, Borre M, Paludan SR, et al. In vivo CRISPR inactivation of Fos promotes prostate cancer progression by altering the associated AP-1 subunit Jun. Oncogene. 2021;40(13):2437–47.
43. Riedel M, Cai H, Stoltze IC, Vendelbo MH, Wagner EF, Bakiri L, Thomsen MK. Targeting AP-1 transcription factors by CRISPR in the prostate. Oncotarget. 2021;12(19):1956–61.
44. Ye R, Pi M, Cox JV, Nishimoto SK, Quarles LD. CRISPR/Cas9 targeting of GPRC6A suppresses prostate cancer tumorigenesis in a human xenograft model. J Exp Clin Cancer Res. 2017;36(1):90.
45. Park JJ, Kim JE, Jeon Y, Lee MR, Choi JY, Song BR, et al. Deletion of NKX3.1 via CRISPR/Cas9 Induces Prostatic Intraepithelial Neoplasia in C57BL/6 Mice. Technol Cancer Res Treat. 2020;19:1533033820964425.
46. Jinek M, Chylinski K, Fonfara I, Hauer M, Doudna JA, Charpentier E. A programmable dual-RNA-guided DNA endonuclease in adaptive bacterial immunity. Science. 2012;337(6096):816–21.
47. Anzalone AV, Koblan LW, Liu DR. Genome editing with CRISPR-Cas nucleases, base editors, transposases and prime editors. Nat Biotechnol. 2020;38(7):824–44.
48. Doudna JA, Charpentier E. Genome editing. The new frontier of genome engineering with CRISPR-Cas9. Science. 2014;346(6213):1258096.
49. Witz A, Dardare J, Francois A, Husson M, Rouyer M, Demange J, et al. CRISPR/Cas9-mediated knock-in of BRCA1/2 mutations restores response to olaparib in pancreatic cancer cell lines. Sci Rep. 2023;13(1):18741.
50. Tsujino T, Takai T, Hinohara K, Gui F, Tsutsumi T, Bai X, et al. CRISPR screens reveal genetic determinants of PARP inhibitor sensitivity and resistance in prostate cancer. Nat Commun. 2023;14(1):252.
51. O'Donnell L, Panier S, Wildenhain J, Tkach JM, Al-Hakim A, Landry MC, et al. The MMS22L-TONSL complex mediates recovery from replication stress and homologous recombination. Mol Cell. 2010;40(4):619–31.
52. Abida W, Patnaik A, Campbell D, Shapiro J, Bryce AH, McDermott R, et al. Rucaparib in men with metastatic castration-resistant prostate

cancer harboring a BRCA1 or BRCA2 gene alteration. Journal of Clinical Oncology. 2020;38(32):3763–72.
53. Lord CJ, Ashworth A. BRCAness revisited. Nat Rev Cancer. 2016;16(2):110–20.
54. Lei H, Wang Z, Jiang D, Liu F, Liu M, Lei X, et al. CRISPR screening identifies CDK12 as a conservative vulnerability of prostate cancer. Cell Death Dis. 2021;12(8):740.
55. Liu J, Zhao Y, He D, Jones KM, Tang S, Allison DB, et al. A kinome-wide CRISPR screen identifies CK1α as a target to overcome enzalutamide resistance of prostate cancer. Cell Rep Med. 2023;4(4):101015.
56. Robinson D, Van Allen EM, Wu YM, Schultz N, Lonigro RJ, Mosquera JM, et al. Integrative clinical genomics of advanced prostate cancer. Cell. 2015;161(5):1215–28.
57. Arriaga JM, Ronaldson-Bouchard K, Picech F, Nunes de Almeida F, Afari S, Chhouri H, et al. In vivo genome-wide CRISPR screening identifies CITED2 as a driver of prostate cancer bone metastasis. Oncogene. 2024;43(17):1303–15.
58. Gilbert LA, Horlbeck MA, Adamson B, Villalta JE, Chen Y, Whitehead EH, et al. Genome-Scale CRISPR-Mediated Control of Gene Repression and Activation. Cell. 2014;159(3):647–61.
59. Shin SH, Lee GY, Lee M, Kang J, Shin HW, Chun YS, Park JW. Aberrant expression of CITED2 promotes prostate cancer metastasis by activating the nucleolin-AKT pathway. Nat Commun. 2018; 9(1):4113.
60. Liu C, Kelnar K, Liu B, Chen X, Calhoun-Davis T, Li H, et al. The microRNA miR-34a inhibits prostate cancer stem cells and metastasis by directly repressing CD44. Nat Med. 2011;17(2):211–5.
61. Abdelaal AM, Sohal IS, Iyer SG, Sudarshan K, Orellana EA, Ozcan KE, et al. Selective targeting of chemically modified miR-34a to prostate cancer using a small molecule ligand and an endosomal escape agent. Mol Ther Nucleic Acids. 2024;35(2):102193.
62. Li WJ, Wang Y, Liu X, Wu S, Wang M, Turowski SG, et al. Developing Folate-Conjugated miR-34a Therapeutic for Prostate Cancer: Challenges and Promises. Int J Mol Sci. 2024;25(4):2123.
63. Camargo JA, Viana NI, Pimenta R, Guimarães VR, Dos Santos GA, Candido P, et al. The Effect of Gene Editing by CRISPR-Cas9 of miR-21 and the Indirect Target MMP9 in Metastatic Prostate Cancer. Int J Mol Sci. 2023;24(19):14847.

64. Gong Y, Chippada-Venkata UD, Oh WK. Roles of matrix metalloproteinases and their natural inhibitors in prostate cancer progression. Cancers (Basel). 2014;6(3):1298–327.
65. Kim K, Kim HH, Lee CH, Kim S, Cheon GJ, Kang KW, et al. Therapeutic efficacy of modified anti-miR21 in metastatic prostate cancer. Biochem Biophys Res Commun. 2020;529(3):707–13.
66. Coppola V, Musumeci M, Patrizii M, Cannistraci A, Addario A, Maugeri-Saccà M, et al. BTG2 loss and miR-21 upregulation contribute to prostate cell transformation by inducing luminal markers expression and epithelial-mesenchymal transition. Oncogene. 2013;32(14):1843–53.
67. Li T, Li D, Sha J, Sun P, Huang Y. MicroRNA-21 directly targets MARCKS and promotes apoptosis resistance and invasion in prostate cancer cells. Biochem Biophys Res Commun. 2009;383(3):280–5.
68. Ding Y, Li N, Dong B, Guo W, Wei H, Chen Q, et al. Chromatin remodeling ATPase BRG1 and PTEN are synthetic lethal in prostate cancer. J Clin Invest. 2019;129(2):759–73.
69. Lee B, Gries K, Valimukhametova AR, McKinney RL, Gonzalez-Rodriguez R, Topkiran UC, et al. In Vitro Prostate Cancer Treatment via CRISPR-Cas9 Gene Editing Facilitated by Polyethyleneimine-Derived Graphene Quantum Dots. Adv Funct Mater. 2023;33(48):2305506.
70. Gao S, Wang S, Zhao Z, Zhang C, Liu Z, Ye P, et al. TUBB4A interacts with MYH9 to protect the nucleus during cell migration and promotes prostate cancer via GSK3β/β-catenin signalling. Nat Commun. 2022;13(1):2792.
71. Wang C, Ke Y, Liu S, Pan S, Liu Z, Zhang H, et al. Ectopic fibroblast growth factor receptor 1 promotes inflammation by promoting nuclear factor-κB signaling in prostate cancer cells. J Biol Chem. 2018;293(38):14839–49.
72. Behan FM, Iorio F, Picco G, Gonçalves E, Beaver CM, Migliardi G, et al. Prioritization of cancer therapeutic targets using CRISPR-Cas9 screens. Nature. 2019;568(7753):511–6.
73. Dorff TB, Blanchard MS, Adkins LN, Luebbert L, Leggett N, Shishido SN, et al. PSCA-CAR T cell therapy in metastatic castration-resistant prostate cancer: a phase 1 trial. Nat Med. 2024;30(6):1636–44.
74. Wei W, Chen ZN, Wang K. CRISPR/Cas9: A Powerful Strategy to Improve CAR-T Cell Persistence. Int J Mol Sci. 2023;24(15):12317.

75. Zhou J, Bobbin ML, Burnett JC, Rossi JJ. Current progress of RNA aptamer-based therapeutics. Front Genet. 2012;3:234.
76. Sheridan C. The world's first CRISPR therapy is approved: who will receive it? Nat Biotechnol. 2024;42(1):3–4.
77. Porter LH, Zhu JJ, Lister NL, Harrison SG, Keerthikumar S, Goode DL, et al. Low-dose carboplatin modifies the tumor microenvironment to augment CAR T cell efficacy in human prostate cancer models. Nat Commun. 2023;14(1):5346.
78. Nishimura H, Minato N, Nakano T, Honjo T. Immunological studies on PD-1 deficient mice: implication of PD-1 as a negative regulator for B cell responses. Int Immunol. 1998;10(10):1563–72.
79. Dötsch S, Svec M, Schober K, Hammel M, Wanisch A, Gökmen F, et al. Long-term persistence and functionality of adoptively transferred antigen-specific T cells with genetically ablated PD-1 expression. Proc Natl Acad Sci U S A. 2023;120(10):e2200626120.
80. Zhang Y, Zhang X, Cheng C, Mu W, Liu X, Li N, et al. CRISPR-Cas9 mediated LAG-3 disruption in CAR-T cells. Front Med. 2017; 11(4):554–62.
81. Wang JY, Doudna JA. CRISPR technology: A decade of genome editing is only the beginning. Science. 2023;379(6629):eadd8643.

https://doi.org/10.1142/9789819826759_0009

CHAPTER 9

CRISPR/Cas9 in the Treatment of Bladder Cancer

Mehrdad Hashemi[1,2], *Alireza Khosravinejad*[1,3], *Mina Alimohammadi*[4], *Neda Zali*[3], *Kimia Sadat Esfahani*[1,3], *Reza Mohajer Shirazi*[1,3], *Behdokht Jamali*[5], *Ali Shirazi*[1,3], *Rojin Ghannad Zadeh*[1,6], *Faranak Jamshidian*[1,7], *Najma Farahani*[1,*], *Afshin Taheriazam*[1,8,*], *Payman Rahimzadeh*[9,*], *Maliheh Entezari*[1,2,*]

[1]Farhikhtegan Medical Convergent Sciences Research Center, Farhikhtegan Hospital, Faculty of Medicine, TeMs. C., Islamic Azad University, Tehran, Iran

[2]Department of Genetics, Faculty of Advanced Sciences and Technology, TeMs. C, Islamic Azad University, Tehran, Iran

[3]Basic and Molecular Epidemiology of Gastrointestinal Disorders Research Center, Research Institute for Gastroenterology and Liver Diseases, Shahid Beheshti University of Medical Sciences, Tehran, Iran

[4]Department of Immunology, School of Medicine, Shahid Beheshti University of Medical Sciences, Tehran, Iran

[5]Department of Microbiology and Genetics, Kherad Institute of Higher Education, Bushehr, Iran

* **Corresponding authors:** Najmafarahani@gmail.com (N.F.); a.taheriazam@iautmu.ac.ir (A.T.); P.rahimzadeh76@gmail.com (P.R.); mentezari@iautmu.ac.ir (M.E.)

[6]Department of Art & Sciences, Faculty of Biology, University of North Florida, Jacksonville, Florida, USA
[7]Department of Biology, ET.C., Islamic Azad University, Tehran, Iran
[8]Department of Orthopedics, Faculty of Medicine, TeMs. C, Islamic Azad University, Tehran, Iran
[9]Surgical Research Society (SRS), Students' Scientific Research Center, Tehran University of Medical Sciences, Tehran, Iran

Abstract

CRISPR/Cas9 has rapidly transformed functional genomics and oncology by enabling precise, scalable interrogation of genetic dependencies that govern tumor initiation, progression, and therapeutic resistance, positioning gene editing as a cornerstone of emergent precision medicine in bladder cancer. Building on limitations of earlier nuclease platforms, CRISPR/Cas systems combine efficiency, modularity, and cost-effectiveness to accelerate target discovery, subtype-specific vulnerability mapping, and rational combination strategies in both non-muscle-invasive and muscle-invasive disease. In muscle-invasive bladder cancer, a clinically heterogeneous entity with poor five-year survival and limited durable benefit from current standards of care and approved second-line agents, CRISPR screening and perturbation studies illuminate drug resistance mechanisms, cell cycle regulators, oncogene/tumor-suppressor circuitry, and context-specific liabilities across molecular subtypes. These insights enable hypothesis-driven development of targeted therapeutics, syntheticlethal approaches, and immunogenetic strategies that may overcome intra- and inter-tumoral heterogeneity. This chapter synthesizes how CRISPR/Cas9 has advanced understanding of bladder cancer biology and outlines translational pathways spanning target validation, biomarker-guided patient selection, and delivery innovation required to convert these genomic insights into clinically meaningful treatments.

Keywords: CRISPR/Cas9; bladder cancer; muscle-invasive bladder cancer; precision oncology; functional genomics screens; target discovery; gene editing delivery

9.1 Introduction

Recent progress in genetic modification techniques has revealed extensive insights into how genetic alterations influence cancer development, progression, spread, and treatment resistance, emphasizing the importance of personalized therapeutic strategies based on specific tumor genetic profiles [1]. These gene modification tools allow researchers to examine gene functions both individually and across the entire genome. While zinc finger nucleases and transcription activator-like effector nucleases were previously the primary methods for genetic alterations [1], they have now been superseded by CRISPR-Cas systems, which offer greater efficiency, cost-effectiveness, and simpler design principles [2]. CRISPR-Cas has emerged as an invaluable scientific instrument for investigating various cancer aspects, including genetic factors driving tumor formation, invasiveness, and treatment resistance, potentially identifying new treatment targets [3–5]. Bladder cancer ranks as the 11th most prevalent cancer across both genders in the United Kingdom, but rises to the 8th position among men, with annual UK diagnoses exceeding 10,000 cases [6]. While non-muscle-invasive bladder cancer (NMIBC) typically has favorable treatment outcomes and survival rates [7], recurrence is frequent. Additionally, approximately 20% of NMIBC cases advance to MIBC, which has a significantly lower five-year survival rate of 45% [6], and once the disease spreads to lymph nodes or other organs, it becomes incurable. The established treatment protocol for MIBC encompasses chemotherapy, complete bladder removal (radical cystectomy), or radiation therapy combined with radiosensitizing agents, while immunotherapy is utilized for metastatic cases [8, 9]. Although targeted therapeutic options for bladder cancer remain sparse, certain treatments such as PDL1 and FGFR3 inhibitors have received approval for use as secondary treatment options when initial therapies fail [10]. Nevertheless, these alternative treatments show limited effectiveness due to persistent resistance issues [10–12]. Research has identified six distinct molecular classifications of MIBC: luminal papillary, luminal non-specified, luminal unstable, stroma-rich, basal-squamous, and neuroendocrine-like [6, 13, 14]. Each subtype exhibits unique treatment response patterns and inherent therapy resistance, significantly impacting patient survival. This highlights the urgent need for new therapeutic approaches to tackle both within-tumor and between-tumor diversity in bladder cancer, an area where CRISPR technologies could provide crucial insights. This article examines how CRISPR-Cas9 genetic modification tools have enhanced our comprehension of MIBC for identifying novel therapeutic targets, and explores potential future applications to enhance treatment outcomes.

9.2 Molecular and Genetic Landscape of Bladder Cancer

Advanced sequencing technologies have enabled comprehensive molecular profiling of bladder cancer patient tumors. Analysis of whole-transcriptome mRNA from patient samples has established a molecular classification system [15–18], though some variations exist in subtype classifications due to patient selection criteria, methodological differences [19–21], and clinical-pathological parameters [22]. Among human cancers, bladder cancer shows one of the highest mutation frequencies, ranking third after lung and skin cancers [23, 24]. Notably, mutations in the TERT promoter region are particularly prevalent, occurring in 70–80% of bladder cancer patients [25–28]. These genetic findings have spurred the development of innovative therapeutic strategies and improved surveillance methods, including urine and blood-based monitoring for early detection and treatment response assessment.

Clinical statistics show that NMIBC accounts for approximately 80% of bladder cancer diagnoses, with generally favorable prognosis (>85% 5-year survival rate [29]) and low progression risk to invasive disease [30, 31]. However, despite scientific and clinical advances, NMIBC's five-year survival rates have remained relatively stagnant, and its high recurrence rate continues to burden healthcare systems [29, 32, 33]. Genetic studies have revealed several key alterations in NMIBC, including chromosome 9 deletions (affecting CDKN2A), mutations in FGFR3 and PI3K genes, and TERT promoter modifications, which appear early in urothelial cancer development [34–36]. A comprehensive transcriptional analysis by Hedegaard et al. (UROMOL study) examined 460 early-stage NMIBC patients (345 Ta stage, 112 T1 stage, 3 carcinoma *in situ*) and 16 MIBC patients, identifying three main subclasses with basal-like and luminal-like characteristics, each showing distinct clinical outcomes [37].

Research shows Class 1 tumors are characterized by early cell cycle gene expression and favorable outcomes. Class 2 tumors, displaying elevated late cell cycle gene expression, are typically associated with high-risk NMIBC. Both Class 1 and 2 tumors demonstrate high uroplakin expression, indicating luminal/umbrella cell characteristics. Class 3 tumors show increased expression of KRT5 and KRT15 (basal cell markers) and elevated long non-coding RNA (lncRNA) levels. Class 2 tumors correlate with reduced survival rates compared to Classes 1 and 3. Significantly, the classification of 14 out of 16 MIBC cases as Class 2 demonstrates the similarity between MIBC and high-risk NMIBC.

A proteomic analysis of 117 patient samples (98 NMIBC, 19 MIBC) identified three NMIBC proteomic subtypes (NPS) [38]. NPS1, comprising 17% (17/98) of cases, primarily consisted of T1 grade 3 high-risk samples with enhanced immune/inflammatory profiles. NPS2 (43%, 42/98) displayed immune-infiltrated/mesenchymal characteristics. NPS3 (40%, 39/98) showed enrichment of luminal differentiation markers (KRT20, CDH1, uroplakins) and undifferentiation markers (KRT5, ITGA6/ITGB4), similar to UROMOL study's Classes 1 and 3. NPS3 patients demonstrated better survival outcomes within the lowest risk group. Future research aims to integrate genomic, transcriptomic, and proteomic classifications while improving data collection feasibility for informed clinical decisions.

For MIBC, where cancer has invaded the muscle layer beyond the epithelium, understanding molecular signatures and subtypes is crucial. Multiple classification studies culminated in a consensus MIBC molecular classification system integrating six distinct subtypes [39]: luminal papillary (LumP), luminal non-specified (LumNS), luminal unstable (LumU), stroma-rich, basal/squamous (Ba/Sq), and neuroendocrine-like (NE-like). This unified classification system aligns well with previous classification studies [39].

The consensus classification reveals that luminal tumors (LumP, LumNS, LumU) demonstrate urothelial differentiation characteristics, activated PPARG and GATA3 regulons, and FGFR3 genetic modifications. LumP represents the most favorable subtype, typically occurring in younger patients with lower-stage (T2) disease. These tumors frequently show FGFR3 mutations and enhanced FGFR3 regulon activity, suggesting potential responsiveness to FGFR3 inhibitors. LumP tumors also feature KDM6A mutations and CDKN2A deletions, while maintaining wild-type TP53.

LumNS tumors often present with micropapillary features and carcinoma *in situ*, showing PPARG amplification, increased PPARG target gene expression, and ELF3 mutations. LumU tumors demonstrate significant genomic instability, copy number variations, and increased APOBEC family mutations. They also show the highest frequency of TP53 and ERCC2 mutations, with ERCC2 mutations linked to chemotherapy sensitivity.

The stroma-rich subtype shows moderate urothelial differentiation with notable stromal cell infiltration and elevated smooth muscle, endothelial, fibroblast, and myofibroblast signatures, along with increased T and B cell markers. Ba/Sq tumors express high levels of basal cell markers (KRT14, KRT5, KRT6) while lacking luminal markers (GATA3, FOXA1). These aggressive tumors, more common in female patients, frequently show TP53 and RB1 mutations, with activated STAT3, HIF1A, and EGFR regulons.

The NE-like subtype is highly uniform, with 81% showing neuroendocrine features and immune infiltration. These tumors universally carry TP53 mutations alongside RB1 mutations and deletions, representing the most aggressive subtype with only 1-year median overall survival. While current MIBC molecular subtyping primarily focuses on mRNA expression (less than 2% of total transcription), Robertson et al. examined non-coding RNA expression patterns, including lncRNAs and microRNAs [18].

Analysis of lncRNA patterns identified a distinct tumor group characterized by high purity, papillary morphology, and organ-confined disease [18], findings later confirmed in subsequent research [40]. These tumors exhibited enhanced activity in pathways involving FGFR3, Sonic hedgehog, and wild-type p53 proteins [18]. Given that protein-coding regions comprise only 1.1% of the human genome, with the majority consisting of intronic (24%) and intergenic (75%) DNA [41], alterations in these non-coding regions are relatively common. Researchers studying bladder cancer have focused on specific mutation patterns, particularly APOBEC-associated C>T and C>G mutations [42]. Notably, MIBC shows the highest concentration of APOBEC-specific mutations among all cancer types. The most well-documented example of APOBEC-specific mutations occurs in the TERT gene promoter region, with bladder cancer showing the highest mutation frequency in this area [43].

9.3 Targeting Oncogenes or Restoring Tumor Suppressor Gene Functions in Bladder Cancer with CRISPR/Cas9

Research utilizing CRISPR-Cas technology has enhanced our understanding of both tumor suppressors and oncogenes. Studies have revealed that the transcription factor KLF4 exhibits tissue-specific effects in different cancers [47]. Reduced KLF4 expression correlates with disease progression and enhanced epithelial-mesenchymal transition (EMT), while increased KLF4 levels are linked to reduced tumor advancement in later-stage disease [47].

Scientists employed CRISPR-mediated KLF4 activation in T24 MIBC cells to investigate its antitumor mechanisms [48]. Their findings demonstrated that enhanced KLF4 expression inhibits T24 cell growth by modulating AKT-p21 signaling pathways, resulting in G1 phase cell cycle arrest. Additionally, KLF4 upregulation diminished the cells' invasive and migratory capabilities while suppressing EMT. The researchers proposed that this CRISPR activation approach could potentially serve as an innovative therapeutic strategy for MIBC, pending clinical validation [48].

Recent research has highlighted the significant role of epigenetic regulators as tumor suppressors across various cancers [49]. These genes influence cancer development through their effects on cell proliferation, differentiation, and metastatic potential [49, 50].

Research using CRISPR-Cas9 to eliminate these epigenetic regulators in bladder cancer cell lines, either individually or together, resulted in markedly increased cell proliferation, with dual knockout showing the most pronounced effect. The histone demethylases UTX and UTY, located on the X and Y chromosomes respectively, frequently display mutations and copy number alterations in bladder cancer [51]. These laboratory findings align with clinical observations from MIBC and high-grade bladder cancer patients, who often exhibit decreased UTX/UTY copy numbers and truncating mutations, supporting their tumor-suppressive function [51]. This research also emphasizes the importance of X-Y gene pairs in cancer development, particularly relevant in bladder cancer where male patients show higher incidence rates [51].

Subsequent investigations explored therapeutic targeting possibilities of UTX loss of function. Research revealed that UTX counteracts EZH2, a methyltransferase involved in histone modification [52]. UTX deletion produces effects similar to EZH2 overexpression [52]. Studies demonstrated that inhibiting EZH2 both delayed tumor formation and reduced tumor growth in xenograft mouse models using UTX-knockout cells and patient-derived tumors [52]. This suggests potential therapeutic applications of EZH2 inhibitors for bladder cancer patients with UTX mutations [52].

However, UTX's role as part of the COMPASS histone H3K4 methylase family necessitates further investigation into other complex components, including frequently mutated MLL3 and MLL4 proteins, as the complete role of COMPASS in cancer development remains unclear [53].

Alternative CRISPR applications have also shown promise. For instance, the RNA-targeting Cas13 system was employed to degrade MYC mRNA oncogene, resulting in decreased MYC protein and mRNA levels, leading to reduced bladder cancer cell growth and enhanced cell death [54]. The advantage of this approach lies in its direct targeting of cytoplasmic mRNA, enabling faster gene expression reduction without DNA alterations [55]. While promising for MIBC treatment, *in vivo* validation remains necessary.

CRISPR-Cas9 has proven valuable in identifying functions of potential oncogenes and tumor suppressors. lncRNAs, despite lacking protein-coding capacity, influence various cellular processes including transcriptional regulation, epigenetic control, and chromosome stability [56]. Their role in cancer has gained increasing attention, with CRISPR-Cas9 helping elucidate their effects.

Research has shown that lncRNA SNHG3 contributes to bladder cancer progression, showing elevated expression in tumor tissues and correlating with poor outcomes. CRISPR-Cas9-mediated SNHG3 elimination in MIBC cell lines decreased cell proliferation, migration, invasion, and angiogenesis [57]. Studies revealed that SNHG3 stabilizes BMI1 through MYC binding, inhibiting cell senescence and correlating with poor prognosis across multiple cancers [57]. These findings suggest the SNHG3-MYC-BMI1 pathway as a potential therapeutic target for controlling MIBC tumor growth and metastasis [57].

The effectiveness of CRISPR screens relies heavily on functional assays that can distinguish and enrich different cellular behavioral patterns. While many assays utilize simple survival-based responses to drug treatments or other challenges, more sophisticated approaches combine CRISPR and homology-directed repair to generate reporter systems. These systems often involve inserting fluorescent protein genes into specific genetic locations, allowing cell population separation based on fluorescence intensity that corresponds to gene activity.

A 2023 investigation demonstrated this approach by using CRISPR-Cas9 to insert eGFP into the PPARγ gene locus [58]. PPARγ, a transcription factor known to promote tumor growth, shows increased expression in luminal bladder cancers [58]. Following a whole-genome CRISPR screen (WGCS), researchers could separate cells based on PPARγ expression levels, enabling identification of genes controlling PPARγ expression [58].

The study identified and validated several genes as potential PPARγ expression regulators, including GATA3, SPT6, SMC1A, and RAD21, suggesting these as possible therapeutic targets for luminal bladder cancer treatment [58]. While these findings were supported by TCGA mRNA expression data, it's important to note that mRNA levels may not accurately reflect protein expression and activity. Furthermore, the lack of *in vivo* validation raises questions about the clinical applicability of these targets (**Table 9.1**).

This methodology highlights the evolving sophistication of CRISPR-based screening approaches, while also emphasizing the importance of comprehensive validation before clinical translation.

9.4 CRISPR/Cas9 in Overcoming Drug Resistance

In MIBC patients, chemotherapy resistance is a common challenge, primarily resulting from adaptive mechanisms within tumors, such as increased drug efflux pump expression, enhanced anti-apoptotic signaling, and heightened DNA repair capabilities [59–61]. While these resistance mechanisms are recognized, their complete understanding remains incomplete, leading to treatment failures. CRISPR screening has emerged as a valuable tool for identifying genetic factors involved in these resistance mechanisms.

WGCS revealed multiple genes influencing chemotherapy response in MIBC. Given cisplatin's role as a primary MIBC treatment [8], understanding resistance mechanisms and genetic factors affecting treatment sensitivity is crucial. A significant WGCS finding demonstrated that eliminating SLFN11 induces chemotherapy resistance [62]. This discovery was confirmed through both animal models and patient tumor analysis [62]. Research showed that following cisplatin-induced DNA damage, SLFN11 regulates cell cycle progression through interaction with MDC1 protein [62].

These findings suggest that elevated SLFN11 expression could predict favorable responses to neoadjuvant chemotherapy [63]. Given SLFN11's chemosensitizing effects across various cancers [63], researchers have proposed using epigenetic modifications to

Table 9.1 CRISPR applications in bladder cancer research.

Target Gene or Pathway	CRISPR-based Technique Used	Biological Function	Observed Effects	Therapeutic Implication	References
KLF4	CRISPR activation	Transcription factor with dual roles in cancer	Suppressed proliferation, reduced invasion/ migration, inhibited EMT via AKT-p21 signaling	Novel therapeutic strategy for MIBC through KLF4 activation	[47, 48]
UTX/UTY	CRISPR/Cas9 knockout	Histone demethylases (epigenetic regulators)	Increased cell proliferation, tumor suppressor role identified	EZH2 inhibition as therapeutic approach for UTX-mutated cancers	[51]
EZH2	Not specified (inhibition study)	Histone methyltransferase	Delayed tumor onset, suppressed tumor growth in UTX knockout models	Targeted therapy for UTX-mutant bladder cancers	[52]
MYC oncogene	Cas13 RNA-targeting	Oncogene regulation	Reduced mRNA/protein expression, decreased proliferation, increased apoptosis	Targeted RNA degradation therapy for MIBC	[54]
SNHG3 lncRNA	CRISPR-Cas9 knockout	Non-coding RNA regulation	Reduced proliferation, migration, invasion, angiogenesis; stabilized BMI1 via MYC binding	Targeting SNHG3-MYC-BMI1 axis for tumor growth regulation	[57]
PPARγ regulatory network	CRISPR/Cas9 with eGFP knockin	Transcription factor driving tumor growth	Identified GATA3, SPT6, SMC1A, RAD21 as PPARγ regulators	Potential druggable targets for luminal bladder cancer therapy	[58]

increase SLFN11 expression as a strategy to restore cisplatin sensitivity in resistant tumors [64]. Clinical trials investigating various epigenetic modulator inhibitors targeting DNA methyltransferases, histone lysine methyltransferases, and histone lysine acetyltransferases have shown promising results when combined with standard treatments across different cancer types [65], suggesting potential therapeutic applications.

Research suggests that reduced DNA-damage response likely occurs through MSH2's role in recruiting ERCC1, a known cisplatin resistance indicator, during DNA mismatch repair processes [66]. Clinical data shows that reduced MSH2 expression in MIBC patient tumors correlates with shorter survival times and worse outcomes, suggesting MSH2's potential as a cisplatin sensitivity biomarker. Additional resistance mechanisms involve circLIFR, a circular RNA that triggers apoptosis through MSH2 interaction [65].

WGCS research identified HNRNPU as a key factor in cisplatin resistance in T24 MIBC cells. HNRNPU elimination decreased cell proliferation and migration while enhancing cisplatin-induced apoptosis [67]. This effect occurs through regulation of NF1, a tumor suppressor gene involved in chemotherapy sensitivity. CRISPR-Cas9 removal of HNRNPU increases NF1 expression in T24 cells, enhancing cisplatin sensitivity [67]. Importantly, eliminating NF1 reverses the increased chemosensitivity seen in HNRNPU-knockout cells, confirming NF1's role in mediating HNRNPU's effects [67]. Analysis of TCGA data revealed that elevated HNRNPU expression correlates with reduced survival in MIBC patients [67], suggesting HNRNPU inhibition as a potential strategy for restoring cisplatin sensitivity [67].

While CRISPR technology has helped identify various chemotherapy resistance factors, further *in vivo* validation is necessary before clinical trials can begin. Current research has focused primarily on cisplatin resistance, despite the use of multiple chemotherapy agents in bladder cancer treatment. This suggests an opportunity for additional CRISPR screening studies to identify genetic factors influencing responses to other chemotherapeutic agents.

9.5 CRISPR/Cas9 and Immunotherapy

Immunotherapy has significantly enhanced bladder cancer treatment, proving effective for MIBC in both initial and subsequent treatment phases, with considerable potential for expanded applications [68]. CRISPR-Cas systems have become vital tools for understanding and identifying new immunotherapy targets.

Various immunotherapeutic approaches are under clinical investigation for MIBC treatment, with particular focus on inhibitors targeting PD1, PDL1, and CTLA4. A notable clinical trial demonstrated that combining the PD1 inhibitor nivolumab with gemcitabine and cisplatin chemotherapy improved complete response rates, reducing the necessity for radical cystectomy in MIBC patients [69]. While these inhibitors function by preventing T cell-mediated tumor killing suppression, CRISPR gene editing could provide deeper insights into these mechanisms, though this approach remains underutilized in bladder cancer studies.

Research examining immune checkpoint protein expression in tumors and circulating blood lymphocytes has yielded important findings. A comparative study of peripheral blood mononuclear cells from bladder cancer patients and healthy individuals revealed elevated PD1 and CTLA4 expression in MIBC patients [70]. In experiments co-culturing MIBC cells with CTLs, CRISPR-Cas9-mediated CTLA4 deletion in CTLs enhanced their anti-tumor activity by increasing MIBC cell apoptosis, demonstrating CTLA4's role in immune evasion [70]. These findings were further validated in mouse bladder cancer models [70].

The development of checkpoint inhibitor resistance in tumors has prompted researchers to use CRISPR technology to investigate resistance mechanisms, particularly regarding PD1. A significant study demonstrated that simultaneously eliminating both PDCD1 (which encodes PD1) and the lncRNA UCA1 using CRISPR-Cas9 enhanced PD1-based antitumor effects in bladder cancer cells, both in laboratory conditions and animal models, resulting in decreased tumor growth and extended survival [71].

Experiments using humanized severe combined immunodeficient mice implanted with PD1 and UCA1-knockout human bladder cancer cells revealed a transformation in the tumor microenvironment from immunosuppressive to stimulatory. This change occurred through increased expression of immune-stimulating genes associated with T helper 1 cells [72]. These findings suggest potential benefits of combination approaches to enhance PD1 immunotherapy effectiveness.

However, this combined PD1-UCA1 targeting strategy awaits clinical testing. Additionally, therapeutic approaches based on lncRNAs face challenges in development, particularly due to patient-to-patient variations in lncRNA expression patterns [73].

Collectively, **Figure 9.1** represents an illustrative view of the substantial role of CRISPR/Cas9 in bladder cancer drug resistance and immunotherapy.

9.6 Preclinical Insights into CRISPR/Cas9-based Gene Therapy

While CRISPR gene editing shows tremendous potential for cancer treatment, several obstacles prevent its direct therapeutic application through gene therapy. Currently, CRISPR-Cas gene editing has found successful therapeutic use primarily in monogenic disorders, such as sickle cell disease, using hematopoietic stem and progenitor cell transplantation [74]. This approach involves eliminating existing stem cells through chemotherapy before introducing CRISPR-Cas9-modified stem cells to rebuild blood and immune systems [74]. Cancer's complexity, involving multiple patient-specific genetic mutations, presents a stark contrast to simpler monogenic disorders.

Nevertheless, CRISPR has enhanced existing cancer treatments, notably CAR-T cell therapy. While effective against acute lymphoblastic leukemia, traditional CAR-T cell therapy faces delays due to patient-specific cell requirements. Researchers addressed this by using CRISPR-Cas9 to modify CD19 and CD22-targeting CAR-T cells, disrupting TRAC region and CD52 gene to prevent rejection.

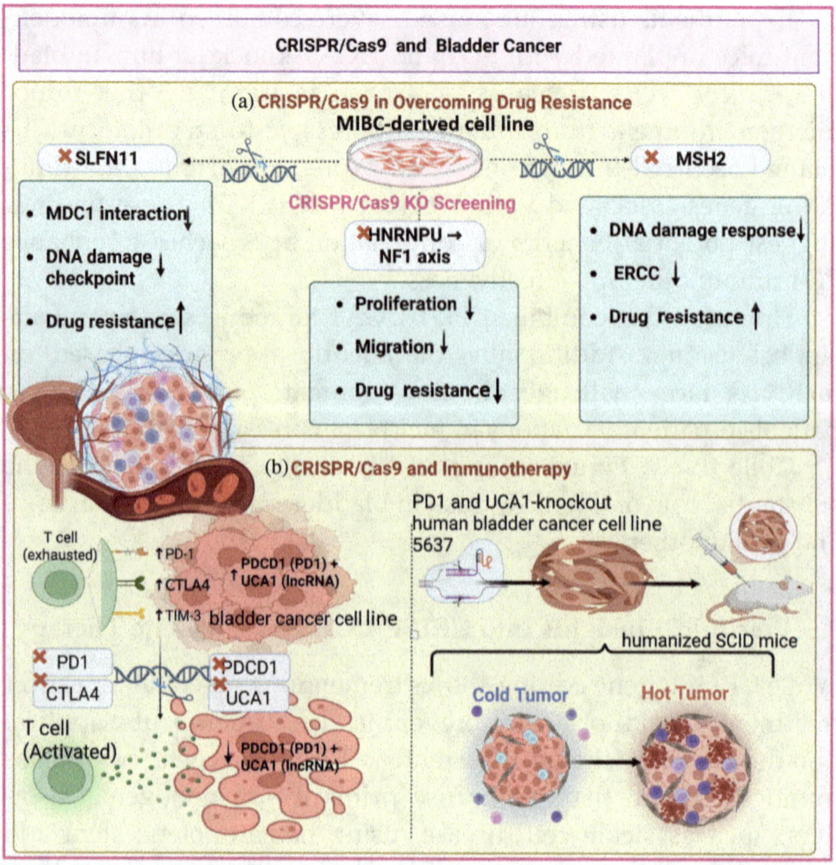

Figure 9.1 CRISPR/Cas9 applications in bladder cancer: drug resistance and immunotherapy enhancement. Two major applications of CRISPR/Cas9 technology in bladder cancer management, focusing on overcoming chemotherapy resistance and enhancing immunotherapy efficacy, are summarized here. **(a) Drug resistance:** CRISPR/Cas9 knockout screening in MIBC-derived cell lines identifies

These modified cells demonstrated positive anticancer responses with minimal side effects when administered to patients [75].

Though successful in blood cancers, adapting these CRISPR-mediated therapies to solid tumors, including bladder cancer, remains challenging. However, preclinical studies show promise, particularly in T cell receptor (TCR) therapy development. This approach uses genetically modified T cells designed to recognize

Figure 9.1 (*Continued on facing page*) critical genes mediating cisplatin resistance. SLFN11 knockout confers chemotherapy resistance through decreased MDC1 (mediator of DNA damage checkpoint 1) interaction, attenuating DNA damage checkpoint activation and reducing drug-induced apoptosis. SLFN11 functions as a potent mediator of cisplatin sensitivity, and its loss represents a mechanism of acquired resistance to platinum-based chemotherapy in bladder cancer. Conversely, WGCS identified MSH2 as the most significantly enriched gene promoting cisplatin resistance. MSH2 knockout reduces cisplatin-mediated apoptosis, diminishes DNA damage response signaling, and impairs ERCC pathway activity, collectively increasing drug resistance. Clinical validation demonstrated that bladder tumors with low MSH2 protein levels exhibit poorer survival when treated with cisplatin- or carboplatin-based therapy, establishing MSH2 as a predictive biomarker for platinum-based chemotherapy response. HNRNPU represents another critical determinant of cisplatin sensitivity identified through CRISPR screening. HNRNPU knockout activates the NF1 axis, decreasing cell proliferation, migration, and drug resistance in bladder cancer cells. RNA sequencing analysis revealed that HNRNPU knockout rewires the transcriptome by downregulating cancer-related pathways (TGF-beta, oncostatin M, focal adhesion) while upregulating DNA repair pathways (double-strand break repair, ATM pathway) and cell cycle checkpoints, sensitizing cells to cisplatin treatment. **(b) Immunotherapy:** CRISPR/Cas9-mediated dual targeting of immune checkpoints and oncogenic lncRNAs demonstrates synergistic antitumor effects in bladder cancer. Combined knockout of PD-1 and UCA1 in 5,637 human bladder cancer cells induces superior therapeutic responses compared to single-agent approaches. UCA1 knockout promotes apoptosis of bladder cancer cells, while PD-1 gene ablation achieved through electroporation of gRNA/Cas9 complexes enhances T cell activation. In humanized severe combined immunodeficient mouse xenograft models, CRISPR/Cas9 treatment upregulates dendritic cell maturation markers (CD80, CD83, CD86) and increases pro-inflammatory cytokine expression (IL-6, IL-12, IL-23, TNF-α). Co-administration of anti-PD-1 and anti-UCA1 treatment suppresses tumor growth and significantly improves survival by transforming immunologically "cold" tumors with minimal T cell infiltration into "hot" tumors characterized by robust immune activation. The combination therapy increases interferon-gamma production by T cells, enhances Th1-associated immune-stimulating gene expression, reduces regulatory/suppressive immune gene transcription, and reshapes the tumor microenvironment from an immunosuppressive to a stimulatory state. Additionally, anti-UCA1 treatment induces interferon-gamma-dependent PD-L1 expression within xenograft tumors, providing mechanistic rationale for checkpoint blockade synergy. This dual-targeting CRISPR strategy also affects CTLA-4 and TIM-3 checkpoint molecules on exhausted T cells, with combined genetic and antibody-based blockade demonstrating potent synergistic effects that support the translational potential of combination immunotherapy for clinical bladder cancer treatment.

specific tumor markers [76], aiming to target cancer cells while sparing healthy tissue.

Initial success in patient-derived xenograft tumors led to clinical trials testing TCR therapy across various cancers, including lung, renal cell, and gastrointestinal cancers, with varying outcomes [77, 78]. A 2023 study developed patient-specific TCR therapy using peripheral blood mononuclear cells from solid tumor patients [79]. This method compared germline and tumor DNA to identify patient-specific mutations, followed by CRISPR-Cas9 modification of T cells to target tumor-specific neoantigens [79].

The process involved eliminating endogenous TRAC and TRBC genes while introducing engineered neoantigen-specific TCRs [79]. Researchers used DNA plasmids designed for homologous recombination with the TRAC site to express neoantigens on T cell surfaces. After reintroduction into patients, these modified T cells successfully targeted tumor sites [79]. Remarkably, some patients with treatment-resistant cancers, who had previously undergone six therapy rounds, showed disease stabilization or tumor reduction within 28 days post-infusion [79]. These results demonstrated both the safety and potential therapeutic value of transgenic T cells in treating various solid tumors.

While CAR-T cell therapy offers powerful and rapid tumor elimination, its effectiveness decreases as target antigen expression increases [80]. In contrast, TCR therapy maintains high proliferation rates even in antigen-rich environments, sustaining effective tumor clearance [80]. This suggests that combining TCR therapy with CRISPR-Cas9 modifications might prove more effective across diverse tumor antigen presentations than CAR-T cell approaches [80].

A key challenge in drug effectiveness involves penetrating the extracellular matrix to reach tumor cells. Researchers addressed this in 5A2-SC8 liver cells by using liquid nanoparticles to simultaneously deliver extracellular matrix-degrading focal adhesion kinase-targeting siRNA along with Cas9 mRNA and PDL1-targeting single-guide RNA [81].

The introduction of focal adhesion kinase-targeting siRNA reduced extracellular matrix density, producing two significant results: it enhanced CRISPR-mediated gene editing efficiency tenfold in tumor spheroid models and improved immune cell penetration, leading to reduced tumor growth in mouse studies [81]. These findings suggest promising potential for developing novel CRISPR-Cas9 therapies for solid tumors, including bladder cancer applications.

Several CRISPR-based therapeutic trials are currently underway. One phase I/II trial is recruiting metastatic gastrointestinal epithelial cancer patients to test CRISPR-Cas9-modified neoantigen-specific tumor infiltrating lymphocytes targeting the CISH immune checkpoint [82]. Another phase I/II trial is evaluating CRISPR-Cas9-edited CAR-T cells in patients with treatment-resistant solid tumors [83]. However, these trials remain in early stages, primarily focusing on safety and dosage optimization, with considerable research needed before clinical implementation.

Despite these limitations, progress in translating these therapies to solid tumors offers hope for treating bladder tumors using gene editing approaches. TCR therapies designed for specific tumor neoantigens could prove particularly valuable in bladder cancer, where tumor heterogeneity poses a significant challenge. The high tumor mutational burden of bladder tumors makes them especially suitable for TCR therapies, as increased tumor mutational burden provides more targetable neo-antigens, potentially improving treatment outcomes [84].

9.7 Challenges and Ethical Considerations

A significant limitation in cancer-focused CRISPR research is the predominance of *in vitro* studies over *in vivo* investigations. While CRISPR-Cas9 screening has proven valuable for identifying potential therapeutic targets, clinical translation remains crucial. This necessitates development of more accessible *in vivo* CRISPR-Cas9 methodologies to validate screening results and accelerate clinical implementation. Such models could encompass animal studies, tumor xenografts, and conditional tissue-specific knockouts for examining gene functions at the tissue level.

Regarding CRISPR-based therapeutic development, safe delivery systems remain a major challenge. These treatments must specifically target tumor cells while avoiding damage to healthy cells and preventing off-target effects — a critical consideration for clinical translation [85]. Off-target modifications could have severe consequences, potentially triggering new cancer-causing mutations.

However, current preclinical and clinical trials combining CRISPR-Cas9-based therapeutics with various systemic treatments have shown minimal off-target effects, suggesting that CRISPR-Cas9 gene editing maintains high targeting specificity. This encouraging finding supports the potential for expanding these therapies into larger-scale clinical trials [86].

GUIDE-seq technology has revolutionized the detection of off-target effects by employing double-stranded oligodeoxynucleotides to locate double-strand breaks, thereby enabling comprehensive genome-wide analysis of unintended CRISPR modifications [87]. Current applications of CRISPR-Cas therapeutic approaches are primarily focused on conditions where genetic markers are well-defined or where edited components can be easily delivered to target cells. In the context of sickle cell disease treatment, the process is relatively straightforward since it involves *ex vivo* manipulation, where hematopoietic stem and progenitor cells are removed, modified, and then reintroduced to patients [74].

The ability to reach specific tissues or organs remains a critical challenge in gene editing. While some organs, such as the liver, have shown accessibility through lipid nanoparticle delivery systems for treating conditions like transthyretin amyloidosis [88], targeting bladder cancer cells *in situ* continues to pose significant challenges [88, 89]. Progress in CRISPR-based treatments for MIBC depends on developing effective delivery methods that minimize off-target effects.

The implementation of CRISPR-Cas gene editing in clinical settings raises various ethical concerns. These include considerations regarding both somatic cell modifications and the introduction of CRISPR-edited cells into patients. Given the nascent stage of these technologies, limited long-term data restricts their widespread clinical adoption [90]. Public understanding and openness about CRISPR-Cas therapies will be essential for their successful clinical integration [91]. The ethical implications are less concerning when modifying an individual's own cells, as the effects remain limited to the patient, unlike germline modifications which could impact future generations [92]. However, since the complete long-term effects of CRISPR-Cas9 human genome editing remain uncertain, strict regulatory oversight is essential to maintain patient safety.

9.8 Future Perspectives

To identify both subtype-specific vulnerabilities and shared pathway dependencies, comprehensive CRISPR-based knockout and activation screening should be implemented across different bladder cancer subtypes, which could inform biomarker-guided clinical trials.

CRISPR modification techniques should be employed to investigate resistance mechanisms against various treatments, including chemotherapy, radiation therapy with sensitizing agents, FGFR3 inhibitors, and PD(L)1 immune checkpoint blockade. This approach would help identify effective combination strategies to prevent or overcome treatment resistance, particularly focusing on DNA damage response pathways, ERBB/PI3K signaling interactions, and EMT/stemness regulatory networks.

A combined approach utilizing base and prime editing for specific allele modification, along with CRISPRi/a for adjustable gene regulation, should be implemented to evaluate therapeutic candidates based on their efficacy and safety profiles. This strategy would be particularly valuable for developing degrader-compatible targets or identifying opportunities for antisense/siRNA interventions when conventional drug binding sites are limited.

Novel delivery methods targeting the bladder should be developed, including specialized nanoparticles for intravesical administration, urothelium-specific viral vectors, and sustained-release hydrogel systems. These approaches should aim to enhance editing efficiency while reducing systemic exposure, and incorporate lineage tracing methods to evaluate therapeutic effectiveness in patients.

CRISPR-derived biomarkers should be incorporated into future clinical studies to guide patient selection and monitor treatment responses. When possible, minimal editing approaches or temporary editor systems should be used, with thorough evaluation of off-target effects, immune responses, and potential germline impacts.

The development of CRISPR-modified immune cells, such as PD-1 edited or enhanced T/NK cells, should be pursued in combination with intravesical treatments and strategies to induce tumor antigen expression, aiming to enhance immune cell infiltration and killing capacity within the bladder microenvironment.

9.9 Conclusion

CRISPR/Cas9 provides a versatile, high-resolution toolkit to deconvolute the genetic architecture of bladder cancer and to expose therapeutically tractable weaknesses that are invisible to bulk transcriptomics or single-agent pharmacology. By aligning subtype-specific functional genomics with delivery-conscious, biomarker-guided development, the field is poised to convert CRISPR-enabled discoveries into targeted and combination therapies that improve durability of response beyond current standards for MIBC and relapsing NMIBC. The next phase will hinge on disciplined target validation, refined local delivery, and ethically grounded clinical implementation, steps that can translate the promise of gene editing into tangible patient benefit.

References

1. Gaj T, Gersbach CA, Barbas CF, 3rd. ZFN, TALEN, and CRISPR/Cas-based methods for genome engineering. Trends Biotechnol. 2013;31(7):397–405.

2. Xiao-Jie L, Hui-Ying X, Zun-Ping K, Jin-Lian C, Li-Juan J. CRISPR-Cas9: a new and promising player in gene therapy. J Med Genet. 2015;52(5):289–96.
3. Awwad SW, Serrano-Benitez A, Thomas JC, Gupta V, Jackson SP. Revolutionizing DNA repair research and cancer therapy with CRISPR-Cas screens. Nat Rev Mol Cell Biol. 2023;24(7):477–94.
4. Das S, Bano S, Kapse P, Kundu GC. CRISPR based therapeutics: a new paradigm in cancer precision medicine. Mol Cancer. 2022;21(1):85.
5. Wang M, Chen M, Wu X, Huang X, Yu B. CRISPR applications in cancer diagnosis and treatment. Cell Mol Biol Lett. 2023;28(1):73.
6. Koutros S, Kiemeney LA, Pal Choudhury P, Milne RL, Lopez de Maturana E, Ye Y, et al. Genome-wide Association Study of Bladder Cancer Reveals New Biological and Translational Insights. Eur Urol. 2023;84(1):127–37.
7. Chang SS, Boorjian SA, Chou R, Clark PE, Daneshmand S, Konety BR, et al. Diagnosis and Treatment of Non-Muscle Invasive Bladder Cancer: AUA/SUO Guideline. J Urol. 2016;196(4):1021–9.
8. Nadal R, Bellmunt J. Management of metastatic bladder cancer. Cancer Treat Rev. 2019;76:10–21.
9. Perera J, Hoskin P. The role of radiotherapy in metastatic bladder cancer. J Cancer Metastasis Treat. 2022;8:4.
10. Stenehjem DD, Tran D, Nkrumah MA, Gupta S. PD1/PDL1 inhibitors for the treatment of advanced urothelial bladder cancer. Onco Targets Ther. 2018;11:5973–89.
11. Lopez-Beltran A, Cimadamore A, Blanca A, Massari F, Vau N, Scarpelli M, et al. Immune Checkpoint Inhibitors for the Treatment of Bladder Cancer. Cancers (Basel). 2021;13(1):131.
12. Massari F, Di Nunno V, Cubelli M, Santoni M, Fiorentino M, Montironi R, et al. Immune checkpoint inhibitors for metastatic bladder cancer. Cancer Treat Rev. 2018;64:11–20.
13. Fong MHY, Feng M, McConkey DJ, Choi W. Update on bladder cancer molecular subtypes. Transl Androl Urol. 2020;9(6):2881–9.
14. McConkey DJ, Choi W. Molecular Subtypes of Bladder Cancer. Curr Oncol Rep. 2018;20(10):77.
15. Choi W, Porten S, Kim S, Willis D, Plimack ER, Hoffman-Censits J, et al. Identification of distinct basal and luminal subtypes of muscle-invasive bladder cancer with different sensitivities to frontline chemotherapy. Cancer Cell. 2014;25(2):152–65.

16. Damrauer JS, Hoadley KA, Chism DD, Fan C, Tiganelli CJ, Wobker SE, et al. Intrinsic subtypes of high-grade bladder cancer reflect the hallmarks of breast cancer biology. Proc Natl Acad Sci U S A. 2014;111(8):3110–5.
17. Lindgren D, Frigyesi A, Gudjonsson S, Sjödahl G, Hallden C, Chebil G, et al. Combined gene expression and genomic profiling define two intrinsic molecular subtypes of urothelial carcinoma and gene signatures for molecular grading and outcome. Cancer Res. 2010;70(9):3463–72.
18. Robertson AG, Kim J, Al-Ahmadie H, Bellmunt J, Guo G, Cherniack AD, et al. Comprehensive molecular characterization of muscle-invasive bladder cancer. Cell. 2017;171(3):540–56.e25.
19. Marzouka NA, Eriksson P, Rovira C, Liedberg F, Sjödahl G, Höglund M. A validation and extended description of the Lund taxonomy for urothelial carcinoma using the TCGA cohort. Sci Rep. 2018;8(1):3737.
20. Seiler R, Ashab HAD, Erho N, van Rhijn BWG, Winters B, Douglas J, et al. Impact of Molecular Subtypes in Muscle-invasive Bladder Cancer on Predicting Response and Survival after Neoadjuvant Chemotherapy. Eur Urol. 2017;72(4):544–54.
21. Tan TZ, Rouanne M, Tan KT, Huang RY, Thiery JP. Molecular Subtypes of Urothelial Bladder Cancer: Results from a Meta-cohort Analysis of 2411 Tumors. Eur Urol. 2019;75(3):423–32.
22. Morera DS, Hasanali SL, Belew D, Ghosh S, Klaassen Z, Jordan AR, et al. Clinical Parameters Outperform Molecular Subtypes for Predicting Outcome in Bladder Cancer: Results from Multiple Cohorts, Including TCGA. J Urol. 2020;203(1):62–72.
23. Alexandrov LB, Nik-Zainal S, Wedge DC, Aparicio SA, Behjati S, Biankin AV, et al. Signatures of mutational processes in human cancer. Nature. 2013;500(7463):415–21.
24. Lawrence MS, Stojanov P, Polak P, Kryukov GV, Cibulskis K, Sivachenko A, et al. Mutational heterogeneity in cancer and the search for new cancer-associated genes. Nature. 2013;499(7457):214–8.
25. Allory Y, Beukers W, Sagrera A, Flández M, Marqués M, Márquez M, et al. Telomerase reverse transcriptase promoter mutations in bladder cancer: high frequency across stages, detection in urine, and lack of association with outcome. Eur Urol. 2014;65(2):360–6.
26. Kurtis B, Zhuge J, Ojaimi C, Ye F, Cai D, Zhang D, et al. Recurrent TERT promoter mutations in urothelial carcinoma and potential clinical applications. Ann Diagn Pathol. 2016;21:7–11.

27. Leão R, Lee D, Figueiredo A, Hermanns T, Wild P, Komosa M, et al. Combined genetic and epigenetic alterations of the TERT promoter affect clinical and biological behavior of bladder cancer. Int J Cancer. 2019;144(7):1676–84.
28. Rachakonda PS, Hosen I, de Verdier PJ, Fallah M, Heidenreich B, Ryk C, et al. TERT promoter mutations in bladder cancer affect patient survival and disease recurrence through modification by a common polymorphism. Proc Natl Acad Sci U S A. 2013;110(43):17426–31.
29. Berdik C. Unlocking bladder cancer. Nature. 2017;551(7679):S34-s5.
30. Babjuk M, Böhle A, Burger M, Capoun O, Cohen D, Compérat EM, et al. EAU Guidelines on Non-Muscle-invasive Urothelial Carcinoma of the Bladder: Update 2016. Eur Urol. 2017;71(3):447–61.
31. Knowles MA, Hurst CD. Molecular biology of bladder cancer: new insights into pathogenesis and clinical diversity. Nat Rev Cancer. 2015;15(1):25–41.
32. Abdollah F, Gandaglia G, Thuret R, Schmitges J, Tian Z, Jeldres C, et al. Incidence, survival and mortality rates of stage-specific bladder cancer in United States: a trend analysis. Cancer Epidemiol. 2013;37(3):219–25.
33. James AC, Gore JL. The costs of non-muscle invasive bladder cancer. Urol Clin North Am. 2013;40(2):261–9.
34. Hartmann A, Moser K, Kriegmair M, Hofstetter A, Hofstaedter F, Knuechel R. Frequent genetic alterations in simple urothelial hyperplasias of the bladder in patients with papillary urothelial carcinoma. Am J Pathol. 1999;154(3):721–7.
35. Hernández S, López-Knowles E, Lloreta J, Kogevinas M, Amorós A, Tardón A, et al. Prospective study of FGFR3 mutations as a prognostic factor in nonmuscle invasive urothelial bladder carcinomas. J Clin Oncol. 2006;24(22):3664–71.
36. López-Knowles E, Hernández S, Malats N, Kogevinas M, Lloreta J, Carrato A, et al. PIK3CA mutations are an early genetic alteration associated with FGFR3 mutations in superficial papillary bladder tumors. Cancer Res. 2006;66(15):7401–4.
37. Hedegaard J, Lamy P, Nordentoft I, Algaba F, Høyer S, Ulhøi BP, et al. Comprehensive Transcriptional Analysis of Early-Stage Urothelial Carcinoma. Cancer Cell. 2016;30(1):27–42.
38. Stroggilos R, Mokou M, Latosinska A, Makridakis M, Lygirou V, Mavrogeorgis E, et al. Proteome-based classification of Nonmuscle Invasive Bladder Cancer. Int J Cancer. 2020;146(1):281–94.

39. Kamoun A, de Reyniès A, Allory Y, Sjödahl G, Robertson AG, Seiler R, et al. A Consensus Molecular Classification of Muscle-invasive Bladder Cancer. Eur Urol. 2020;77(4):420–33.
40. de Jong JJ, Liu Y, Robertson AG, Seiler R, Groeneveld CS, van der Heijden MS, et al. Long non-coding RNAs identify a subset of luminal muscle-invasive bladder cancer patients with favorable prognosis. Genome Med. 2019;11(1):60.
41. Venter JC, Adams MD, Myers EW, Li PW, Mural RJ, Sutton GG, et al. The sequence of the human genome. Science. 2001;291(5507):1304–51.
42. Roberts SA, Lawrence MS, Klimczak LJ, Grimm SA, Fargo D, Stojanov P, et al. An APOBEC cytidine deaminase mutagenesis pattern is widespread in human cancers. Nat Genet. 2013;45(9):970–6.
43. Vinagre J, Almeida A, Pópulo H, Batista R, Lyra J, Pinto V, et al. Frequency of TERT promoter mutations in human cancers. Nat Commun. 2013;4:2185.
44. Liu J, Zhang Y, Zeng Q, Zeng H, Liu X, Wu P, et al. Delivery of RIPK4 small interfering RNA for bladder cancer therapy using natural halloysite nanotubes. Sci Adv. 2019;5(9):eaaw6499.
45. Chen SH, Zhaori G. Potential clinical applications of siRNA technique: benefits and limitations. Eur J Clin Invest. 2011;41(2):221–32.
46. Isazadeh H, Oruji F, Shabani S, Behroozi J, Nasiri H, Isazadeh A, Akbari M. Advances in siRNA delivery approaches in cancer therapy: challenges and opportunities. Mol Biol Rep. 2023;50(11):9529–43.
47. He Z, He J, Xie K. KLF4 transcription factor in tumorigenesis. Cell Death Discov. 2023;9(1):118.
48. Xu X, Li J, Zhu Y, Xie B, Wang X, Wang S, et al. CRISPR-ON-Mediated KLF4 overexpression inhibits the proliferation, migration and invasion of urothelial bladder cancer in vitro and in vivo. Oncotarget. 2017;8(60):102078–87.
49. Chen LJ, Xu XY, Zhong XD, Liu YJ, Zhu MH, Tao F, et al. The role of lysine-specific demethylase 6A (KDM6A) in tumorigenesis and its therapeutic potentials in cancer therapy. Bioorg Chem. 2023;133:106409.
50. Matar M, Prince G, Hamati I, Baalbaky M, Fares J, Aoude M, et al. Implication of KDM6A in bladder cancer. Pharmacogenomics. 2023;24(9):509–22.
51. Ahn J, Kim KH, Park S, Ahn YH, Kim HY, Yoon H, et al. Target sequencing and CRISPR/Cas editing reveal simultaneous loss of UTX and UTY in urothelial bladder cancer. Oncotarget. 2016;7(39):63252–60.

52. Ler LD, Ghosh S, Chai X, Thike AA, Heng HL, Siew EY, et al. Loss of tumor suppressor KDM6A amplifies PRC2-regulated transcriptional repression in bladder cancer and can be targeted through inhibition of EZH2. Sci Transl Med. 2017;9(378):eaai8312.
53. Lang A, Yilmaz M, Hader C, Murday S, Kunz X, Wagner N, et al. Contingencies of UTX/KDM6A Action in Urothelial Carcinoma. Cancers (Basel). 2019;11(4):481.
54. Zhuang C, Zhuang C, Zhou Q, Huang X, Gui Y, Lai Y, Yang S. Engineered CRISPR/Cas13d Sensing hTERT Selectively Inhibits the Progression of Bladder Cancer In Vitro. Front Mol Biosci. 2021;8:646412.
55. Hillary VE, Ceasar SA. A Review on the Mechanism and Applications of CRISPR/Cas9/Cas12/Cas13/Cas14 Proteins Utilized for Genome Engineering. Mol Biotechnol. 2023;65(3):311–25.
56. Zhang R, Xia LQ, Lu WW, Zhang J, Zhu JS. LncRNAs and cancer. Oncol Lett. 2016;12(2):1233–9.
57. Xie J, Ni J, Shi H, Wang K, Ma X, Li W, Peng B. LncRNA SNHG3 enhances BMI1 mRNA stability by binding and regulating c-MYC: Implications for the carcinogenic role of SNHG3 in bladder cancer. Cancer Med. 2023;12(5):5718–35.
58. Tortora D, Roberts ME, Kumar G, Kotapalli SS, Ritch E, Scurll JM, et al. A genome-wide CRISPR screen maps endogenous regulators of PPARG gene expression in bladder cancer. iScience. 2023;26(5):106525.
59. Liu S, Chen X, Lin T. Emerging strategies for the improvement of chemotherapy in bladder cancer: Current knowledge and future perspectives. J Adv Res. 2022;39:187–202.
60. Massari F, Santoni M, Ciccarese C, Brunelli M, Conti A, Santini D, et al. Emerging concepts on drug resistance in bladder cancer: Implications for future strategies. Crit Rev Oncol Hematol. 2015; 96(1):81–90.
61. Yu HM, Wang TC. Mechanism of cisplatin resistance in human urothelial carcinoma cells. Food Chem Toxicol. 2012;50(5):1226–37.
62. Kumar G, Ritch E, Oo H, Wang C, Tortora D, Thaper D, et al., editors. Genome-wide CRISPR screen reveals SLFN11 as a potent mediator of cisplatin sensitivity in muscle-invasive bladder cancer. Urol Oncol Semin Orig Invest. 2020;38(12):905.
63. Luan J, Gao X, Hu F, Zhang Y, Gou X. SLFN11 is a general target for enhancing the sensitivity of cancer to chemotherapy (DNA-damaging agents). J Drug Target. 2020;28(1):33–40.

64. Zhang B, Ramkumar K, Cardnell RJ, Gay CM, Stewart CA, Wang WL, et al. A wake-up call for cancer DNA damage: the role of Schlafen 11 (SLFN11) across multiple cancers. Br J Cancer. 2021;125(10):1333–40.
65. Zhang H, Xiao X, Wei W, Huang C, Wang M, Wang L, et al. CircLIFR synergizes with MSH2 to attenuate chemoresistance via MutSα/ATM-p73 axis in bladder cancer. Mol Cancer. 2021;20(1):70.
66. Lan L, Hayashi T, Rabeya RM, Nakajima S, Kanno S, Takao M, et al. Functional and physical interactions between ERCC1 and MSH2 complexes for resistance to cis-diamminedichloroplatinum(II) in mammalian cells. DNA Repair (Amst). 2004;3(2):135–43.
67. Shi ZD, Hao L, Han XX, Wu ZX, Pang K, Dong Y, et al. Targeting HNRNPU to overcome cisplatin resistance in bladder cancer. Mol Cancer. 2022;21(1):37.
68. Rhea LP, Mendez-Marti S, Kim D, Aragon-Ching JB. Role of immunotherapy in bladder cancer. Cancer Treat Res Commun. 2021;26:100296.
69. Galsky MD, Daneshmand S, Izadmehr S, Gonzalez-Kozlova E, Chan KG, Lewis S, et al. Gemcitabine and cisplatin plus nivolumab as organ-sparing treatment for muscle-invasive bladder cancer: a phase 2 trial. Nat Med. 2023;29(11):2825–34.
70. Zhang W, Shi L, Zhao Z, Du P, Ye X, Li D, et al. Disruption of CTLA-4 expression on peripheral blood CD8+T cell enhances anti-tumor efficacy in bladder cancer. Cancer Chemother Pharmacol. 2019;83(5):911–20.
71. Zhen S, Lu J, Chen W, Zhao L, Li X. Synergistic Antitumor Effect on Bladder Cancer by Rational Combination of Programmed Cell Death 1 Blockade and CRISPR-Cas9-Mediated Long Non-Coding RNA Urothelial Carcinoma Associated 1 Knockout. Hum Gene Ther. 2018; 29(12):1352–63.
72. Zhen S, Hua L, Liu YH, Sun XM, Jiang MM, Chen W, et al. Inhibition of long non-coding RNA UCA1 by CRISPR/Cas9 attenuated malignant phenotypes of bladder cancer. Oncotarget. 2017;8(6):9634–46.
73. Nandwani A, Rathore S, Datta M. LncRNAs in cancer: Regulatory and therapeutic implications. Cancer Lett. 2021;501:162–71.
74. Frangoul H, Bobruff Y, Cappellini MD, Corbacioglu S, Fernandez CM, De la Fuente J, et al. Safety and efficacy of CTX001 in patients with transfusion-dependent β-thalassemia and sickle cell disease: early results from the climb THAL-111 and climb SCD-121 studies of autologous CRISPR-CAS9-modified CD34+ hematopoietic stem and progenitor cells. Blood. 2020;136:3–4.

75. Hu Y, Zhou Y, Zhang M, Ge W, Li Y, Yang L, et al. CRISPR/Cas9-Engineered Universal CD19/CD22 Dual-Targeted CAR-T Cell Therapy for Relapsed/Refractory B-cell Acute Lymphoblastic Leukemia. Clin Cancer Res. 2021;27(10):2764–72.
76. Tsimberidou AM, Van Morris K, Vo HH, Eck S, Lin YF, Rivas JM, Andersson BS. T-cell receptor-based therapy: an innovative therapeutic approach for solid tumors. J Hematol Oncol. 2021;14(1):102.
77. He J, Xiong X, Yang H, Li D, Liu X, Li S, et al. Defined tumor antigen-specific T cells potentiate personalized TCR-T cell therapy and prediction of immunotherapy response. Cell Res. 2022;32(6):530–42.
78. Tan E, Gakhar N, Kirtane K. TCR gene-engineered cell therapy for solid tumors. Best Pract Res Clin Haematol. 2021;34(3):101285.
79. Foy SP, Jacoby K, Bota DA, Hunter T, Pan Z, Stawiski E, et al. Non-viral precision T cell receptor replacement for personalized cell therapy. Nature. 2023;615(7953):687–96.
80. Wachsmann TLA, Wouters AK, Remst DFG, Hagedoorn RS, Meeuwsen MH, van Diest E, et al. Comparing CAR and TCR engineered T cell performance as a function of tumor cell exposure. Oncoimmunology. 2022;11(1):2033528.
81. Zhang D, Wang G, Yu X, Wei T, Farbiak L, Johnson LT, et al. Enhancing CRISPR/Cas gene editing through modulating cellular mechanical properties for cancer therapy. Nat Nanotechnol. 2022;17(7):777–87.
82. Lou E, Choudhry MS, Starr TK, Folsom TD, Bell J, Rathmann B, et al. Targeting the intracellular immune checkpoint CISH with CRISPR-Cas9-edited T cells in patients with metastatic colorectal cancer: a first-in-human, single-centre, phase 1 trial. Lancet Oncol. 2025;26(5):559–70.
83. Pal SK, Reimers MA, Garmezy B, Xu W, Hoimes CJ, Weinstein M, et al. A phase 1/2, open-label, multicenter, dose escalation and cohort expansion study of the safety and efficacy of anti-CD70 allogeneic CRISPR-Cas9–engineered T cells (CTX131) in adult patients with relapsed or refractory solid tumors. J Clin Oncol. 2024;42(16 suppl):TPS2676.
84. Jardim DL, Goodman A, de Melo Gagliato D, Kurzrock R. The Challenges of Tumor Mutational Burden as an Immunotherapy Biomarker. Cancer Cell. 2021;39(2):154–73.
85. Yang Y, Xu J, Ge S, Lai L. CRISPR/Cas: Advances, Limitations, and Applications for Precision Cancer Research. Front Med (Lausanne). 2021;8:649896.

86. Wang SW, Gao C, Zheng YM, Yi L, Lu JC, Huang XY, et al. Current applications and future perspective of CRISPR/Cas9 gene editing in cancer. Mol Cancer. 2022;21(1):57.
87. Tsai SQ, Zheng Z, Nguyen NT, Liebers M, Topkar VV, Thapar V, et al. GUIDE-seq enables genome-wide profiling of off-target cleavage by CRISPR-Cas nucleases. Nat Biotechnol. 2015;33(2):187–97.
88. Gillmore JD, Gane E, Taubel J, Kao J, Fontana M, Maitland ML, et al. CRISPR-Cas9 In Vivo Gene Editing for Transthyretin Amyloidosis. N Engl J Med. 2021;385(6):493–502.
89. Aimo A, Castiglione V, Rapezzi C, Franzini M, Panichella G, Vergaro G, et al. RNA-targeting and gene editing therapies for transthyretin amyloidosis. Nat Rev Cardiol. 2022;19(10):655–67.
90. Go SW. Germline Gene Therapy in the Era of Precise Genome Editing: How Far Should We Go?. In: Soniewicka M, editor. The Ethics of Reproductive Genetics: Between Utility, Principles, and Virtues. Springer; 2018. pp. 157–71.
91. Jiang F, Doudna JA. CRISPR-Cas9 Structures and Mechanisms. Annu Rev Biophys. 2017;46:505–29.
92. Brokowski C, Adli M. CRISPR Ethics: Moral Considerations for Applications of a Powerful Tool. J Mol Biol. 2019;431(1):88–101.

https://doi.org/10.1142/9789819826759_0010

CHAPTER 10

CRISPR/Cas9 in the Treatment of HPV Cancers, Primarily Cervical Cancer

Mehrdad Hashemi[1,2], *Alireza Khosravinejad*[1,3], *Mina Alimohammadi*[4], *Reza Mohajer Shirazi*[1,3], *Rojin Ghannad Zadeh*[1,5], *Behdokht Jamali*[6], *Neda Zali*[3], *Kimia Sadat Esfahani*[1,3], *Ali Shirazi*[1,3], *Faranak Jamshidian*[1,7], *Najma Farahani*[1,*], *Afshin Taheriazam*[1,8,*], *Payman Rahimzadeh*[9,*], *Maliheh Entezari*[1,2,*]

[1]Farhikhtegan Medical Convergent Sciences Research Center, Farhikhtegan Hospital, Faculty of Medicine, TeMs. C., Islamic Azad University, Tehran, Iran
[2]Department of Genetics, Faculty of Advanced Sciences and Technology, TeMs. C, Islamic Azad University, Tehran, Iran
[3]Basic and Molecular Epidemiology of Gastrointestinal Disorders Research Center, Research Institute for Gastroenterology and Liver Diseases, Shahid Beheshti University of Medical Sciences, Tehran, Iran
[4]Department of Immunology, School of Medicine, Shahid Beheshti University of Medical Sciences, Tehran, Iran
[5]Department of Art & Sciences, Faculty of Biology, University of North Florida, Jacksonville, Florida, USA

* **Corresponding authors:** Najmafarahani@gmail.com (N.F.); a.taheriazam@iautmu.ac.ir (A.T.); P.rahimzadeh76@gmail.com (P.R.); mentezari@iautmu.ac.ir (M.E.)

[6]Department of Microbiology and Genetics, Kherad Institute of Higher Education, Bushehr, Iran
[7]Department of Biology, ET.C., Islamic Azad University, Tehran, Iran
[8]Department of Orthopedics, Faculty of Medicine, TeMs. C, Islamic Azad University, Tehran, Iran
[9]Surgical Research Society (SRS), Students' Scientific Research Center, Tehran University of Medical Sciences, Tehran, Iran

Abstract

High-risk human papillomaviruses (HPV) are etiologically linked to cervical and other anogenital cancers through persistent expression of the viral oncogenes E6 and E7, which neutralize the tumor suppressors p53 and pRb to drive uncontrolled proliferation and malignant transformation. Conventional therapies for HPV-associated disease including cryotherapy, laser, electrosurgery, chemotherapy, and radiation are largely ablative or non-specific; although effective in the short term, they remain invasive and exhibit meaningful recurrence rates, and prophylactic vaccines do not clear established infections. CRISPR/Cas9 genome editing enables direct, sequence-specific disruption of E6/E7, restoring p53/pRb pathways, triggering apoptosis, and inhibiting tumor growth in preclinical cervical cancer models, including adeno-associated virus-delivered systems and multi-guide designs targeting integrated viral DNA. Complementary precision modality immunotherapies and RNA-based therapeutics also target the HPV oncogenic program, but nuclear localization of many non-coding RNAs and delivery barriers limit durable silencing, bolstering the rationale for DNA-level editing. This chapter synthesizes mechanistic and translational advances in CRISPR/Cas9-mediated inactivation of HPV oncogenes, evaluates delivery technologies, on-target efficacy, and safety considerations, and outlines development priorities for clinical translation in cervical cancer and related HPV-driven malignancies.

Keywords: CRISPR/Cas9; human papillomavirus; cervical cancer; p53; genome editing therapy; therapeutic vaccines

10.1 Introduction

High-risk human papillomavirus (HPV) infections have been linked to various human cancers, particularly cervical cancer [1]. These viruses continuously produce E6 and E7 oncoproteins, which disrupt crucial tumor suppressors like p53 and retinoblastoma protein (pRb), leading to uncontrolled cellular proliferation and cancer development [2]. Current treatments for ano-genital HPV infections primarily rely on destructive or ablative methods. Various therapeutic options for treating genital warts include cryotherapy, surgical removal with scissors, laser procedures, and electrosurgical techniques. While ablative treatments such as cryotherapy initially show high success rates of 70–80%, they often face recurrence rates between 25–39%, even after multiple treatment sessions [3]. Despite the effectiveness of preventive vaccines, they cannot eliminate existing infections. Traditional treatments such as chemotherapy, radiotherapy, and surgical interventions are often invasive and lack specificity, highlighting the necessity for innovative, targeted therapeutic approaches against HPV-associated cancers [4]. Recent developments have introduced novel therapeutic strategies designed to specifically target HPV-infected cells while preserving healthy tissue. These include immunotherapeutic approaches, such as therapeutic vaccines and immune checkpoint blockade, which have demonstrated promise in enhancing immune responses against HPV-related cancers [5]. Additionally, RNA-targeted therapies, including antisense oligonucleotides and small interfering RNAs (siRNAs), offer mechanisms to suppress viral oncogene expression [6]. While these RNA-based strategies show potential for improving treatment outcomes in patients with HPV-driven cancers, targeting nuclear-localized non-coding RNAs through RNA-based interventions presents significant technical challenges [6, 7].

Research is exploring epigenetic interventions as a therapeutic strategy against HPV-induced cancer development, focusing on modifications to DNA methylation patterns and histone modifications that influence gene expression. Through the creation of specific DNA double-strand breaks, CRISPR-Cas9 can effectively inhibit E6 and E7 gene expression, thereby reactivating p53 and pRb tumor suppressor pathways, promoting cell death, and inhibiting cancerous growth [8]. The current investigation explores the potential application of CRISPR-Cas9 as a targeted therapeutic tool for HPV-associated cancers, specifically through its ability to deactivate viral oncogenes E6 and E7 [9]. This chapter evaluates the therapeutic potential of CRISPR-Cas9 technology by analyzing its capacity to restore tumor suppressor functions (p53 and pRb), while also examining the associated challenges and possible clinical applications in HPV treatment.

10.2 Molecular and Genetic Landscape of Cervical Cancer

Cervical cancer ranks among the top four most frequently diagnosed cancers affecting women globally, with HPV infection serving as the primary driver of its development and progression [10]. Scientists have currently identified more than 400 different HPV variants [11]. High-risk HPVs are responsible for over 90% of cervical cancer cases and are also implicated, though less frequently, in other anogenital cancers and head and neck malignancies [12]. During high-risk HPV-related cancer progression, viral DNA typically becomes incorporated into the host cell chromosomes, with viral proteins playing crucial roles in carcinogenesis. While most HPV infections are naturally cleared within months, some persist chronically. These enduring infections continuously express viral oncogenes that suppress tumor suppressor proteins p53 and Rb, leading to increased genomic instability, accumulation of mutations, and potential viral integration into host DNA. High-risk HPVs specifically target tumor cells rather than stromal cells, making them the exclusive carriers of E6 and E7 viral oncogenes [13].

HPV's E1 and E2 proteins serve as key factors in identifying replication origins, while E4 and E5 proteins contribute to viral life cycle regulation. The primary oncogenic activity is carried out by E6 and E7 proteins. E6 protein promotes carcinogenesis primarily through inducing p53 degradation and activating telomerase, resulting in decreased expression of apoptosis-inhibiting genes [14]. E6 may also collaborate with oncogenic kinases, including EGFR and tyrosine-protein kinase Met, to enhance epigenetic regulation. The E7 protein influences multiple signaling cascades, particularly by interfering with pRb and the cell cycle regulator p21 [15, 16]. Both pRb and p21 play vital roles in epithelial regulation and function as tumor suppressors [17].

High-risk HPV types, specifically HPV16 and HPV18, produce E7 proteins that demonstrate particularly strong binding to pRb. A crucial biochemical function of pRb involves its interaction with E2F family transcription factors, which primarily suppress genes associated with replication enzymes. This interaction is fundamental to pRb's tumor-suppressing capabilities [18]. Recent studies have shown that while the HPV16 genome displays numerous amino acid-altering variations during infection, the E7 protein maintains remarkable genetic consistency [19].

Continuous expression of E6 and E7 viral oncoproteins results in enhanced genomic instability, facilitating mutation accumulation. This process compromises normal cell growth regulation, ultimately fostering cancer development [20]. A distinctive feature of cervical cancer is the persistent expression of E6 and E7, which occurs following the integration of viral genetic material into the host's chromosomal DNA [21]. Researchers have explored various therapeutic approaches targeting E6 and E7 proteins, including the development of small-molecule compounds, peptide-based treatments, and therapeutic vaccines for specific cervical cancer intervention [22]. An alternative therapeutic strategy for HPV-associated cancers involves using targeted mutagenesis to permanently inactivate viral E6 and/or E7 genes, with the anticipated outcome of eliminating HPV-transformed cells [21].

10.3 Current Approaches in Cervical Cancer Therapy

The primary cause of cervical cancer is persistent infection with high-risk HPV strains [23]. Research has demonstrated that sustained infection with high-risk HPV variants, most notably types

16 and 18, accounts for approximately 90% of cervical cancer occurrences [22]. Scientific investigations have conclusively shown that viral oncogenes E6 and E7 are fundamental to cervical cancer initiation and advancement, displaying cancer-promoting characteristics essential for maintaining the malignant state of cancer cells [14, 24]. Early and precise identification of HPV infections is vital for optimal disease control and prevention of HPV-associated cancers [25].

Various surgical techniques are employed to treat HPV-induced cervical precancerous lesions. These include local anesthesia-based excisional procedures, cryosurgery (using freezing methods), electrosurgical approaches such as cone biopsy (conization) and loop electrosurgical excision procedure, and laser-based treatments [26]. To combat the rising incidence of HPV-related cancers, particularly cervical cancer, vaccination programs have been enhanced. Three FDA-approved preventive vaccines — Gardasil, Gardasil 9 (by Merck Sharp & Dohme-MSD), and Cervarix (by GlaxoSmithKline-GSK) — demonstrate nearly 100% effectiveness in preventing cervical cancer. These vaccines contain virus-like particles derived from recombinantly produced L1 protein [27]. Contemporary treatment protocols for cervical cancer encompass surgical procedures, combination therapy involving adjuvant or neoadjuvant chemotherapy with radiation, and complete or radical hysterectomy [28].

Treatment protocols are customized according to several factors including disease progression, tumor characteristics, and individual patient factors. The therapeutic approach may involve radiation therapy, chemotherapy, or their combination, either as standalone treatments or in conjunction with surgery [29, 30]. For early disease stages, modified radical hysterectomy (extra-fascial hysterectomy) is typically recommended, though this surgical intervention can impact fertility and is invasive [31]. For patients with underlying health conditions or functional limitations, radiation therapy may be preferred over surgical intervention [32].

Radiotherapy remains fundamental in cervical cancer treatment across all stages, encompassing whole pelvic radiation, brachytherapy, and intracavitary radiation techniques. While particularly effective for stage 1A patients unsuitable for surgery and those with advanced tumors, radiotherapy can produce adverse effects [33]. Though chemotherapy alone plays a limited role, its combination with radiotherapy has emerged as the preferred treatment approach [34].

Although HPV is implicated in virtually all cervical cancer cases, viral presence alone does not guarantee malignancy development. Cancer progression typically requires extended time and additional carcinogenic mechanisms, particularly immune system evasion [35]. This understanding has led to increased interest in immunotherapeutic approaches for treating HPV-induced cancers [36].

CRISPR technology has revolutionized targeted modification of E6 and E7 genes in HPV types 6, 11, 16, and 18. Research has confirmed CRISPR/Cas9's antiviral effectiveness in various laboratory cell cultures and HPV-positive tumor xenograft models. E6 and E7 gene disruption resulted in decreased viral protein levels and restored p53 and pRb tumor suppressor functionality [37, 38]. The potential synergy between CRISPR/Cas9 and conventional chemotherapy or radiotherapy could establish novel therapeutic strategies and enhance treatment outcomes for cervical cancer patients [9].

10.4 Targeting HPV Oncogenes with CRISPR/Cas9

Research utilizing CRISPR/Cas targeting of the HPV16 E7 oncogene in cervical cancer cells revealed selective effects: mutational changes triggered cell death and growth inhibition specifically in HPV16-positive cells, while HPV16-negative cells remained unaffected. The successful disruption of E7 gene expression and subsequent elimination of E7 oncoprotein restored pRb tumor suppressor function, indicating the therapeutic potential of HPV16-E7 gRNA-guided CRISPR/Cas approaches for cervical cancer [36].

Further investigations have demonstrated that CRISPR/Cas9 targeting of E6/E7 promoter and open reading frame (ORF) regions leads to multiple beneficial effects: decreased E6 and E7 mRNA levels, enhanced P53 protein expression, reduced pRb levels, increased apoptosis, and inhibited SiHa cell proliferation. The therapeutic efficacy was further validated *in vivo*, where CRISPR/Cas9-modified cells showed reduced growth [36].

Modified CRISPR/Cas9 systems specifically targeting HPV16 and HPV18 E6/E7 mRNA have demonstrated significant tumor growth reduction and apoptosis induction through intratumoral administration, suggesting potential use as complementary therapy [39]. Laboratory experiments and mechanistic studies indicate that direct CRISPR/Cas9 delivery to HPV-positive tumors, particularly through intratumoral administration, could effectively suppress tumor growth and induce cell death. While current evidence is primarily limited to cellular models, these findings provide foundation for developing direct injection-based treatments [36].

Preclinical studies in mouse models have shown that intratumoral CRISPR/Cas9 administration targeting E7 effectively reduces tumor growth and promotes apoptosis in HPV-positive tumors [40]. While research and clinical trials demonstrate that intratumoral injection can successfully deliver CRISPR-Cas9 components to tumor cells with improved precision and potentially reduced off-target effects, clinical implementation remains in early stages. Concerns persist regarding potential local toxicity and immune responses [41, 42].

While intratumoral administration has demonstrated effectiveness in both preclinical and clinical research for localized cancers, offering benefits such as concentrated therapeutic delivery, minimized systemic effects, and enhanced tumor targeting [43], clinical implementation faces several obstacles. Tumor heterogeneity significantly impacts therapeutic agent distribution, with poorly vascularized or necrotic tumor regions showing reduced treatment response. Furthermore, accurate delivery to deep-seated or difficult-to-access tumors presents technical challenges.

Nevertheless, successful applications of intratumoral delivery in clinical trials, particularly with oncolytic viruses and immune checkpoint inhibitors for melanoma and other skin cancers, have yielded positive outcomes [44]. Although large-scale clinical trials validating direct CRISPR/Cas system delivery for cancer treatment are pending, preliminary data is encouraging [38].

Complementary research has explored multiple single-guide RNAs (sgRNAs) designed to target E6 and E7 oncogene promoters and transcripts. This strategy successfully enhanced p53 and pRb expression levels, supporting CRISPR/Cas9's therapeutic potential in cervical cancer treatment [40]. A significant *in vivo* investigation demonstrated that systemic delivery of E6 and E7 sgRNA through a CRISPR/Cas9 vector effectively induced tumor cell apoptosis in mouse models. This study provided valuable understanding of post-editing cellular responses within tumors, reinforcing CRISPR/Cas9's therapeutic value [45]. These combined findings suggest that oncogene-targeted genome editing approaches show substantial promise for clinical cancer treatment applications.

During HPV-induced cancer development, viral genetic material typically becomes integrated into the host cell's chromosomal DNA, with viral protein expression playing a crucial role in cancer formation [13]. The field of cervical cancer research has seen numerous advances over recent decades, with significant early progress focusing on HPV-related mechanisms. Additional research has explored cervical cancer prevention and treatment strategies as a model for addressing other HPV-associated malignancies [46].

CRISPR-Cas9, representing the most sophisticated genome editing technology currently available, originated as a bacterial adaptive defense system [47]. Its key advantage lies in its programmability using short RNA sequences, making it more user-friendly compared to alternative genome editing technologies such as transcription activator-like effector nucleases and zinc finger nucleases. Scientists have demonstrated CRISPR-Cas9's ability to target and modify human chromosomal DNA [48, 49]. This research culminated in a milestone achievement in 2020 with the completion of a phase I clinical trial utilizing CRISPR-Cas9 in advanced non-small cell lung cancer patients, marking its debut in clinical oncology [50].

In recent years, CRISPR-Cas9 has been extensively applied to target HPV genes implicated in cervical cancer development [47]. Research has increasingly demonstrated that E6 and E7 genes play fundamental roles in triggering cell cycle arrest and apoptosis [51], leading researchers to focus extensively on these genes as primary therapeutic targets [8, 52, 53]. The first application of CRISPR-Cas9 targeting HPV16-E7 for treating HPV-positive cervical cancer was reported in 2014 [39]. That same year, another study revealed that CRISPR-Cas9 targeting of E6 and E7 loci significantly elevated p53 and p21 levels, resulting in marked reduction of cervical cancer cell proliferation in laboratory conditions [40].

Subsequent studies demonstrated that E6 and E7 gene suppression produced various effects, including decreased cervical cancer cell proliferation. A 2016 investigation revealed that targeted HPV16 E6/E7 gene silencing could enhance sensitivity to cisplatin chemotherapy in cervical cancer, suggesting new possibilities for gene therapy approaches [54]. In 2019, the same research group discovered synergistic anticancer effects when combining HPV16 E6/E7 inhibition with PD-1 pathway blockade [55].

Beyond E6/E7-targeted therapy, researchers have explored other HPV oncogenic mechanisms using CRISPR-Cas9. A 2017 study demonstrated SIRT1's crucial role in HPV16 replication through CRISPR-Cas9-mediated silencing [56]. This research extended into 2020, examining the SIRT1-WRN axis's regulatory function and revealing viral replication's dependence on Werner syndrome protein (WRN) [57].

Recent research has expanded to investigate host proteins interacting with E6/E7 gene products. A 2020 study showed that HPV16 and HPV18 E7 oncoprotein suppresses cell differentiation genes by binding to host tumor suppressor PTPN14. CRISPR-Cas9-mediated PTPN14 mutation in cervical cancer cells significantly reduced their oncogenic potential, highlighting PTPN14's importance in suppressing high-risk HPV-induced tumor development (see **Table 10.1** and **Figure 10.1**) [58]. Research continues to explore various applications of CRISPR-Cas9-based gene therapy.

Table 10.1 CRISPR/Cas9 studies targeting HPV in cervical cancer.

Focus Area	Target Gene(s)	Main Outcomes	Reference
CRISPR/Cas9 targeting HPV16 E7 oncogene	E7 (HPV16)	Induced apoptosis, inhibited cell growth in HPV16+ cells; restored pRb expression	[36]
CRISPR/Cas9 targeting E6/E7 promoter and ORF	E6/E7 transcripts	Reduced E6/E7 mRNA; increased P53; decreased pRb; enhanced apoptosis; inhibited SiHa growth	[39]
Engineered CRISPR/Cas9 for HPV16/18 E6/E7 mRNA	E6/E7 mRNA (HPV16/18)	Significantly reduced tumor growth; induced apoptosis *in vivo*	[39]
Preclinical intratumoral administration	E7 oncogene	Suppressed tumor growth; induced apoptosis in HPV+ tumors	[40]
sgRNAs targeting E6/E7 promoters and transcripts	E6/E7 oncogenes	Marked increase in p53 and pRb expression	[40]
Systemic administration of E6/E7 sgRNA	E6/E7 genes	Effective induction of tumor cell death through apoptosis	[45]
Targeting E6/E7 loci	E6/E7 genes	Increased p53 and p21; reduced cell proliferation	[40]
HPV16 E6/E7 gene silencing with cisplatin	HPV16 E6/E7	Potential sensitizer for cisplatin chemotherapy	[54]
HPV16 E6/E7 inhibition with PD-1 pathway	E6/E7 + PD-1	Synergistic anticancer effects	[55]
SIRT1 gene silencing	SIRT1 gene	Demonstrated importance for HPV16 replication control	[56]
SIRT1-WRN axis regulation	SIRT1-WRN	Viral replication cycle dependence on WRN	[57]
PTPN14 gene mutation	**PTPN14 gene**	**Reduced oncogenic potential; crucial role in tumor suppression**	**[58]**

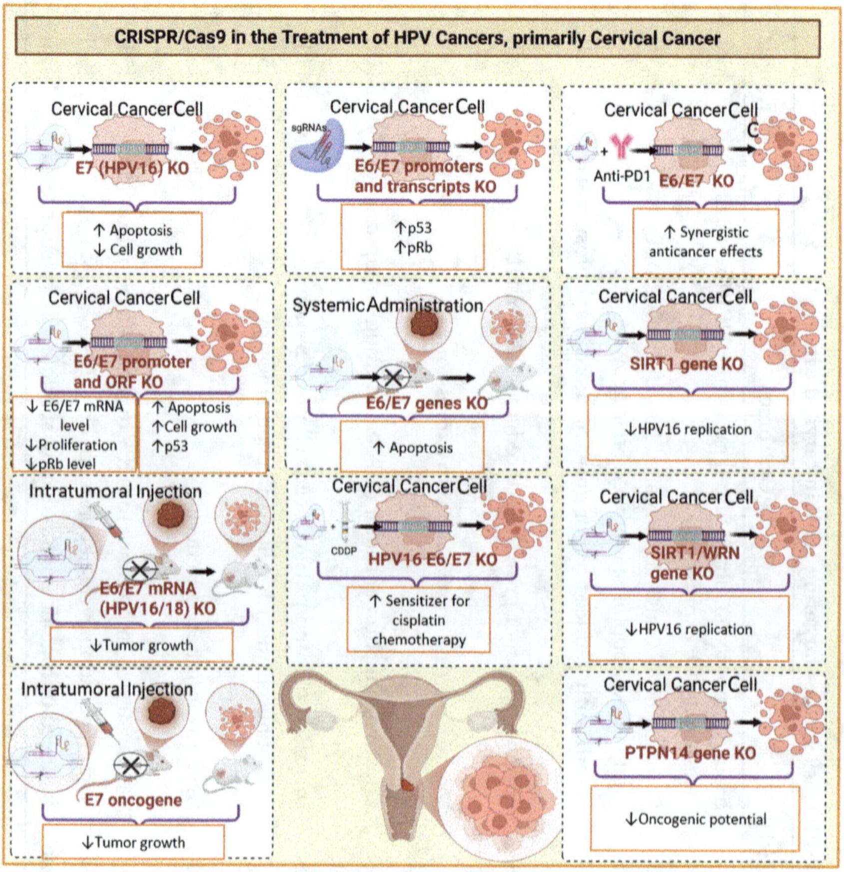

Figure 10.1 CRISPR/Cas9 applications in HPV-driven cervical cancer treatment: therapeutic strategies targeting viral oncogenes. The scheme illustrates multiple CRISPR/Cas9-mediated therapeutic strategies for treating cervical cancer driven by HPV, primarily HPV16 and HPV18. **Direct E7 oncogene targeting:** CRISPR/Cas9-mediated knockout of HPV16 E7 oncogene induces apoptosis and inhibits cell growth in HPV-positive cervical cancer cells (SiHa and CaSki) while sparing HPV-negative cells. E7 protein disruption directly leads to downregulation of E7 oncoprotein and restoration of tumor suppressor pRb expression, triggering cell cycle arrest and apoptotic cell death. This approach demonstrates specificity for HPV-transformed cells without affecting normal tissue, establishing E7 as a critical therapeutic target. **E6/E7 promoter and transcript targeting:** CRISPR/Cas9 targeting of E6/E7 promoters and transcripts using sgRNAs achieves dual disruption of both oncogenes, resulting in simultaneous upregulation of p53 and pRb tumor suppressors. Gene-targeting approaches using

Figure 10.1 (*Continued on facing page*) non-viral liposome delivery systems demonstrate that double-targeting E6 and E7 increases p53 protein expression significantly compared to single-gene targeting. Both *in vitro* and *in vivo* experiments confirm that E6/E7 knockout induces apoptosis, inhibits cell proliferation, and suppresses tumor growth through reactivation of p53/p21 and pRb pathways. **E6/E7 promoter and ORF targeting:** CRISPR/Cas9 targeting of both E6/E7 promoters and ORFs achieves comprehensive disruption of viral oncogene expression. This strategy reduces E6/E7 mRNA levels, decreases cellular proliferation, and downregulates pRb levels while inducing cellular senescence characterized by increased cell surface area, senescence-associated β-galactosidase activity, loss of lamin B1 protein, and cytoplasmic chromatin fragments. Adeno-associated virus type 2 vector-mediated delivery of CRISPR/Cas9 targeting E6 demonstrates high tumor-suppressing effects *in vivo* with minimal side effects, as E6-targeting CRISPR/Cas9 specifically affects cervical cancer cells without damaging normal tissue. **Systemic administration for E6/E7 gene knockout:** Systemic administration of CRISPR/Cas9 targeting E6/E7 genes induces widespread apoptosis in cervical cancer cells and organoids. This delivery approach enables therapeutic genome editing beyond local tumor sites, providing potential for treating metastatic or disseminated disease. **SIRT1 gene knockout:** CRISPR/Cas9-mediated knockout of SIRT1 (sirtuin 1) reduces HPV16 replication in cervical cancer cells. SIRT1 controls the recruitment of WRN to E1-E2 replicating DNA, and SIRT1 depletion results in mutagenic HPV16 E1-E2 DNA replication. Clinical cervical cytology samples demonstrate that SIRT1 expression positively correlates with cervical disease progression from CIN1 to CIN3, establishing SIRT1 as a therapeutic target for preventing disease advancement. **Combined SIRT1/WRN gene knockout:** Dual knockout of SIRT1 and WRN genes synergistically reduces HPV16 replication efficiency. CRISPR/Cas9 editing demonstrates that WRN, like SIRT1, regulates both the quantity and fidelity of E1-E2 replication. The SIRT1-WRN axis represents a critical regulatory mechanism for viral DNA replication in cervical cancer cells, and disruption of this axis impairs viral genome maintenance. **HPV16 E6/E7 knockout with cisplatin sensitization:** CRISPR/Cas9-mediated HPV16 E6/E7 knockout delivered via cationic delivery of DNA and peptides enhances sensitivity to cisplatin chemotherapy in cervical cancer cells. This combination approach overcomes drug resistance by restoring p53 and pRb tumor suppressor function, which amplifies chemotherapy-induced apoptosis and cell cycle arrest. **Intratumoral injection of E6/E7 mRNA knockout:** Direct intratumoral injection of CRISPR/Cas9 targeting E6/E7 mRNA in HPV16/18-positive cervical tumors reduces tumor growth in preclinical models. This local delivery strategy achieves high concentrations of genome-editing machinery at the tumor site while minimizing systemic exposure and potential off-target effects. **E7 oncogene intratumoral injection:** Intratumoral injection of CRISPR/Cas9 specifically targeting the E7 oncogene reduces tumor growth and suppresses

Figure 10.1 (*Continued*) malignant phenotype. Genetic deletion of HPV E7 oncogene effectively regresses established tumors and sensitizes HPV-positive cancers to additional therapeutic interventions. **PTPN14 gene knockout:** CRISPR/Cas9-mediated knockout of PTPN14 reduces oncogenic potential in cervical cancer cells. While germline loss-of-function variants in PTPN14 confer increased risk of cervical cancer development, somatic PTPN14 mutations in established tumors paradoxically associate with improved survival outcomes. CRISPR-Cas9 mutation targeting PTPN14 in cervical cancer cells significantly reduces proliferation and oncogenic signaling, suggesting context-dependent roles for PTPN14 in cervical carcinogenesis. **Combined anti-PD-1 and E6/E7 knockout immunotherapy:** Combination therapy using CRISPR/Cas9-mediated E6/E7 knockout with anti-PD-1 immune checkpoint blockade demonstrates synergistic antitumor effects in humanized SCID mouse models. CRISPR/Cas9 targeting of HPV16 E6/E7 induces apoptosis, triggers autophagy, and releases damage-associated molecular patterns that activate dendritic cells and CD8+ T cells. Administration of gRNA-PD-1 together with gRNA-HPV16 E6/E7 improves survival and suppresses tumor growth by increasing infiltration of dendritic cells, CD4+ and CD8+ T lymphocytes. This combination therapy enhances Th1-associated immune-stimulating gene expression while reducing transcription of regulatory/suppressive immune genes, transforming the tumor microenvironment from immunosuppressive ("cold" tumor) to immunologically activated ("hot" tumor). HPV knockout increases PD-1 blockade efficacy by reversing immunosuppression and promoting immune memory with sustained tumor regression.

10.5 CRISPR/Cas9 in Overcoming Drug Resistance

Patients diagnosed with HPV-driven cancers typically undergo traditional treatments such as chemotherapy, radiotherapy, or concurrent chemoradiotherapy. However, a significant challenge in cancer treatment is the development of drug resistance by cancer cells, which compromises the effectiveness of chemotherapy.

A groundbreaking study in 2016 introduced the first application of CRISPR-Cas9 targeting HPV16 E6/E7, demonstrating its potential as an effective enhancer for cisplatin chemotherapy in cervical cancer treatment [54]. The research showed particular effectiveness when combined with cisplatin for HPV16-positive cervical cancer cases. Further investigations revealed the significance of mixed lineage leukemia 5 (MLL5) in HPV-positive cervical cancer cell development [65]. Studies demonstrated that eliminating MLL5 significantly enhanced cisplatin's therapeutic efficacy in cells containing HPV-18. Research also showed that targeting MLL5 through CRISPR-Cas9 exhibited greater anticancer properties compared to targeting E6.

In treating head and neck squamous cell carcinoma (HNSCC), radiation therapy remains one of the primary and most successful treatment options. However, research has shown that different HPV types respond differently to radiotherapy, particularly noting that cervical cancer patients with HPV-18 DNA show distinct treatment responses [66]. Recent advancements include the development of a specialized CRISPR-Cas9 screening system to determine optimal radiation sensitization strategies for both HPV-positive and HPV-negative HNSCC [67]. Evidence suggests that combining radiotherapy with CRISPR-Cas9-based suppression of genetic repair mechanisms could enhance treatment outcomes for HNSCC patients [67].

10.6 CRISPR/Cas9 and Immunotherapy Modulation

The introduction of immune checkpoint inhibitors has revolutionized cancer treatment, making immunotherapy one of the most encouraging therapeutic approaches. Recent applications of CRISPR-Cas9 have focused on developing immune-based therapeutic agents, including chimeric antigen receptor T (CAR-T) cells and targeting the programmed cell death protein-1 (PD-1) and its ligand (PD-L1) [68].

PD-1 and PD-L1 function as suppressors of T cell immune responses [69]. These proteins, found on cervical T cells and dendritic cells, have been recently linked to high-risk HPV infection, with their expression levels increasing in correlation with advancing stages of cervical intraepithelial neoplasia [70]. To investigate the relationship between HPV16 E6 and PD-1 expression, scientists developed a modified C33 cell line that continuously produces HPV16 E6/E7 (SiHa-E6/E7). Using a SiHa cervical cancer mouse model, researchers explored whether combining targeted therapy with immunotherapy could produce enhanced therapeutic effects. The results demonstrated synergistic benefits when CRISPR-Cas9 was used to simultaneously target HPV16 E6/E7 and block PD-1 [55].

Research has demonstrated that EZH2, which functions as a catalytic component in PRC2, inhibits the downregulation of the PD-1/PD-L1 pathway [71]. Studies have shown that elevated EZH2 expression correlates with enhanced tumor progression, including increased cell division, invasive behavior, and metastatic potential, making it clinically significant [71]. Experimental studies in mouse models of endometriosis have explored the effects of suppressing or eliminating EZH2 activity, revealing its role in promoting epithelial-mesenchymal transition in cancer development [72]. Additionally, investigations have identified EZH2 as a promising therapeutic candidate in HNSCC, particularly for enhancing immune response and antigen presentation [73]. Scientists suggest that combining EZH2 inhibitors with PD-1 blockade could offer therapeutic benefits for HNSCC patients, though additional preclinical investigation is needed.

Clinical researchers have conducted trials utilizing CRISPR-Cas9 technology to delete PD-1 in T cells for treating various cancers. Notable success has been achieved in NSCLC treatment using this approach [50]. However, current literature lacks studies specifically examining CRISPR-Cas9-mediated deletion of CAR-T or PD-1 as an immunotherapeutic strategy for HPV-associated malignancies.

10.7 CRISPR/Cas9 in HPV Detection

The significance of nucleic acid detection methods has become particularly evident during the COVID-19 pandemic. While various genetic testing approaches exist, the CRISPR-Cas9 platform offers distinct benefits in detection applications, beyond its established role in gene manipulation and control. The widespread adoption of polymerase chain reaction (PCR) stems from its capacity to exponentially amplify DNA targets with remarkable sensitivity. This has made PCR the preferred method for DNA analysis and genotyping, exemplified by its use in SARS-CoV-2 detection during the COVID-19 crisis. The integration of PCR and CRISPR technologies has opened new possibilities in nucleic acid detection methodologies [74].

A breakthrough came in 2018 when Qiao and Beibei introduced CRISPR-Cas9-associated reverse PCR. This technique involves circularizing Cas9-cleaved target DNA followed by reverse PCR amplification, achieving high sensitivity through its specialized detection approach [74]. Building on this foundation, they later developed ctPCR, a novel Cas9-based DNA detection and typing method [75]. This streamlined process can be completed in approximately 3–4 hours using qPCR equipment. While ctPCR proved valuable for DNA analysis, it initially required comparing Ct values and DNA quantities between two quantitative PCR reactions. This limitation was addressed in a subsequent iteration that enabled single-reaction detection, eliminating the need for comparative analysis [76]. The improved protocol could be performed entirely within PCR instruments without intermediate sample handling.

Beyond PCR-based approaches, researchers developed CRISPR-Cas9-assisted DNA detection [77]. This innovative method offers several advantages over existing techniques, including simplicity, speed, and the elimination of pre-amplification steps. It incorporates fluorescent hybridization chain reaction and can deliver results in under 30 minutes.

10.8 Future Perspectives and Conclusion

For the past two decades, scientists have pursued the development of reliable and cost-effective techniques for precise genomic modifications in living cells. Genome editing technology has shown promising applications across multiple fields. For instance, genetic disorders in humans could potentially be treated by eliminating disease-causing genes through gene therapy [78].

CRISPR-based methodologies have gained widespread acceptance in the scientific community due to their ability to efficiently target and modify DNA in living cells across numerous species, including humans and other eukaryotic organisms [79]. This precision editing technology shows potential in personalized gene therapy for treating inherited single-gene disorders and targeting specific pathogenic sequences to combat infectious diseases, among other applications. However, implementing CRISPR faces several practical and technical challenges, primarily related to delivery strategies, repair pathway control, off-target and on-target effects, and important ethical considerations [80].

The CRISPR/Cas genome editing platform represents a promising therapeutic alternative that could potentially supplement or replace conventional treatments like radiation, chemotherapy, and surgical interventions. The extensive research conducted on CRISPR/Cas indicates its potential as a revolutionary approach to cancer treatment [26]. However, these techniques require further optimization for effectiveness, safety, and precision before clinical implementation. The outlook for precise gene therapy in cervical cancer treatment appears promising as our understanding of programmable Cas nucleases continues to expand. CRISPR technology may soon play a crucial role in treating genetic disorders [81].

The primary challenge hindering widespread clinical application of CRISPR/Cas9 in human medicine remains the development of safe and effective *in vivo* delivery systems. While viral vectors are currently the predominant choice in clinical trials, concerns regarding immunogenicity, cytotoxicity, and carcinogenicity still need to be addressed [82].

Nanotechnology's rapid advancement has enhanced the potential of lipids and carrier polymers. Nanocarriers demonstrate several advantages, including reduced off-target effects, efficient packaging and protection of CRISPR/Cas9 components, and improved blood circulation, cellular uptake, and targeting precision through surface modifications. However, developing sustained-release nanocarrier systems for tumor-specific CRISPR/Cas editing still faces numerous physical barriers [83]. While current nanocarrier technology may not meet all requirements for widespread clinical use, ongoing developments in biomaterials are expected to expand therapeutic applications of genome editing [84].

CRISPR screening, though in its early stages, shows promise in identifying crucial cancer genes and potential therapeutic targets. Earlier research utilized CRISPR screening to explore immune cell functions and their interactions with cancer cells, with future studies expected to focus on other immune regulatory cells to uncover novel regulatory pathways in the tumor microenvironment. The ability to create allogeneic T cells with enhanced anti-cancer properties and fewer adverse effects through CRISPR gene editing has enabled broader clinical applications of universal CAR-T cells, marking significant progress in immuno-oncology [85]. The CRISPR/Cas9 system has also shown promise in targeting cancer-causing viruses. Studies targeting HPV18-E6 or HPV16-E6 demonstrated reduced proliferation and increased apoptosis specifically in HPV-positive cervical cancer cells, while sparing HPV-negative cells, suggesting a novel therapeutic approach [86].

Recent technological advances in CRISPR are enabling more precise and safer applications. Base editing and prime editing systems offer more refined alternatives to traditional CRISPR-Cas9, allowing specific nucleotide modifications without double-stranded breaks, potentially reducing off-target effects [87]. Advancing delivery methods remains crucial, with ongoing development of viral vectors, lipid nanoparticles, and extracellular vesicle-based systems potentially improving clinical gene editing specificity and efficiency [88, 89]. The combination of CRISPR-mediated gene editing with immune checkpoint inhibitors or engineered T-cell therapies could enhance treatment outcomes for HPV-associated cancers [90, 91]. Future clinical research must focus on safety evaluation, long-term effectiveness, and personalized CRISPR approaches based on individual tumor genomics to realize this technology's full potential [92].

Targeted disruption of HPV E6/E7 with CRISPR/Cas9 directly reverses the core oncogenic lesion of HPV-driven cancers, primarily cervical cancer, by restoring p53 and pRb functions, inducing apoptosis, and constraining tumor growth, thereby offering a rational and potentially disease-modifying alternative to ablative or non-specific therapies. Early preclinical studies using viral and non-viral delivery systems demonstrate on-target activity and proof-of-concept efficacy, while the limitations of existing ablative treatments and the inability of vaccines to clear established infections highlight the therapeutic opportunity for genome editing. Realizing clinical impact will depend on advances in delivery, specificity, and durability, and on rational combinations with immunotherapy and conventional modalities that leverage restored tumor suppressor pathways and host immunity against HPV-associated malignancies.

References

1. Yeo-Teh NSL, Ito Y, Jha S. High-Risk Human Papillomaviral Oncogenes E6 and E7 Target Key Cellular Pathways to Achieve Oncogenesis. Int J Mol Sci. 2018;19(6):1706.
2. Moody CA, Laimins LA. Human papillomavirus oncoproteins: pathways to transformation. Nat Rev Cancer. 2010;10(8):550–60.
3. Stanley MA. Genital human papillomavirus infections: current and prospective therapies. J Gen Virol. 2012;93(Pt 4):681–91.
4. Stanley M, Pinto LA, Trimble C. Human papillomavirus vaccines--immune responses. Vaccine. 2012;30 Suppl 5:F83–7.
5. Yang A, Farmer E, Wu TC, Hung CF. Perspectives for therapeutic HPV vaccine development. J Biomed Sci. 2016;23(1):75.
6. Casarotto M, Fanetti G, Guerrieri R, Palazzari E, Lupato V, Steffan A, et al. Beyond MicroRNAs: Emerging Role of Other Non-Coding RNAs in HPV-Driven Cancers. Cancers (Basel). 2020;12(5):1246.
7. Heydarnia E, Dorostgou Z, Hedayati N, Mousavi V, Yahyazadeh S, Alimohammadi M, et al. Circular RNAs and cervical cancer: friends or foes? A landscape on circRNA-mediated regulation of key signaling pathways involved in the onset and progression of HPV-related cervical neoplasms. Cell Commun Signal. 2024;22(1):107.
8. Inturi R, Jemth P. CRISPR/Cas9-based inactivation of human papillomavirus oncogenes E6 or E7 induces senescence in cervical cancer cells. Virology. 2021;562:92–102.

9. Zhen S, Li X. Oncogenic Human Papillomavirus: Application of CRISPR/Cas9 Therapeutic Strategies for Cervical Cancer. Cell Physiol Biochem. 2017;44(6):2455–66.
10. Díaz L, Bernadez-Vallejo SV, Vargas-Castro R, Avila E, Gómez-Ceja KA, García-Becerra R, et al. The Phytochemical α-Mangostin Inhibits Cervical Cancer Cell Proliferation and Tumor Growth by Downregulating E6/E7-HPV Oncogenes and KCNH1 Gene Expression. Int J Mol Sci. 2023;24(3):3055.
11. Mlynarczyk-Bonikowska B, Rudnicka L. HPV Infections-Classification, Pathogenesis, and Potential New Therapies. Int J Mol Sci. 2024;25(14):7616.
12. Pešut E, Đukić A, Lulić L, Skelin J, Šimić I, Milutin Gašperov N, et al. Human Papillomaviruses-Associated Cancers: An Update of Current Knowledge. Viruses. 2021;13(11):2234.
13. Integrated genomic and molecular characterization of cervical cancer. Nature. 2017;543(7645):378–84.
14. Scheffner M, Huibregtse JM, Vierstra RD, Howley PM. The HPV-16 E6 and E6-AP complex functions as a ubiquitin-protein ligase in the ubiquitination of p53. Cell. 1993;75(3):495–505.
15. Münger K, Werness BA, Dyson N, Phelps WC, Harlow E, Howley PM. Complex formation of human papillomavirus E7 proteins with the retinoblastoma tumor suppressor gene product. Embo J. 1989; 8(13):4099–105.
16. Spangle JM, Münger K. The human papillomavirus type 16 E6 oncoprotein activates mTORC1 signaling and increases protein synthesis. J Virol. 2010;84(18):9398–407.
17. Saiz-Ladera C, Lara MF, Garín M, Ruiz S, Santos M, Lorz C, et al. p21 suppresses inflammation and tumorigenesis on pRB-deficient stratified epithelia. Oncogene. 2014;33(37):4599–612.
18. Bhattacharjee R, Das SS, Biswal SS, Nath A, Das D, Basu A, et al. Mechanistic role of HPV-associated early proteins in cervical cancer: Molecular pathways and targeted therapeutic strategies. Crit Rev Oncol Hematol. 2022;174:103675.
19. Mirabello L, Yeager M, Yu K, Clifford GM, Xiao Y, Zhu B, et al. HPV16 E7 Genetic Conservation Is Critical to Carcinogenesis. Cell. 2017; 170(6):1164–74.e6.
20. Vats A, Trejo-Cerro O, Thomas M, Banks L. Human papillomavirus E6 and E7: What remains? Tumour Virus Res. 2021;11:200213.
21. Pal A, Kundu R. Human Papillomavirus E6 and E7: The Cervical Cancer Hallmarks and Targets for Therapy. Front Microbiol. 2019;10:3116.

22. Ling K, Dou Y, Yang N, Deng L, Wang Y, Li Y, et al. Genome editing mRNA nanotherapies inhibit cervical cancer progression and regulate the immunosuppressive microenvironment for adoptive T-cell therapy. J Control Release. 2023;360:496–513.
23. Ling K, Yang L, Yang N, Chen M, Wang Y, Liang S, et al. Gene Targeting of HPV18 E6 and E7 Synchronously by Nonviral Transfection of CRISPR/Cas9 System in Cervical Cancer. Hum Gene Ther. 2020;31(5–6):297–308.
24. Walboomers JM, Jacobs MV, Manos MM, Bosch FX, Kummer JA, Shah KV, et al. Human papillomavirus is a necessary cause of invasive cervical cancer worldwide. J Pathol. 1999;189(1):12–9.
25. Williams J, Kostiuk M, Biron VL. Molecular Detection Methods in HPV-Related Cancers. Front Oncol. 2022;12:864820.
26. Khairkhah N, Bolhassani A, Najafipour R. Current and future direction in treatment of HPV-related cervical disease. J Mol Med (Berl). 2022;100(6):829–45.
27. Williamson AL. Recent Developments in Human Papillomavirus (HPV) Vaccinology. Viruses. 2023;15(7):1440.
28. Marchetti C, Fagotti A, Tombolini V, Scambia G, De Felice F. Survival and toxicity in neoadjuvant chemotherapy plus surgery versus definitive chemoradiotherapy for cervical cancer: A systematic review and meta-analysis. Cancer Treat Rev. 2020;83:101945.
29. Chang CW, Yang ST, Liu HH, Chang WH, Lee WL, Wang PH. Surgery-based radiation-free multimodality treatment for locally advanced cervical cancer. Taiwan J Obstet Gynecol. 2024;63(5):651–64.
30. Marquina G, Manzano A, Casado A. Targeted Agents in Cervical Cancer: Beyond Bevacizumab. Curr Oncol Rep. 2018;20(5):40.
31. Angeles MA, Martínez-Gómez C, Migliorelli F, Voglimacci M, Figurelli J, Motton S, et al. Novel Surgical Strategies in the Treatment of Gynecological Malignancies. Curr Treat Options Oncol. 2018;19(12):73.
32. Cohen PA, Jhingran A, Oaknin A, Denny L. Cervical cancer. Lancet. 2019;393(10167):169–82.
33. Chargari C, Deutsch E, Blanchard P, Gouy S, Martelli H, Guérin F, et al. Brachytherapy: An overview for clinicians. CA Cancer J Clin. 2019;69(5):386–401.
34. Duenas-Gonzalez A, Gonzalez-Fierro A. Pharmacodynamics of current and emerging treatments for cervical cancer. Expert Opin Drug Metab Toxicol. 2019;15(8):671–82.

35. Smola S. Immunopathogenesis of HPV-Associated Cancers and Prospects for Immunotherapy. Viruses. 2017;9(9):254.
36. Hu Z, Ma D. The precision prevention and therapy of HPV-related cervical cancer: new concepts and clinical implications. Cancer Med. 2018;7(10):5217–36.
37. Mali P, Yang L, Esvelt KM, Aach J, Guell M, DiCarlo JE, et al. RNA-guided human genome engineering via Cas9. Science. 2013; 339(6121):823–6.
38. Zahedipour F, Zahedipour F, Zamani P, Jaafari MR, Sahebkar A. Harnessing CRISPR technology for viral therapeutics and vaccines: from preclinical studies to clinical applications. Virus Res. 2024;341:199314.
39. Kennedy EM, Kornepati AV, Goldstein M, Bogerd HP, Poling BC, Whisnant AW, et al. Inactivation of the human papillomavirus E6 or E7 gene in cervical carcinoma cells by using a bacterial CRISPR/Cas RNA-guided endonuclease. J Virol. 2014;88(20):11965–72.
40. Zhen S, Hua L, Takahashi Y, Narita S, Liu YH, Li Y. In vitro and in vivo growth suppression of human papillomavirus 16-positive cervical cancer cells by CRISPR/Cas9. Biochem Biophys Res Commun. 2014;450(4):1422–6.
41. He C, Jaffar Ali D, Xu H, Kumaravel S, Si K, Li Y, et al. Epithelial cell-derived microvesicles: A safe delivery platform of CRISPR/Cas9 conferring synergistic anti-tumor effect with sorafenib. Exp Cell Res. 2020;392(2):112040.
42. Li C, Yang T, Weng Y, Zhang M, Zhao D, Guo S, et al. Ionizable lipid-assisted efficient hepatic delivery of gene editing elements for oncotherapy. Bioact Mater. 2022;9:590–601.
43. Hong WX, Haebe S, Lee AS, Westphalen CB, Norton JA, Jiang W, Levy R. Intratumoral Immunotherapy for Early-stage Solid Tumors. Clin Cancer Res. 2020;26(13):3091–9.
44. Andtbacka RH, Kaufman HL, Collichio F, Amatruda T, Senzer N, Chesney J, et al. Talimogene Laherparepvec Improves Durable Response Rate in Patients With Advanced Melanoma. J Clin Oncol. 2015;33(25):2780–8.
45. Jubair L, Fallaha S, McMillan NAJ. Systemic Delivery of CRISPR/Cas9 Targeting HPV Oncogenes Is Effective at Eliminating Established Tumors. Mol Ther. 2019;27(12):2091–9.
46. Alsbeih G. HPV Infection in Cervical and Other Cancers in Saudi Arabia: Implication for Prevention and Vaccination. Front Oncol. 2014;4:65.

47. Wei Y, Zhao Z, Ma X. Description of CRISPR-Cas9 development and its prospects in human papillomavirus-driven cancer treatment. Front Immunol. 2022;13:1037124.
48. Jinek M, Chylinski K, Fonfara I, Hauer M, Doudna JA, Charpentier E. A programmable dual-RNA-guided DNA endonuclease in adaptive bacterial immunity. Science. 2012;337(6096):816–21.
49. Jinek M, East A, Cheng A, Lin S, Ma E, Doudna J. RNA-programmed genome editing in human cells. Elife. 2013;2:e00471.
50. Lu Y, Xue J, Deng T, Zhou X, Yu K, Deng L, et al. Safety and feasibility of CRISPR-edited T cells in patients with refractory non-small-cell lung cancer. Nat Med. 2020;26(5):732–40.
51. Mittal S, Banks L. Molecular mechanisms underlying human papillomavirus E6 and E7 oncoprotein-induced cell transformation. Mutat Res Rev Mutat Res. 2017;772:23–35.
52. Bortnik V, Wu M, Julcher B, Salinas A, Nikolic I, Simpson KJ, et al. Loss of HPV type 16 E7 restores cGAS-STING responses in human papilloma virus-positive oropharyngeal squamous cell carcinomas cells. J Microbiol Immunol Infect. 2021;54(4):733–9.
53. Xiong J, Tan S, Yu L, Shen H, Qu S, Zhang C, et al. E7-Targeted Nanotherapeutics for Key HPV Afflicted Cervical Lesions by Employing CRISPR/Cas9 and Poly (Beta-Amino Ester). Int J Nanomedicine. 2021;16:7609–22.
54. Zhen S, Lu JJ, Wang LJ, Sun XM, Zhang JQ, Li X, et al. In Vitro and In Vivo Synergistic Therapeutic Effect of Cisplatin with Human Papillomavirus16 E6/E7 CRISPR/Cas9 on Cervical Cancer Cell Line. Transl Oncol. 2016;9(6):498–504.
55. Zhen S, Lu J, Liu YH, Chen W, Li X. Synergistic antitumor effect on cervical cancer by rational combination of PD1 blockade and CRISPR-Cas9-mediated HPV knockout. Cancer Gene Ther. 2020;27(3–4):168–78.
56. Das D, Smith N, Wang X, Morgan IM. The Deacetylase SIRT1 Regulates the Replication Properties of Human Papillomavirus 16 E1 and E2. J Virol. 2017;91(10):e00102–17.
57. James CD, Das D, Morgan EL, Otoa R, Macdonald A, Morgan IM. Werner Syndrome Protein (WRN) Regulates Cell Proliferation and the Human Papillomavirus 16 Life Cycle during Epithelial Differentiation. mSphere. 2020;5(5):e00858–20.
58. Hatterschide J, Brantly AC, Grace M, Munger K, White EA. A Conserved Amino Acid in the C Terminus of Human Papillomavirus

E7 Mediates Binding to PTPN14 and Repression of Epithelial Differentiation. J Virol. 2020;94(17):e01024–20.

59. Hyakusoku H, Sano D, Takahashi H, Hatano T, Isono Y, Shimada S, et al. JunB promotes cell invasion, migration and distant metastasis of head and neck squamous cell carcinoma. J Exp Clin Cancer Res. 2016;35:6.
60. Broutian TR, Jiang B, Li J, Akagi K, Gui S, Zhou Z, et al. Human papillomavirus insertions identify the PIM family of serine/threonine kinases as targetable driver genes in head and neck squamous cell carcinoma. Cancer Lett. 2020;476:23–33.
61. Zhong S, Zhang Y, Yin X, Di W. CDK7 inhibitor suppresses tumor progression through blocking the cell cycle at the G2/M phase and inhibiting transcriptional activity in cervical cancer. Onco Targets Ther. 2019;12:2137–47.
62. Abboodi F, Buckhaults P, Altomare D, Liu C, Hosseinipour M, Banister CE, et al. HPV-inactive cell populations arise from HPV16-transformed human keratinocytes after p53 knockout. Virology. 2021;554:9–16.
63. Leung TH, Tang HW, Siu MK, Chan DW, Chan KK, Cheung AN, Ngan HY. Human papillomavirus E6 protein enriches the CD55(+) population in cervical cancer cells, promoting radioresistance and cancer aggressiveness. J Pathol. 2018;244(2):151–63.
64. Leung TH, Tang HW, Siu MK, Chan DW, Chan KK, Cheung AN, Ngan HY. CD71(+) Population Enriched by HPV-E6 Protein Promotes Cancer Aggressiveness and Radioresistance in Cervical Cancer Cells. Mol Cancer Res. 2019;17(9):1867–80.
65. Pirouzfar M, Amiri F, Dianatpour M, Takhshid MA. CRISPR/Cas9-mediated knockout of MLL5 enhances apoptotic effect of cisplatin in HeLa cells in vitro. Excli j. 2020;19:170–82.
66. Bachtiary B, Obermair A, Dreier B, Birner P, Breitenecker G, Knocke TH, et al. Impact of multiple HPV infection on response to treatment and survival in patients receiving radical radiotherapy for cervical cancer. Int J Cancer. 2002;102(3):237–43.
67. Dok R, Bamps M, Glorieux M, Zhao P, Sablina A, Nuyts S. Radiosensitization approaches for HPV-positive and HPV-negative head and neck squamous carcinomas. Int J Cancer. 2020;146(4):1075–85.
68. Xia AL, He QF, Wang JC, Zhu J, Sha YQ, Sun B, Lu XJ. Applications and advances of CRISPR-Cas9 in cancer immunotherapy. J Med Genet. 2019;56(1):4–9.

69. Ishida Y. PD-1: Its Discovery, Involvement in Cancer Immunotherapy, and Beyond. Cells. 2020;9(6):1376.
70. Yang W, Song Y, Lu YL, Sun JZ, Wang HW. Increased expression of programmed death (PD)-1 and its ligand PD-L1 correlates with impaired cell-mediated immunity in high-risk human papillomavirus-related cervical intraepithelial neoplasia. Immunology. 2013;139(4):513–22.
71. Fang J, Zhang M, Li Q. Enhancer of zeste homolog 2 expression is associated with tumor cell proliferation and invasion in cervical cancer. Am J Med Sci. 2011;342(3):198–204.
72. Zhang Q, Dong P, Liu X, Sakuragi N, Guo SW. Enhancer of Zeste homolog 2 (EZH2) induces epithelial-mesenchymal transition in endometriosis. Sci Rep. 2017;7(1):6804.
73. Zhou L, Mudianto T, Ma X, Riley R, Uppaluri R. Targeting EZH2 Enhances Antigen Presentation, Antitumor Immunity, and Circumvents Anti-PD-1 Resistance in Head and Neck Cancer. Clin Cancer Res. 2020;26(1):290–300.
74. Zhang B, Wang Q, Xu X, Xia Q, Long F, Li W, et al. Detection of target DNA with a novel Cas9/sgRNAs-associated reverse PCR (CARP) technique. Anal Bioanal Chem. 2018;410(12):2889–900.
75. Wang Q, Zhang B, Xu X, Long F, Wang J. CRISPR-typing PCR (ctPCR), a new Cas9-based DNA detection method. Sci Rep. 2018;8(1):14126.
76. Gao J, Wu L, Yang D, Gong W, Wang J. A One-Pot CRISPR/Cas9-Typing PCR for DNA Detection and Genotyping. J Mol Diagn. 2021;23(1):46–60.
77. Xu X, Luo T, Gao J, Lin N, Li W, Xia X, Wang J. CRISPR-Assisted DNA Detection: A Novel dCas9-Based DNA Detection Technique. Crispr J. 2020;3(6):487–502.
78. Liu W, Li L, Jiang J, Wu M, Lin P. Applications and challenges of CRISPR-Cas gene-editing to disease treatment in clinics. Precis Clin Med. 2021;4(3):179–91.
79. Kozovska Z, Rajcaniova S, Munteanu P, Dzacovska S, Demkova L. CRISPR: History and perspectives to the future. Biomed Pharmacother. 2021;141:111917.
80. Young SA, Aitken RJ, Ikawa M. Advantages of using the CRISPR/Cas9 system of genome editing to investigate male reproductive mechanisms using mouse models. Asian J Androl. 2015;17(4):623–7.
81. Stefanoudakis D, Kathuria-Prakash N, Sun AW, Abel M, Drolen CE, Ashbaugh C, et al. The Potential Revolution of Cancer Treatment with CRISPR Technology. Cancers (Basel). 2023;15(6):1813.

82. Bulcha JT, Wang Y, Ma H, Tai PWL, Gao G. Viral vector platforms within the gene therapy landscape. Signal Transduct Target Ther. 2021;6(1):53.
83. Xu X, Liu C, Wang Y, Koivisto O, Zhou J, Shu Y, Zhang H. Nanotechnology-based delivery of CRISPR/Cas9 for cancer treatment. Adv Drug Deliv Rev. 2021;176:113891.
84. Wang SW, Gao C, Zheng YM, Yi L, Lu JC, Huang XY, et al. Current applications and future perspective of CRISPR/Cas9 gene editing in cancer. Mol Cancer. 2022;21(1):57.
85. Elmas E, Saljoughian N, de Souza Fernandes Pereira M, Tullius BP, Sorathia K, Nakkula RJ, et al. CRISPR Gene Editing of Human Primary NK and T Cells for Cancer Immunotherapy. Front Oncol. 2022;12:834002.
86. Ehrke-Schulz E, Heinemann S, Schulte L, Schiwon M, Ehrhardt A. Adenoviral Vectors Armed with PAPILLOMAVIRUs Oncogene Specific CRISPR/Cas9 Kill Human-Papillomavirus-Induced Cervical Cancer Cells. Cancers (Basel). 2020;12(7):1934.
87. Anzalone AV, Randolph PB, Davis JR, Sousa AA, Koblan LW, Levy JM, et al. Search-and-replace genome editing without double-strand breaks or donor DNA. Nature. 2019;576(7785):149–57.
88. Glass Z, Lee M, Li Y, Xu Q. Engineering the Delivery System for CRISPR-Based Genome Editing. Trends Biotechnol. 2018;36(2):173–85.
89. Lino CA, Harper JC, Carney JP, Timlin JA. Delivering CRISPR: a review of the challenges and approaches. Drug Deliv. 2018;25(1):1234–57.
90. Eyquem J, Mansilla-Soto J, Giavridis T, van der Stegen SJ, Hamieh M, Cunanan KM, et al. Targeting a CAR to the TRAC locus with CRISPR/Cas9 enhances tumour rejection. Nature. 2017;543(7643):113–7.
91. Stadtmauer EA, Fraietta JA, Davis MM, Cohen AD, Weber KL, Lancaster E, et al. CRISPR-engineered T cells in patients with refractory cancer. Science. 2020;367(6481):eaba7365.
92. Doudna JA, Charpentier E. Genome editing. The new frontier of genome engineering with CRISPR-Cas9. Science. 2014;346(6213):1258096.

https://doi.org/10.1142/9789819826759_0011

CHAPTER 11

CRISPR/Cas9 in the Treatment of Ovarian Cancer

Mehrdad Hashemi[1,2], *Alireza Khosravinejad*[1,3], *Mina Alimohammadi*[4], *Kimia Sadat Esfahani*[1,3], *Ali Shirazi*[1,3], *Reza Mohajer Shirazi*[1,3], *Behdokht Jamali*[5], *Rojin Ghannad Zadeh*[1,6], *Faranak Jamshidian*[1,7], *Neda Zali*[3], *Najma Farahani*[1,*], *Afshin Taheriazam*[1,8,*], *Payman Rahimzadeh*[9,*], *Maliheh Entezari*[1,2,*]

[1]Farhikhtegan Medical Convergent Sciences Research Center, Farhikhtegan Hospital, Faculty of Medicine, TeMs. C., Islamic Azad University, Tehran, Iran
[2]Department of Genetics, Faculty of Advanced Sciences and Technology, TeMs. C, Islamic Azad University, Tehran, Iran
[3]Basic and Molecular Epidemiology of Gastrointestinal Disorders Research Center, Research Institute for Gastroenterology and Liver Diseases, Shahid Beheshti University of Medical Sciences, Tehran, Iran
[4]Department of Immunology, School of Medicine, Shahid Beheshti University of Medical Sciences, Tehran, Iran
[5]Department of Microbiology and Genetics, Kherad Institute of Higher Education, Bushehr, Iran

* **Corresponding authors:** Najmafarahani@gmail.com (N.F.); a.taheriazam@iautmu.ac.ir (A.T.); P.rahimzadeh76@gmail.com (P.R.); mentezari@iautmu.ac.ir (M.E.)

[6]Department of Art & Sciences, Faculty of Biology, University of North Florida, Jacksonville, Florida, USA
[7]Department of Biology, ET.C., Islamic Azad University, Tehran, Iran
[8]Department of Orthopedics, Faculty of Medicine, TeMs. C, Islamic Azad University, Tehran, Iran
[9]Surgical Research Society (SRS), Students' Scientific Research Center, Tehran University of Medical Sciences, Tehran, Iran

Abstract

CRISPR/Cas9 offers a coherent framework to translate the molecular understanding of ovarian cancer into targeted interventions by directly interrogating and modulating the genes that drive late diagnosis, chemoresistance, recurrence, and metastatic progression. As a comparatively simple, efficient, and flexible platform relative to transcription activator-like effector nucleases and zinc finger nucleases, CRISPR/Cas9 enables functional mapping of oncogenic pathways, systematic identification of drug resistance mechanisms, and therapeutic editing either by gene knockout, transcriptional interference/activation, or RNA-targeted degradation to restore drug sensitivity and suppress malignant phenotypes. In ovarian cancer, where the standard combination of surgical debulking and platinum-based chemotherapy is undermined by acquired resistance and relapse, CRISPR/Cas9 serves both as a discovery engine and a therapeutic candidate: it can validate and disable culpable biomolecules, create nonfunctional protein products, eliminate pathogenic transcripts, and rationally prioritize biomarkers and targets for precision treatment. This chapter synthesizes how the CRISPR/Cas systems have matured from research tools to translational approaches in ovarian cancer, emphasizing applications that bridge mechanistic insight with clinically relevant endpoints.

Keywords: CRISPR/Cas9; ovarian cancer; gene knockout; chemoresistance; functional genomics; precision oncology; gene silencing; therapeutics

11.1 Introduction

Among gynecological cancers, ovarian cancer ranks as the third most prevalent and stands as the second most frequent cause of death from cancer in the female population [1] .The disease's high fatality rate among gynecological malignancies is particularly concerning. Due to non-specific symptoms and a lack of reliable diagnostic indicators, approximately 70% of ovarian cancer cases are identified at advanced stages [2]. While current treatment protocols typically involve surgical tumor removal combined with platinum-based chemotherapy, this approach proves successful in only 70–80% of patients, largely due to chemotherapy resistance. This resistance significantly diminishes the chances of five-year survival. The high mortality rates observed in ovarian cancer patients can be attributed to three main factors: delayed diagnosis, resistance to chemotherapy, and frequent disease recurrence [3]. The scientific breakthrough of CRISPR/Cas technology has transformed genetic modification and regulation, marking it as one of the most significant discoveries of our time [4]. When compared to traditional genetic modification methods like transcription activator-like effector nucleases and zinc finger nucleases, CRISPR/Cas offers superior benefits, including cost-effectiveness, straightforward design, and the capability to precisely target specific DNA sequences or multiple sites simultaneously within cells [5]. Over the last ten years, CRISPR/Cas has transformed cancer research, enhancing our knowledge of ovarian cancer development pathways and helping address persistent challenges such as tumor recurrence, treatment resistance, metastatic spread, and tumor heterogeneity.

This revolutionary technology has enabled researchers to examine cancer biology from multiple angles and has revealed previously unknown therapeutic targets. Despite current limitations in ovarian cancer treatment options, therapeutic strategies continue to advance [6]. Scientists persistently seek innovative therapeutic approaches for ovarian cancer, and CRISPR/Cas9 technology presents a promising avenue by enabling genetic code modification [7]. The implementation of CRISPR/Cas9 in various cancer treatments [8] has opened new possibilities for ovarian cancer therapy, including the identification and screening of oncogenes and drug-resistance genes, as well as their potential elimination. This review examines how CRISPR/Cas systems have evolved as research tools in ovarian cancer studies and their adaptation for enhanced cancer diagnosis and treatment strategies.

Researchers utilize gene editing through knockout and gene silencing via CRISPR/Cas to investigate the molecular mechanisms underlying various aspects of this cancer. Once identified, the molecules responsible for cancer development are targeted using CRISPR/Cas through several approaches: creating non-functional truncated proteins, destroying defective mRNA [9], or interrupting oncogene expression [10] in cancer cells. Our analysis focuses on evaluating CRISPR/Cas9's applications in ovarian cancer research, particularly its contribution to understanding chemoresistance mechanisms and identifying novel therapeutic targets. Additionally, we explore the practical challenges and limitations encountered when implementing this technique in clinical settings.

11.2 Molecular Landscape and Pathogenesis of Ovarian Cancer

The complete understanding of ovarian cancer pathogenesis remains elusive, with no universally accepted theory. A major challenge in understanding its development lies in the disease's heterogeneous composition, encompassing multiple histological types with distinct characteristics and behaviors [11]. While non-epithelial tumors constitute 40% of ovarian growths, they represent only 10% of ovarian malignancies [12, 13].

The traditional theory suggested that ovarian cancers originated exclusively from the ovarian surface epithelium. According to this model, the repetitive physical trauma to epithelial cells during ovulation, followed by immediate repair processes throughout a woman's reproductive years, leads to cumulative DNA damage. These damaged epithelial cells become vulnerable to transformation and may invaginate into the cortical stroma. These invaginations eventually form isolated spherical structures called cortical inclusion cysts within the stroma. The epithelial cells within these cysts, when exposed to ovarian hormones, undergo increased proliferation and eventual malignant transformation [14, 15].

This hypothesis aligns with epidemiological evidence linking the number of ovulatory cycles to ovarian cancer risk. However, it fails to account for several critical factors: the diverse histological types of ovarian cancer and their varying prognoses [16], the lack of morphological similarity between ovarian surface epithelium (mesothelium) and various cell types (serous, endometrioid, mucinous, clear cells, or transitional cells) [15], and the paradoxically increased ovarian cancer risk in polycystic ovary syndrome patients despite their reduced ovulatory cycles [14, 15].

The historical focus on the ovary as the primary site of cancer origin led to limited investigation of precursor lesions in other locations [15]. A significant breakthrough came with the discovery of frequent epithelial dysplasia (50%) in the fallopian tubes of women carrying BRCA1/2 mutations who underwent preventive salpingo-oophorectomy. This dysplasia, termed tubal intraepithelial carcinoma (TIC), shared characteristics with high-grade serous ovarian carcinoma (HGSOC). Further research revealed histological similarities between ovarian cancer and high-grade serous peritoneal cancer, independent of BRCA status. Notably, examinations of the unaffected ovary in ovarian cancer patients showed either normal tissue or changes unlike high-grade serous neoplasms [15]. These findings suggest the fallopian tube as the likely origin of ovarian cancer precursor lesions, which subsequently spread to nearby ovarian tissue.

TIC specimens consistently show TP53 gene mutations. Immunohistochemical analysis of normal fallopian tubes revealed that TP53 expression patterns in secretory cells matched those found in serous ovarian cancer. However, not all TP53 mutations progress to cancer. These mutations may represent cellular responses to DNA damage caused by cytokine and oxidant exposure in tubal epithelial cells, with approximately 50% of mutations eventually leading to cancer development [11, 14].

The fimbrial region, located at the fallopian tube's distal end, harbors the majority of TICs (70–90%). Though initially disputed, this theory has gained widespread acceptance among experts. The fimbriae's proximity to the ovary exposes them to similar environmental stressors, and their rich vascular network facilitates cancer spread to the ovaries through blood vessels [15].

Kurman and Shih [15] proposed a comprehensive theory integrating histological, clinical, and genetic findings of ovarian cancer, categorizing it into two distinct types. Type I encompasses low-grade serous, mucinous, endometrioid, clear cell, and transitional histologies, while Type II includes high-grade serous, undifferentiated, and carcinosarcoma histologies [15].

Type I ovarian cancers are believed to originate within the ovary itself. These cancers exhibit slow growth patterns, generally remain confined to the ovary at diagnosis, maintain genetic stability, and typically display more benign characteristics [16]. They develop through a gradual progression of morphological changes, transitioning through a borderline phase before becoming malignant. Their pathogenesis follows the conventional pathway: ovarian surface epithelial inclusion cysts undergo transformation due to environmental proliferation stimuli. Type I cancers predominantly feature KRAS and BRAF mutations, which activate the MAPK oncogenic pathway [14, 15].

In contrast, Type II ovarian cancers likely originate outside the ovary, particularly in the fallopian tubes. These aggressive tumors demonstrate genetic instability and are typically diagnosed at advanced stages. Type II cancers frequently exhibit TP53 mutations (50–80%), along with HER2/neu (10–20%) and AKT (12–18%) gene overexpression. Approximately half of Type II cases show BRCA1/2 mutations. The precursor cells, located in the fallopian tubes, undergo neoplastic transformation through a combination of TP53 mutations and environmental stressors, including inflammatory cytokines and reactive oxygen species. Research has linked TP53 mutations to lower parity, suggesting ovulation remains a risk factor for these mutations [15, 16]. While this theory provides a more comprehensive explanation of ovarian cancer pathogenesis compared to previous models, it still leaves gaps in understanding cancers of non-ovarian origin [16].

11.3 Mechanistic Basis of CRISPR/Cas9 in Ovarian Cancer Therapy

The development of ovarian cancer involves complex interactions among multiple cancer-associated genes, including tumor suppressors, oncogenes, and genes related to DNA damage. This process also encompasses various transcription factors, protein molecules, and RNA species. A crucial mechanism driving ovarian cancer metastasis is the epithelial-to-mesenchymal transition (EMT), during which epithelial cells undergo significant changes, losing their cellular connections and experiencing alterations in gene expression patterns [17]. In current ovarian cancer research, scientists are exploring CRISPR/Cas9's potential as a gene-editing tool, with its various applications described in subsequent sections.

11.4 CRISPR/Cas9-based Targeting of Genes in Relation to Ovarian Cancer

The BIRC5 gene produces survivin, a protein that inhibits apoptosis and plays a role in EMT, invasion, and metastasis [18–20]. Irregular survivin expression activates various cancer-promoting pathways. Multiple cancer types, including ovarian cancer, show elevated survivin levels [19]. Traditional therapeutic approaches targeting BIRC5/survivin have shown limited effectiveness [21]. CRISPR-Cas9-mediated targeting of BIRC5 could potentially revolutionize treatment strategies for ovarian cancer and other malignancies.

A major challenge in implementing CRISPR systems clinically is off-target effects. Two strategies have been developed to address this: replacing positively charged amino acids with neutral ones in Cas9's DNA binding domain [22], and using Cas9 nickases, which create single-strand DNA breaks. With nickases, two nearby target sequences are required for a double-strand break, significantly reducing unintended double-strand breaks elsewhere in the genome [23, 24].

Analysis of TCGA datasets, Oncomine database, and patient tissue samples by Zhao et al. revealed high BIRC5/survivin expression in ovarian serous carcinomas, correlating with poor survival outcomes [20]. In a subsequent study, Qi et al. used a biodegradable carrier (ARP-F) to deliver BIRC5-targeting CRISPR-Cas9 plasmid (pCas9-surv) in tumor-bearing mice. Intravenous administration of ARP-F/pCas9-surv significantly reduced tumor growth, with near-complete tumor suppression when combined with temozolomide [25]. The same research team also demonstrated successful treatment in an orthotopic hepatocellular carcinoma mouse model using pCas9-surv (renamed pCas9-survivin) delivered via a lactose-derived branched cationic biopolymer (LBP) [26].

Tail vein administration of LBP/pCas9-survivin resulted in significant tumor reduction. When combined with sorafenib, an anti-cancer medication, the treatment led to near-complete tumor regression after 35 days. Although Qi et al.'s methodology differed from Zhao et al.'s by using a Cas9 double-stranded DNA endonuclease and non-ovarian cancer cells, their results demonstrate the therapeutic potential of CRISPR-Cas9 BIRC5/survivin targeting, particularly when used alongside conventional cancer treatments, for both ovarian and other cancers.

MicroRNA expression patterns are frequently altered in various cancers. miR-21, widely recognized as an oncomiR, shows consistent upregulation across 16 cancer types, including ovarian cancer [27]. This makes it an attractive target for CRISPR-Cas therapeutic interventions applicable to multiple cancers. However, since individual miRNAs can influence numerous gene transcripts, careful consideration must be given to potential unintended effects when targeting these molecules.

Huo et al. investigated miR-21 targeting in SKOV3 and OVCAR3 ovarian cancer cell lines [28]. Their approach utilized a lentiviral delivery system with four distinct guide RNAs (gRNAs): three targeting the pre-miR-21 hairpin structure's stem region and one targeting its loop sequences. They established stable cell lines through puromycin selection following vector integration and analyzed the DNA from vector-transduced cells.

All four CRISPR-Cas9 gRNAs successfully induced mutations in their target sequences, resulting in significantly decreased miR-21 expression and increased PDCD4 (a miR-21 target gene) expression in both SKOV3 and OVCAR3 cell lines. Detailed analysis of cells modified with gRNA2 and gRNA3, which targeted the pre-miR-21 hairpin stem structure, revealed reduced oncogenic characteristics including decreased cell proliferation, migration, and invasion. These modified cells also showed enhanced apoptosis and increased sensitivity to paclitaxel chemotherapy. Additionally, miR-21 disruption inhibited the EMT process. Notably, the stably transduced cells exhibited exclusively anti-oncogenic effects with no observed pro-oncogenic activity, suggesting miR-21 as a promising CRISPR-Cas9 therapeutic target for both ovarian and other cancers.

BMI1 codes for a ring finger protein that serves as a crucial component of the polycomb group complex 1 (PRC1), which regulates gene expression through chromatin modification. Elevated BMI1 expression correlates with multiple cancer-promoting processes: enhanced cell proliferation, migration, invasion, and metastasis; reduced apoptosis; maintenance of cancer stem cell properties; and increased resistance to radiation and chemotherapy treatments. This gene shows high expression across numerous cancer types [29].

Clinical studies of ovarian cancer patients revealed that while high BMI1 expression occurred in a subset of cases, it significantly correlated with histological grade and reduced survival time [30]. Another investigation confirmed the association between elevated BMI1 expression and poor patient survival [31]. Current BMI1-targeted therapies primarily rely on small molecule inhibitors [29]; however, these approaches have limitations: they require continuous administration until disease resolution and lack BMI1-specific targeting [29]. These limitations position BMI1 as an attractive target for CRISPR-Cas ovarian cancer therapy, with potential applications in other cancers. However, given BMI1's broad influence on gene regulation, careful evaluation of potential unintended effects from its knockout is essential. Zhao et al. employed pX330 BbsI vectors to deliver CRISPR-Cas9 components to SKOV3 ovarian cancer cells [32]. Their approach utilized two gRNAs targeting different BMI1 domains to enhance editing efficiency. Following puromycin selection of successfully transfected cells, they achieved complete BMI1 expression elimination. This BMI1 knockout resulted in decreased cell proliferation, migration, and invasion; enhanced apoptosis and platinum sensitivity; reduced tumor formation rate in subcutaneous inoculation (from 100% to 50%); and dramatic reduction in average tumor size (from 1986.7 mm^3 to 5.3 mm^3). Significantly, BMI1 elimination showed no pro-oncogenic effects, supporting its potential as a CRISPR-Cas9 therapeutic target for both ovarian and other cancers.

11.5 CRISPR/Cas9-based Double Knockouts

Walton et al. [33] utilized CRISPR-Cas9 to generate both single (Trp53-/-) and double (Trp53-/-, Brca2-/-) gene deletions in the ID8 murine ovarian carcinoma model. The Trp53-/-, Brca2-/- mutations led to enhanced sensitivity to rucaparib (a PARP inhibitor), reduced orthotopic tumor growth, and the development of intratumoral tertiary lymphoid structures enriched with CD3+ T cells. In a subsequent study, Walton et al. [34] expanded their investigation to include multiple double knockouts (Trp53/Pten, Trp53/Nf1, and Trp53/Brca2) and a triple knockout (Trp53/Brca1/Pten) within the same model. Their findings revealed that Trp53-/-, Pten-/- and Trp53-/-, Nf1-/- mutations increased tumor growth and reduced survival following cisplatin treatment. In contrast, Trp53-/-, Brca1-/- and Trp53-/-, Brca2-/- tumors exhibited compromised homologous recombination and heightened sensitivity to platinum-based and PARP inhibitor therapies. However, PTEN loss in Trp53-/-, Brca2-/- tumors (resulting in Trp53-/-, Brca2-/-, Pten-/-) significantly diminished cisplatin sensitivity. While double knockouts may enhance chemotherapeutic efficacy, further research is necessary to fully elucidate their impact in ovarian cancer. These studies also contribute to the identification of chemoresistance-associated genes, as evidenced by increased cisplatin resistance following SULF1 and ZNF587B knockdown [35].

Figure 11.1 in this regard illustrates CRISPR/Cas9-mediated therapeutic approaches in ovarian cancer, focusing on single-gene targeting and complex multi-gene knockout strategies to understand tumor biology and enhance chemotherapy response.

11.6 CRISPR/Cas9 in Overcoming Drug Resistance

Platinum-based chemotherapy initially shows promising results in treating ovarian cancer, a deadly malignant condition. Unfortunately, nearly all patients experience disease recurrence, making chemotherapy resistance a significant clinical challenge. Traditional research approaches, including candidate gene analysis and genome-wide association studies, were unable to elucidate the mechanisms behind chemotherapy resistance in ovarian cancer [35].

The emergence of CRISPR/Cas9 technology has led to substantial advances in understanding the genetic foundations of chemotherapy resistance in ovarian cancer. This innovative tool has proven valuable in identifying various biomarkers linked to chemotherapy sensitivity. Research demonstrated that disrupting miR-21 activity using lentiviral CRISPR/Cas9 vectors in SKOV3 and OVCAR-3 ovarian cancer cell lines reduced their ability to invade and multiply. Additionally, apoptosis assays revealed enhanced sensitivity of these cancer cells to paclitaxel treatment [28].

Scientists have identified two key proteins through CRISPR/Cas9 research that could potentially overcome drug resistance in ovarian cancer: B7-H3 [36] and HE4 [37]. Using CRISPR/Cas9, researchers examined B7-H3's influence on ovarian cancer development in OVCAR-3 and A2780 cell lines. They found that elevated B7-H3 levels promoted cancer progression by triggering stem cell characteristics, activating PI3K/AKT pathways, and increasing anti-apoptotic BCL-2 protein expression. The relationship between BCL-2 overexpression and resistance to paclitaxel and cisplatin was confirmed through CRISPR/Cas9-mediated BCL-2 knockout in these cell lines [36].

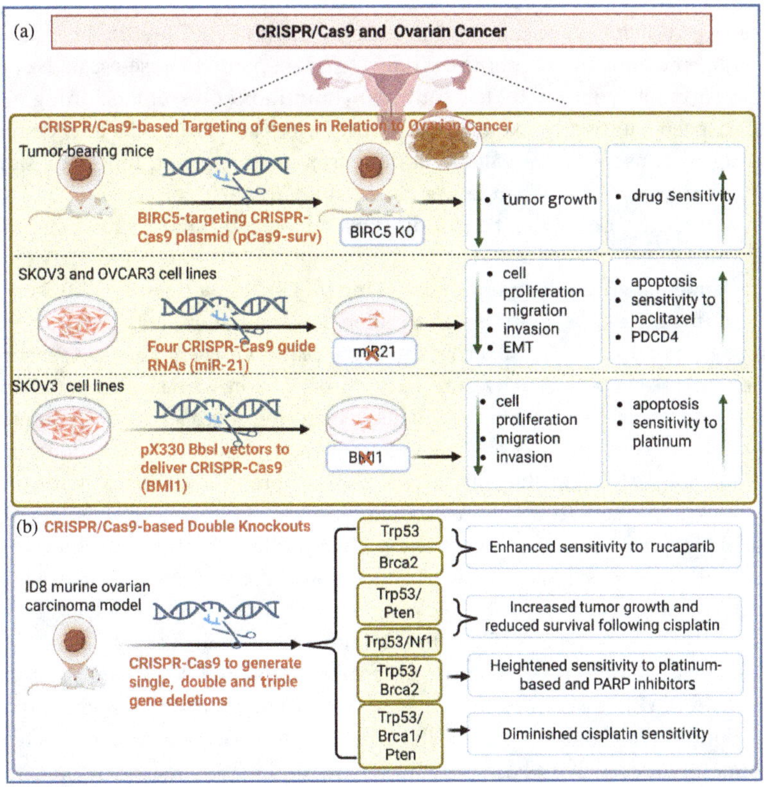

Figure 11.1 CRISPR/Cas9 applications in ovarian cancer: gene targeting and combination knockout strategies. (a) Single-gene targeting; BIRC5 knockout: Lentiviral CRISPR/Cas9 nickase-mediated BIRC5 (survivin) gene editing in tumor-bearing mice and ovarian cancer cell lines (SKOV3 and OVCAR3) inhibits tumor growth and enhances drug sensitivity. BIRC5 knockout suppresses EMT by upregulating epithelial marker cytokeratin 7 and downregulating mesenchymal markers including snail2, β-catenin, and vimentin through attenuation of TGFβ signaling. Cell proliferation, migration, and invasion are significantly inhibited following BIRC5 disruption, and knockout cells demonstrate increased apoptosis and enhanced sensitivity to paclitaxel treatment. Survivin overexpression in ovarian cancer strongly correlates with poor patient survival, chemoresistance, and tumor metastasis, establishing BIRC5 as a critical therapeutic target. **miR-21 knockout:** CRISPR/Cas9-mediated knockout of miR-21 using four gRNAs in SKOV3 and OVCAR3 ovarian cancer cell lines reduces cell proliferation, migration, invasion, and EMT while inducing apoptosis. miR-21 disruption upregulates its target gene PDCD4 (programmed cell death 4), a tumor suppressor that promotes apoptosis. Lentiviral delivery of miR-21 gRNAs sensitizes ovarian cancer cells to

Figure 11.1 (*Continued*) paclitaxel chemotherapy, with CRISPR-edited cells showing significantly enhanced apoptosis induction in response to dose-escalated paclitaxel treatment compared to controls. Immunofluorescent staining with active-caspase-3 antibody confirms that miR-21 loss sensitizes cells to chemotherapy drug response. Clinical validation demonstrates that serum miR-21 is significantly overexpressed in ovarian cancer patients and inversely correlates with PDCD4 levels, supporting miR-21 as both a diagnostic biomarker and therapeutic target. **BMI1 knockout:** CRISPR/Cas9-mediated knockout of BMI1 (B-cell-specific Moloney murine leukemia virus integration site 1) using pX330 BbsI vectors in SKOV3 epithelial ovarian cancer cells reduces cell proliferation, migration, and invasion while promoting apoptosis. BMI1 silencing enhances platinum chemotherapy sensitivity through increased caspase-3 cleavage, reduced Bcl-2 expression, and elevated apoptotic rates (3.3% vs 1.9% in controls). RNA sequencing reveals that BMI1 regulates extracellular matrix structure and angiogenesis through modulation of focal adhesion and PI3K/AKT signaling pathways. BMI1 expression correlates with tumor progression and chemoresistance in ovarian cancer management, establishing it as a potential biomarker and therapeutic target. **(b) Double and triple knockout strategies:** CRISPR/Cas9 technology enables generation of ID8 murine ovarian carcinoma models with single, double, and triple gene deletions to investigate HGSOC biology and chemotherapy responses. **Trp53/Brca2 double knockout:** Trp53-/-; Brca2-/- ID8 cells demonstrate defective homologous recombination and significantly enhanced sensitivity to PARP inhibitor rucaparib *in vitro* compared to Trp53-/- single mutants. These double knockout tumors exhibit slower intraperitoneal growth, increased intratumoral tertiary lymphoid structures rich in CD3+ T cells, and improved response to platinum-based therapy. The model recapitulates key features of BRCA2-deficient HGSOC and validates synthetic lethality approaches using PARP inhibition. **Trp53/Pten double knockout:** Trp53-/-; Pten-/- double mutant cells display increased tumor growth rates *in vivo* and reduced survival following cisplatin chemotherapy compared to Trp53-/- single mutants. Loss of PTEN significantly accelerates Trp53-/-; Brca2-/- tumor growth and reduces platinum sensitivity *in vitro*, indicating that PTEN status modulates chemotherapy response independent of BRCA status. **Trp53/Nf1 double knockout:** Trp53-/-; Nf1-/- cells exhibit accelerated intraperitoneal growth, increased proliferation rates, and decreased survival following cisplatin treatment *in vivo* compared to Trp53-/- controls. These findings suggest that NF1 loss confers aggressive tumor phenotype and chemotherapy resistance in ovarian cancer. **Trp53/Brca2 double knockout with enhanced PARP inhibitor sensitivity:** CRISPR-generated Trp53-/-; Brca2-/- models demonstrate heightened sensitivity to both platinum-based chemotherapy and PARP inhibitors, validating the clinical observation that BRCA2-deficient ovarian cancers respond preferentially to DNA-damaging agents. This model has been instrumental in evaluating combination therapies and

Figure 11.1 (*Continued on facing page*) mechanisms of PARP inhibitor resistance. **Trp53/Brca1/Pten triple knockout:** Trp53-/-; Brca1-/-; Pten-/- triple knockout cells represent advanced HGSOC models with multiple cooperating mutations. These cells maintain defective homologous recombination due to Brca1 loss while exhibiting accelerated growth characteristics conferred by Pten deletion. However, additional PTEN loss significantly reduces cisplatin sensitivity despite retained BRCA1 deficiency, demonstrating complex genotype-phenotype interactions in multi-mutant contexts. The CRISPR/Cas9-generated ID8 derivative models with defined genetic alterations in Trp53, Brca1, Brca2, Pten, and Nf1 provide tractable syngeneic systems to investigate HGSOC biology, tumor-immune interactions, and mechanism-based therapeutic discovery for platinum and PARP inhibitor chemotherapy.

Additionally, studies utilizing CRISPR/Cas double nickase in SKOV3-C1 and OVCAR8 cell lines revealed that HE4 overexpression contributes to chemotherapy resistance by disrupting MAPK signaling and altering tubulin dynamics. Notably, eliminating HE4 in SKOV3-C1 cells showed potential in partially reversing cisplatin resistance [37].

Research utilizing whole genome-scale CRISPR-Cas9 (GeCKO) library has identified ZNF587B and SULF1 as predictive markers for cisplatin resistance in A2780 and SKOV3 ovarian cancer cell lines [35]. To better understand HGSOC, scientists modified the ID8 murine model, which previously lacked typical HGSOC mutations, using CRISPR/Cas9. The modified ID8 models with Trp53−/−; Brca2−/− and Trp53−/−; Brca1−/− showed heightened sensitivity to PARP inhibitors and platinum-based treatments compared to Trp53 deletion alone. Additionally, removing Pten and Nf1 decreased survival rates after cisplatin treatment *in vivo* [34].

Studies demonstrated that CRISPR/Cas9-mediated knockout of P-glycoprotein [10] in ADR/A2780 and CCDC69[38] in A2780cis and SKOV3 cell lines enhanced sensitivity to doxorubicin and cisplatin respectively. The increased cisplatin sensitivity in CCDC69-knockout cells was attributed to mitochondrial Bax redistribution, reduced cMyc expression, and p53 acetylation at K382 [38].

Recent findings show that PLA2G3 expression correlates with poor outcomes, potentially due to its role in lipid droplet formation and ciliation. PLA2G3 knockout using CRISPR/Cas9 reduced tumor growth and increased cellular sensitivity to platinum-based treatments [39]. Similarly, eliminating VASH2, a proangiogenic protein, led to altered expression of tubulin carboxypeptidase and cyclin B1, resulting in improved paclitaxel response [40].

Chemoresistance has been associated with both wild-type and mutant p53. CRISPR/Cas9 studies revealed that loss of p53 phosphorylation at Ser20, caused by Chk2 downregulation, primarily drives cisplatin resistance. This resistance can be overcome using oxaliplatin, which reactivates Ser20 p53 phosphorylation through the MEK1/2 pathway [41].

Additionally, CRISPR/Cas9 research confirmed that chemotherapy can induce point mutations in key redox enzymes, specifically the glutathione peroxidase-1 (GPX1) gene in epithelial ovarian cancer cells, leading to chemoresistance [42]. Overall, CRISPR/Cas9 technology has enabled researchers to identify crucial differences between chemosensitive and chemoresistant cells.

11.7 Preclinical Studies on CRISPR/Cas9 use in Ovarian Cancer Therapy

Several genes, including PRL-R, BMI1, EPHA1, etc., have been identified as key drivers in ovarian cancer initiation and progression [32, 43, 44]. The disease process begins when cells with genetic mutations become resistant to normal growth control mechanisms, leading to abnormal proliferation and tissue invasion. CRISPR-Cas9 technology offers a precise method to eliminate these problematic genes, thereby reducing cellular proliferation, migration, and invasion. For instance, BMI1 deletion using CRISPR-Cas9 promotes cell death and suppresses tumor growth [32].

In their research, Zhao and colleagues examined BMI1 knockout effects in SKNOV3 cell lines using CRISPR-Cas9 [32]. Their findings revealed that BMI1 silencing modified the PI3K/Akt signaling pathway *in vitro* and suppressed tumor cell growth, movement, and invasion in mouse xenograft models. Similarly, Zhu's team employed CRISPR-Cas9 to remove EGFL6 in SKOV3 cells

[45]. This intervention affected multiple genes involved in cancer progression and angiogenesis, notably reducing FGF-2/PDGFB signaling pathway activity and diminishing tumor growth and spread in xenograft studies.

CRISPR-Cas9-mediated APELA knockout in ovarian clear cell carcinoma (OCCC) cell lines increased p53 expression, disrupted cell proliferation, and inhibited cancer development in NOD-SCID mice. Additional studies have demonstrated significant results using CRISPR-Cas9 to target other cancer-associated genes, including BMPR1A, CXCR2, EPHA1, GRHL2, MTF1, MUC16, NANOG, OC-2, PAR2, and PRL-R [10, 46–52].

Furthermore, CRISPR-Cas9 can enhance anti-tumor immunity through PD-L1 gene knockout. Yahata's research team eliminated the PD-L1 gene in ID8 murine ovarian cancer cells using CRISPR-Cas9, resulting in improved anti-tumor immune responses, reduced immunosuppressive cytokine production, and decreased cancer progression in syngeneic mice [53].

Research has shown that CRISPR-Cas9 can be employed to modify genome methylation as a therapeutic approach for ovarian cancer. He and colleagues conducted experiments where they induced ovarian cancers in athymic female nude mice by introducing both paclitaxel-sensitive and paclitaxel-resistant cancer cells into the peritoneal cavity [54]. They then delivered CRISPR-Cas9 targeting DNA methyltransferase 1 (DNMT1) via intraperitoneal liposome injection. This intervention resulted in DNMT1 downregulation and tumor cell necrosis in both types of ovarian cancer tumors.

Multidrug resistance (MDR) presents a significant challenge in ovarian cancer treatment, often arising from increased expression of ATP-binding cassette (ABC) drug transporters. Researchers found that using CRISPR-Cas9 to eliminate the ABCB1 gene (MDR1) in the Adriamycin-resistant A2780/ADR cell line decreased P-glycoprotein expression and enhanced doxorubicin's therapeutic efficacy [10, 55].

Beyond ABCB1 deletion, CRISPR-Cas9 knockout of various other genes has been shown to enhance chemotherapy sensitivity in ovarian cancer cells. For instance, eliminating enhancer of zeste homolog 2 (EZH2) in SK-3rd cells (derived from human epithelial ovarian cancer) reduced CHK1 expression and inhibited both spheroid formation and chemoresistance *in vitro* [56]. Similarly, CRISPR-Cas9-mediated removal of BM1 and BRCA1 genes increased cancer cell susceptibility to chemotherapeutic agents [32, 34].

Research by Walton and colleagues demonstrated that CRISPR-Cas9-mediated elimination of BRCA1 and BRCA2 in ID8 ovarian cancer cells enhanced their responsiveness to platinum-based therapy and PARP inhibitors [33, 34]. Additional studies revealed that targeting BRCA1 using CRISPR-Cas9, either through suppressing TP53-induced glycolysis and apoptosis regulator (TIGAR) [57] or in combination with Trp53 knockout [33], increased tumor cell sensitivity to chemotherapy, promoting cancer cell death and limiting tumor progression.

Combining insights from Walton's [33, 34] and Fang's [57] research suggests that TIGAR gene knockout, which subsequently reduces BRCA1 expression, could be an effective therapeutic strategy. This approach aligns with He and colleagues' work [54], who demonstrated CRISPR-Cas9's potential in targeting genome methylation for ovarian cancer treatment. Their study involved creating ovarian tumors in athymic female nude mice using both paclitaxel-sensitive and resistant cancer cells, followed by CRISPR-Cas9 delivery via liposomes to target DNMT1. This intervention led to DNMT1 downregulation and tumor cell death in both types of cancer.

CRISPR-Cas9 has also proven effective in microRNA modification. Huo and colleagues found that miR-21 knockout increased paclitaxel sensitivity in SKOV3 and OVCAR3 cell lines [28], while miR-137 elimination reduced cisplatin-induced apoptosis in SKOV3 cells [58]. These findings suggest that CRISPR-Cas9 gene editing could represent a promising new approach for targeted molecular therapy.

In a separate investigation, He's team employed a GeCKO (loss-of-function CRISPR-Cas9 knockout library) to identify genes whose absence contributes to chemotherapy resistance (**Table 11.1**)

Table 11.1 CRISPR-Cas9 gene editing targets for ovarian cancer therapy.

Target Gene or Pathway	Biological Role in Cancer	CRISPR-Cas9 Effects	Therapeutic Applications	Cell Lines/ Models Used	Reference
BMI1	Component of PRC1 complex; chromatin remodeling; cell proliferation, migration, invasion	Reduced proliferation, migration, invasion; promoted apoptosis; increased drug sensitivity	Tumor growth inhibition; chemosensitization	SKNOV3 cell lines; mouse xenograft model	[32]
EGFL6	Associated with proliferation, migration, invasion, angiogenesis	Downregulated FGF-2/ PDGFB signaling; reduced tumor growth, metastasis, angiogenesis	Anti-metastatic therapy; anti-angiogenic therapy	SKOV3 cell line; xenograft model	[45]
APELA	Promotes tumor initiation and progression	Induced p53 expression; disrupted cell proliferation; inhibited tumorigenesis	OCCC targeted therapy	OCCC cell lines; NOD-SCID mice	[60]
ABC transporters (ABCB1/MDR1)	Drug efflux pumps; MDR	Reduced P-glycoprotein expression; increased doxorubicin efficacy	Overcoming MDR; chemosensitization	A2780/ADR resistant cell line	[10]

(Continued)

Table 11.1 (*Continued*)

Target Gene or Pathway	Biological Role in Cancer	CRISPR-Cas9 Effects	Therapeutic Applications	Cell Lines/ Models Used	Reference
EZH2	Histone methylation; gene repression	Decreased CHK1 expression; inhibited spheroid formation and chemoresistance	Chemoresistance reversal	SK-3rd epithelial ovarian cancer cell line	[56]
MicroRNAs (miR-21, miR-137)	Gene regulation; oncogenic or tumor suppressor functions	miR-21 knockout: sensitized to paclitaxel; miR-137 knockout: decreased cisplatin-induced apoptosis	MicroRNA-targeted therapy; chemosensitization	SKOV3, OVCAR3 cell lines	[28, 61]
Immunotherapy targets (PD-L1)	Immune checkpoint; immune evasion	Enhanced anti-tumor immunity; downregulated immunosuppressant cytokines	Cancer immunotherapy; immune activation	ID8 murine cell line; syngeneic mice	[53]

[59]. Their research demonstrated that CRISPR-Cas9-mediated DYNLL1 elimination increased chemotherapy resistance in BRCA1-mutant HGSOC.

11.8 CRISPR/Cas9 and Ovarian Cancer Diagnosis or Prognosis

CRISPR/Cas9 technology has revolutionized the identification of oncogenic biomarkers that help predict ovarian cancer susceptibility, assist in diagnosis, and forecast prognosis or metastasis potential. This genetic tool has proven invaluable in examining how various genes influence cancer development and progression.

Using this genome editing technology, researchers identified novel missense variants in BR1P1. When BR1P1 was eliminated using CRISPR/Cas9 in ovarian cancer cells and animal models, increased sensitivity to interstrand crosslinking was observed. These rare variants may indicate elevated ovarian cancer risk, making them valuable for risk assessment and diagnosis [62].

Scientists investigated the role of BCAM-AKT2 fusion gene using CRISPR/Cas9-mediated translocation in HEK-293T and OVCAR8 cell lines. This fusion gene appears in 7% of HGSOC patients, making it a distinctive marker for HGSOC cases [63].

CRISPR/Cas9 also helped identify molecular drivers in granulosa cell tumor. Eliminating miR-10a reduced tumor growth and aggressiveness while affecting chemotherapy response. Research showed that miR-10a influences tumorigenesis and treatment sensitivity by modulating PTEN and Wnt/Akt signaling pathways [64].

Studies using CRISPR/Cas9 to knockout MTF1 (using lentiviral nickase vectors) [65] and ATAD2 (using lentiCRISPRV2 vectors) [66] in ovarian cancer cells revealed their roles in metastasis, cell proliferation, and survival. These findings suggest both genes could serve as biomarkers for early diagnosis, prognosis prediction, and potential therapeutic targets [65, 66].

Researchers used CRISPR/Cas9 to investigate miR137's role in carcinogenesis by creating a knockout model in A2789 ovarian cancer cells. The study revealed that cells lacking miR137 showed increased proliferation rates, establishing miRNA137's function as a tumor suppressor [61].

Similar research identified HCRP1 as a potential metastasis marker in epithelial ovarian cancer, with CRISPR/Cas9 helping to elucidate how its loss of function promotes tumor progression [67]. Studies of DPYSL4 [68] and Dot1L [69] deletion demonstrated their anti-tumor properties: DPYSL4 supports p53's tumor suppression activities [68], while Dot1L loss increases cell invasiveness and promotes cancer stem-like characteristics [69].

CRISPR/Cas9 studies revealed the role of the androgen receptor in ovarian cancer stem cells. In A2780 and SKOV3 cell lines, the androgen receptor was found to promote Nanog (a stem cell marker) overexpression, leading to enhanced proliferation, migration, and tumorigenesis [51].

Additionally, CRISPR/Cas9-mediated modification of various genes — EGFL6 [45], BMPR1A [48], GRHL2 [47], SNAI1 [70], and EIF5A2 [71] — in ovarian cancer cells demonstrated reduced proliferation and migration, indicating their significance in disease prognosis and progression. This technology also contributed to understanding the functions of the mannose receptor LY75.

Research showed that the LY75 receptor plays a crucial role in maintaining epithelial ovarian cancer cell phenotype and potentially influences metastatic capabilities [72]. CRISPR/Cas9 studies revealed a novel chromosomal instability mechanism in HGSOC. Elimination of RBX1 [73], CUL1, and SKP1 [74] genes enhanced chromosomal instability and promoted pre-cancerous cell transformation in ovarian cancer cell lines. Reduced expression of these genes was identified as an early event in HGSOC development.

Scientists also employed CRISPR/Cas9 to investigate the functions of long non-coding RNAs LINK-A and LOC642852 in ovarian cancer cells [75, 76]. LINK-A knockout demonstrated anti-tumor properties by decreasing migration and MMP-9 production [75]. Similarly, LOC642852 inactivation in OVCAR-8 cells and HGSOC clinical samples affected cell signaling pathways. The study revealed that LOC642852 interacts with TLE3 and FGFR3, and its removal significantly decreased cell motility and invasiveness [76].

These studies demonstrate how CRISPR/Cas9's precise gene editing capabilities help establish clear connections between genotype and phenotype in ovarian cancer research [70].

11.9 Challenges and Ethical Considerations

A critical challenge lies in the efficiency of genetic modification and the viability of edited cells. For CRISPR/Cas9-based cancer therapies to be effective, high editing success rates are essential, yet current *in vivo* modification rates remain relatively low, below 10% [77]. The effectiveness of genome editing techniques will enhance as modification rates improve. The editing rate in CRISPR/Cas9 systems is largely determined by how double-strand break repair mechanisms function. Two distinct repair pathways — non-homologous end joining (NHEJ) and homology direct repair (HDR) — result in varying levels of editing success across different cell types and states. While NHEJ operates throughout the cell cycle and proves more versatile for creating indels to disable target genes, HDR occurs exclusively during S/G2 phases. HDR's effectiveness in precise gene modification is limited by both the DNA template types and homology arm length. Enhanced therapeutic outcomes for ovarian cancer could be achieved through strategies that boost both NHEJ and HDR repair efficiencies while reducing unintended modifications [78].

A significant concern is the off-target effect, which occurs when single-guide RNA binds to unintended DNA sequences, creating unwanted cleavage sites. This issue stems from sequence similarities within the human genome and limitations in gRNA target specificity. When gRNA attaches to similar non-target sites, it directs Cas9 to create cleavage points, triggering DNA repair mechanisms that can lead to harmful *in vivo* mutations. Studies have demonstrated that CRISPR/Cas9 frequently generates unintended indels at non-target genomic locations [80, 81]. Several approaches have been developed to minimize Cas9-mediated off-target effects, including high-fidelity Cas9 endonucleases, modified Cas9 nickase, PAM-preference altered Cas9, truncated gRNAs with shorter protospacer complementary sequences, and synthetic switches [82]. Additionally, various computational tools like CasOT, CCTop, Cas-OFFinder, and TagScan help predict potential genome-wide off-target effects [81, 83].

Effective delivery systems represent another crucial challenge in cancer therapy using CRISPR/Cas9. While viral vectors are commonly employed for delivering CRISPR/Cas9 components, adeno-associated virus vectors (AAV) have emerged as the preferred choice for *in vivo* delivery due to their low cytotoxicity, efficient transduction across various cell types, and temporary expression characteristics [84].

A critical concern is cell death triggered by CRISPR/Cas9-induced double-strand DNA repair mechanisms, which can lead to TP53 gene overexpression. While TP53 inhibition can prevent cell death, this approach risks increasing oncogenic potential and off-target effects [87].

The bacterial origin of Cas9 endonuclease poses immunogenicity challenges, triggering pre-existing immune responses that could compromise treatment efficacy and cause adverse effects. This immune response can be reduced through REC1 domain modifications that eliminate T cell-specific immunogenic epitopes [88]. Although AAV vectors show relatively low immunogenicity, they still elicit B and T cell responses against viral components and transgenes, potentially leading to cell destruction, therapeutic neutralization, and complications for future treatments. Non-viral delivery systems, such as liposome-based approaches, may help minimize these immune complications [66].

Additional challenges include CRISPR RNA target site mutations, which can reduce effectiveness as viruses evolve during treatment, though this may be addressed through sequence adjustments [89]. The technology also faces issues with mosaicism [89], RNA instability, and sensitivity to RNA secondary structures [90].

11.10 Future Perspectives

CRISPR/Cas9's advancement from target identification to therapeutic application should proceed through integrated programs that combine robust biomarker strategies with delivery systems tailored to the peritoneal environment. The most promising immediate applications will likely involve targeted editing strategies aligned with specific molecular contexts, including eliminating dominant resistance and survival mechanisms, using base or prime editing to restore sensitivity lost through mutation reversal, and employing CRISPR interference/activation to regulate pathway activity where double-strand breaks would be too risky. Given ovarian cancer's diverse spatial and temporal heterogeneity, future clinical trials should incorporate ongoing molecular analysis across tumor sites, ascites, and circulating DNA to identify suitable editing targets, measure targeting effectiveness, and modify treatment approaches as tumor populations evolve.

To overcome delivery challenges, research should prioritize the development of intraperitoneal, tumor-targeting systems such as ligand-guided lipid nanoparticles, polymeric or extracellular vesicle carriers, and compact viral or hybrid vectors. These systems should be engineered to target ovarian cancer's characteristic expression of folate receptor-α, mesothelin, and αvβ3/αvβ5 integrins. Microenvironment-responsive mechanisms triggered by pH, redox, or enzymatic activity can help concentrate editing activity within malignant areas while minimizing exposure to healthy tissue. Editing components should be temporary and precise, utilizing ribonucleoprotein or mRNA combined with enhanced Cas variants, multiple guide designs to prevent target evasion, and compact nucleases or split systems for size-constrained delivery.

Additional safety measures should include cancer-specific promoters, microRNA response elements to restrict activity to malignant cells, comprehensive off-target analysis, and independent validation to minimize genotoxicity risks, particularly in TP53-deficient contexts.

The most promising therapeutic strategy involves strategic combinations. CRISPR editing can enhance existing treatments in multiple ways: restoring sensitivity to platinum and PARP inhibitors by targeting DNA-repair pathways; improving taxane effectiveness by reducing EMT and stem cell-like properties; and enhancing anti-VEGF treatments by disrupting angiogenic and survival signaling pathways. Immunotherapy combinations show particular promise through elimination of inherent immune checkpoints (such as CISH), enhancement of antigen presentation, and suppression of inhibitory ligands. These approaches could potentially transform unresponsive peritoneal disease into treatment-sensitive states, augmenting checkpoint inhibition or cell-based therapies.

Testing should occur in adaptively designed early-phase trials that utilize intraperitoneal access and measure editing effectiveness, pathway modulation, circulating tumor DNA dynamics, and patient-focused outcomes like ascites management and treatment-free periods. Sustainable clinical implementation requires standardized, GMP-compliant processes for guide selection and editor production, quality control protocols, flexible delivery systems, and adaptable gRNA libraries for addressing emerging resistance.

11.11 Conclusion

Ovarian cancer's high mortality stems from late detection and the persistence of chemoresistant, recurrent disease; within this context, CRISPR/Cas9 provides a timely path to precision by aligning editable genomic lesions with therapeutic intent. Beyond its advantages of design simplicity and multiplexing, the platform's true value lies in its ability to couple mechanism-level edits knocking out resistance drivers, silencing oncogenic programs, or ablating faulty transcripts with measurable restoration of treatment responsiveness and disease control. As delivery technologies, safety engineering, and patient selection frameworks advance, CRISPR/Cas9 can move from mapping vulnerabilities to correcting them, transforming heterogeneous and refractory ovarian cancer into a domain where gene-level interventions augment and personalize existing standards of care.

References

1. Lheureux S, Gourley C, Vergote I, Oza AM. Epithelial ovarian cancer. Lancet. 2019;393(10177):1240–53.

2. Menon U, Karpinskyj C, Gentry-Maharaj A. Ovarian Cancer Prevention and Screening. Obstet Gynecol. 2018;131(5):909–27.
3. Lheureux S, Braunstein M, Oza AM. Epithelial ovarian cancer: Evolution of management in the era of precision medicine. CA Cancer J Clin. 2019;69(4):280–304.
4. Adli M. The CRISPR tool kit for genome editing and beyond. Nat Commun. 2018;9(1):1911.
5. Khan SH. Genome-Editing Technologies: Concept, Pros, and Cons of Various Genome-Editing Techniques and Bioethical Concerns for Clinical Application. Mol Ther Nucleic Acids. 2019;16:326–34.
6. Kurnit KC, Fleming GF, Lengyel E. Updates and New Options in Advanced Epithelial Ovarian Cancer Treatment. Obstet Gynecol. 2021;137(1):108–21.
7. Akram F, Ikram Ul H, Ahmed Z, Khan H, Ali MS. CRISPR-Cas9, A Promising Therapeutic Tool for Cancer Therapy: A Review. Protein Pept Lett. 2020;27(10):931–44.
8. Jiang C, Meng L, Yang B, Luo X. Application of CRISPR/Cas9 gene editing technique in the study of cancer treatment. Clin Genet. 2020;97(1):73–88.
9. Cho SW, Kim S, Kim JM, Kim JS. Targeted genome engineering in human cells with the Cas9 RNA-guided endonuclease. Nat Biotechnol. 2013;31(3):230–2.
10. Norouzi-Barough L, Sarookhani M, Salehi R, Sharifi M, Moghbelinejad S. CRISPR/Cas9, a new approach to successful knockdown of ABCB1/P-glycoprotein and reversal of chemosensitivity in human epithelial ovarian cancer cell line. Iran J Basic Med Sci. 2018;21(2):181–7.
11. Gross AL, Kurman RJ, Vang R, Shih Ie M, Visvanathan K. Precursor lesions of high-grade serous ovarian carcinoma: morphological and molecular characteristics. J Oncol. 2010;2010:126295.
12. Berek JS, Bast Jr RC. Epithelial ovarian cancer. Holland-Frei Cancer Medicine 6th edition: BC Decker; 2003.
13. Prat J. Pathology of cancers of the female genital tract. Int J Gynecol Obstet. 2015;131:S132-S45.
14. Erickson BK, Conner MG, Landen CN, Jr. The role of the fallopian tube in the origin of ovarian cancer. Am J Obstet Gynecol. 2013;209(5):409–14.
15. Kurman RJ, Shih Ie M. The origin and pathogenesis of epithelial ovarian cancer: a proposed unifying theory. Am J Surg Pathol. 2010; 34(3):433–43.

16. Koshiyama M, Matsumura N, Konishi I. Recent concepts of ovarian carcinogenesis: type I and type II. Biomed Res Int. 2014;2014:934261.
17. Jiang F, Zhou K, Ma L, Gressel S, Doudna JA. STRUCTURAL BIOLOGY. A Cas9-guide RNA complex preorganized for target DNA recognition. Science. 2015;348(6242):1477–81.
18. Frazzi R. BIRC3 and BIRC5: multi-faceted inhibitors in cancer. Cell Biosci. 2021;11(1):8.
19. Jaiswal PK, Goel A, Mittal RD. Survivin: A molecular biomarker in cancer. Indian J Med Res. 2015;141(4):389–97.
20. Zhao G, Wang Q, Gu Q, Qiang W, Wei JJ, Dong P, et al. Lentiviral CRISPR/Cas9 nickase vector mediated BIRC5 editing inhibits epithelial to mesenchymal transition in ovarian cancer cells. Oncotarget. 2017;8(55):94666–80.
21. Li F, Aljahdali I, Ling X. Cancer therapeutics using survivin BIRC5 as a target: what can we do after over two decades of study? J Exp Clin Cancer Res. 2019;38(1):368.
22. Slaymaker IM, Gao L, Zetsche B, Scott DA, Yan WX, Zhang F. Rationally engineered Cas9 nucleases with improved specificity. Science. 2016;351(6268):84–8.
23. Ran FA, Hsu PD, Lin CY, Gootenberg JS, Konermann S, Trevino AE, et al. Double nicking by RNA-guided CRISPR Cas9 for enhanced genome editing specificity. Cell. 2013;154(6):1380–9.
24. Shen B, Zhang W, Zhang J, Zhou J, Wang J, Chen L, et al. Efficient genome modification by CRISPR-Cas9 nickase with minimal off-target effects. Nat Methods. 2014;11(4):399–402.
25. Qi Y, Song H, Xiao H, Cheng G, Yu B, Xu FJ. Fluorinated Acid-Labile Branched Hydroxyl-Rich Nanosystems for Flexible and Robust Delivery of Plasmids. Small. 2018;14(42):e1803061.
26. Qi Y, Liu Y, Yu B, Hu Y, Zhang N, Zheng Y, et al. A Lactose-Derived CRISPR/Cas9 Delivery System for Efficient Genome Editing In Vivo to Treat Orthotopic Hepatocellular Carcinoma. Adv Sci (Weinh). 2020;7(17):2001424.
27. Sharma PC, Gupta A. MicroRNAs: potential biomarkers for diagnosis and prognosis of different cancers. Transl Cancer Res. 2020;9(9):5798–818.
28. Huo W, Zhao G, Yin J, Ouyang X, Wang Y, Yang C, et al. Lentiviral CRISPR/Cas9 vector mediated miR-21 gene editing inhibits the epithelial to mesenchymal transition in ovarian cancer cells. J Cancer. 2017;8(1):57–64.

29. Xu J, Li L, Shi P, Cui H, Yang L. The Crucial Roles of Bmi-1 in Cancer: Implications in Pathogenesis, Metastasis, Drug Resistance, and Targeted Therapies. Int J Mol Sci. 2022;23(15):8231.
30. Yang GF, He WP, Cai MY, He LR, Luo JH, Deng HX, et al. Intensive expression of Bmi-1 is a new independent predictor of poor outcome in patients with ovarian carcinoma. BMC Cancer. 2010;10:133.
31. Abd El hafez A, El-Hadaad HA. Immunohistochemical expression and prognostic relevance of Bmi-1, a stem cell factor, in epithelial ovarian cancer. Ann Diagn Pathol. 2014;18(2):58–62.
32. Zhao Q, Qian Q, Cao D, Yang J, Gui T, Shen K. Role of BMI1 in epithelial ovarian cancer: investigated via the CRISPR/Cas9 system and RNA sequencing. J Ovarian Res. 2018;11(1):31.
33. Walton J, Blagih J, Ennis D, Leung E, Dowson S, Farquharson M, et al. CRISPR/Cas9-Mediated Trp53 and Brca2 Knockout to Generate Improved Murine Models of Ovarian High-Grade Serous Carcinoma. Cancer Res. 2016;76(20):6118–29.
34. Walton JB, Farquharson M, Mason S, Port J, Kruspig B, Dowson S, et al. CRISPR/Cas9-derived models of ovarian high grade serous carcinoma targeting Brca1, Pten and Nf1, and correlation with platinum sensitivity. Sci Rep. 2017;7(1):16827.
35. Ouyang Q, Liu Y, Tan J, Li J, Yang D, Zeng F, et al. Loss of ZNF587B and SULF1 contributed to cisplatin resistance in ovarian cancer cell lines based on Genome-scale CRISPR/Cas9 screening. Am J Cancer Res. 2019;9(5):988–98.
36. Zhou L, Zhao Y. B7-H3 Induces Ovarian Cancer Drugs Resistance Through An PI3K/AKT/BCL-2 Signaling Pathway. Cancer Manag Res. 2019;11:10205–14.
37. Ribeiro JR, Schorl C, Yano N, Romano N, Kim KK, Singh RK, Moore RG. HE4 promotes collateral resistance to cisplatin and paclitaxel in ovarian cancer cells. J Ovarian Res. 2016;9(1):28.
38. Cui L, Liang B, Yang Y, Zhu M, Kwong J, Zheng H, Wang CC. Inhibition of coiled coil domain containing protein 69 enhances platinum-induced apoptosis in ovarian cancer cells. Oncotarget. 2017;8(60):101634–48.
39. Ray U, Roy D, Jin L, Thirusangu P, Staub J, Xiao Y, et al. Group III phospholipase A2 downregulation attenuated survival and metastasis in ovarian cancer and promotes chemo-sensitization. J Exp Clin Cancer Res. 2021;40(1):182.

40. Koyanagi T, Saga Y, Takahashi Y, Tamura K, Yoshiba T, Takahashi S, et al. Knockout of vasohibin-2 reduces tubulin carboxypeptidase activity and increases paclitaxel sensitivity in ovarian cancer. Cancer Med. 2021;10(8):2732–9.
41. Bhatt M, Ivan C, Xie X, Siddik ZH. Drug-dependent functionalization of wild-type and mutant p53 in cisplatin-resistant human ovarian tumor cells. Oncotarget. 2017;8(7):10905–18.
42. Fletcher NM, Belotte J, Saed MG, Memaj I, Diamond MP, Morris RT, Saed GM. Specific point mutations in key redox enzymes are associated with chemoresistance in epithelial ovarian cancer. Free Radic Biol Med. 2017;102:122–32.
43. Cui Y, Wu BO, Flamini V, Evans BAJ, Zhou D, Jiang WG. Knockdown of EPHA1 Using CRISPR/CAS9 Suppresses Aggressive Properties of Ovarian Cancer Cells. Anticancer Res. 2017;37(8):4415–24.
44. Karthikeyan S, Russo A, Dean M, Lantvit DD, Endsley M, Burdette JE. Prolactin signaling drives tumorigenesis in human high grade serous ovarian cancer cells and in a spontaneous fallopian tube derived model. Cancer Lett. 2018;433:221–31.
45. Zhu W, Liu C, Lu T, Zhang Y, Zhang S, Chen Q, Deng N. Knockout of EGFL6 by CRISPR/Cas9 Mediated Inhibition of Tumor Angiogenesis in Ovarian Cancer. Front Oncol. 2020;10:1451.
46. Chen X, Li X, Wang X, Zhu Q, Wu X, Wang X. MUC16 impacts tumor proliferation and migration through cytoplasmic translocation of P120-catenin in epithelial ovarian cancer cells: an original research. BMC Cancer. 2019;19(1):171.
47. Faddaoui A, Sheta R, Bachvarova M, Plante M, Gregoire J, Renaud MC, et al. Suppression of the grainyhead transcription factor 2 gene (GRHL2) inhibits the proliferation, migration, invasion and mediates cell cycle arrest of ovarian cancer cells. Cell Cycle. 2017;16(7):693–706.
48. Hirschhorn T, Levi-Hofman M, Danziger O, Smorodinsky NI, Ehrlich M. Differential molecular regulation of processing and membrane expression of Type-I BMP receptors: implications for signaling. Cell Mol Life Sci. 2017;74(14):2645–62.
49. Jiang Y, Lim J, Wu KC, Xu W, Suen JY, Fairlie DP. PAR2 induces ovarian cancer cell motility by merging three signalling pathways to transactivate EGFR. Br J Pharmacol. 2021;178(4):913–32.
50. Kodama M, Kodama T, Newberg JY, Katayama H, Kobayashi M, Hanash SM, et al. In vivo loss-of-function screens identify KPNB1 as

a new druggable oncogene in epithelial ovarian cancer. Proc Natl Acad Sci U S A. 2017;114(35):E7301-e10.

51. Ling K, Jiang L, Liang S, Kwong J, Yang L, Li Y, et al. Nanog interaction with the androgen receptor signaling axis induce ovarian cancer stem cell regulation: studies based on the CRISPR/Cas9 system. J Ovarian Res. 2018;11(1):36.
52. Qin W, Xiong Y, Chen J, Huang Y, Liu T. DC-CIK cells derived from ovarian cancer patient menstrual blood activate the TNFR1-ASK1-AIP1 pathway to kill autologous ovarian cancer stem cells. J Cell Mol Med. 2018;22(7):3364–76.
53. Yahata T, Mizoguchi M, Kimura A, Orimo T, Toujima S, Kuninaka Y, et al. Programmed cell death ligand 1 disruption by clustered regularly interspaced short palindromic repeats/Cas9-genome editing promotes antitumor immunity and suppresses ovarian cancer progression. Cancer Sci. 2019;110(4):1279–92.
54. He ZY, Zhang YG, Yang YH, Ma CC, Wang P, Du W, et al. In Vivo Ovarian Cancer Gene Therapy Using CRISPR-Cas9. Hum Gene Ther. 2018;29(2):223–33.
55. Binkhathlan Z, Lavasanifar A. P-glycoprotein inhibition as a therapeutic approach for overcoming multidrug resistance in cancer: current status and future perspectives. Curr Cancer Drug Targets. 2013;13(3):326–46.
56. Wen Y, Hou Y, Yi X, Sun S, Guo J, He X, et al. EZH2 activates CHK1 signaling to promote ovarian cancer chemoresistance by maintaining the properties of cancer stem cells. Theranostics. 2021;11(4):1795–813.
57. Fang P, De Souza C, Minn K, Chien J. Genome-scale CRISPR knockout screen identifies TIGAR as a modifier of PARP inhibitor sensitivity. Commun Biol. 2019;2:335.
58. Li X, Chen W, Zeng W, Wan C, Duan S, Jiang S. microRNA-137 promotes apoptosis in ovarian cancer cells via the regulation of XIAP. Br J Cancer. 2017;116(1):66–76.
59. He YJ, Meghani K, Caron MC, Yang C, Ronato DA, Bian J, et al. DYNLL1 binds to MRE11 to limit DNA end resection in BRCA1-deficient cells. Nature. 2018;563(7732):522–6.
60. Yi Y, Tsai SH, Cheng JC, Wang EY, Anglesio MS, Cochrane DR, et al. APELA promotes tumour growth and cell migration in ovarian cancer in a p53-dependent manner. Gynecol Oncol. 2017;147(3):663–71.

61. Chen W, Li Q, Du J, Li X, Jiang S, He Y. Establishment of an miR-137-knockout cell model using CRISPR/Cas9 genome editing. Oncol Lett. 2018;16(3):4027–32.
62. Moyer CL, Ivanovich J, Gillespie JL, Doberstein R, Radke MR, Richardson ME, et al. Rare BRIP1 Missense Alleles Confer Risk for Ovarian and Breast Cancer. Cancer Res. 2020;80(4):857–67.
63. Kannan K, Coarfa C, Chao PW, Luo L, Wang Y, Brinegar AE, et al. Recurrent BCAM-AKT2 fusion gene leads to a constitutively activated AKT2 fusion kinase in high-grade serous ovarian carcinoma. Proc Natl Acad Sci U S A. 2015;112(11):E1272–7.
64. Tu J, Cheung HH, Lu G, Chen Z, Chan WY. MicroRNA-10a promotes granulosa cells tumor development via PTEN-AKT/Wnt regulatory axis. Cell Death Dis. 2018;9(11):1076.
65. Ji L, Zhao G, Zhang P, Huo W, Dong P, Watari H, et al. Knockout of MTF1 Inhibits the Epithelial to Mesenchymal Transition in Ovarian Cancer Cells. J Cancer. 2018;9(24):4578–85.
66. Liu Q, Liu H, Li L, Dong X, Ru X, Fan X, et al. ATAD2 predicts poor outcomes in patients with ovarian cancer and is a marker of proliferation. Int J Oncol. 2020;56(1):219–31.
67. Tomasich E, Topakian T, Heller G, Udovica S, Krainer M, Marhold M. Loss of HCRP1 leads to upregulation of PD-L1 via STAT3 activation and is of prognostic significance in EGFR-dependent cancer. Transl Res. 2021;230:21–33.
68. Nagano H, Hashimoto N, Nakayama A, Suzuki S, Miyabayashi Y, Yamato A, et al. p53-inducible DPYSL4 associates with mitochondrial supercomplexes and regulates energy metabolism in adipocytes and cancer cells. Proc Natl Acad Sci U S A. 2018;115(33):8370–5.
69. Wang X, Wang H, Xu B, Jiang D, Huang S, Yu H, et al. Depletion of H3K79 methyltransferase Dot1L promotes cell invasion and cancer stem-like cell property in ovarian cancer. Am J Transl Res. 2019;11(2):1145–53.
70. Haraguchi M, Sato M, Ozawa M. CRISPR/Cas9n-Mediated Deletion of the Snail 1Gene (SNAI1) Reveals Its Role in Regulating Cell Morphology, Cell-Cell Interactions, and Gene Expression in Ovarian Cancer (RMG-1) Cells. PLoS One. 2015;10(7):e0132260.
71. Zhao G, Zhang W, Dong P, Watari H, Guo Y, Pfeffer LM, et al. EIF5A2 controls ovarian tumor growth and metastasis by promoting epithelial to mesenchymal transition via the TGFβ pathway. Cell Biosci. 2021;11(1):70.

72. Faddaoui A, Bachvarova M, Plante M, Gregoire J, Renaud MC, Sebastianelli A, et al. The mannose receptor LY75 (DEC205/CD205) modulates cellular phenotype and metastatic potential of ovarian cancer cells. Oncotarget. 2016;7(12):14125–42.
73. Bungsy M, Palmer MCL, Jeusset LM, Neudorf NM, Lichtensztejn Z, Nachtigal MW, McManus KJ. Reduced RBX1 expression induces chromosome instability and promotes cellular transformation in high-grade serous ovarian cancer precursor cells. Cancer Lett. 2021;500:194–207.
74. Lepage CC, Palmer MCL, Farrell AC, Neudorf NM, Lichtensztejn Z, Nachtigal MW, McManus KJ. Reduced SKP1 and CUL1 expression underlies increases in Cyclin E1 and chromosome instability in cellular precursors of high-grade serous ovarian cancer. Br J Cancer. 2021;124(10):1699–710.
75. Filippov-Levy N, Davidson B, Reich R. The Biological Role of the Long Non-coding RNA LINK-A in Ovarian Carcinoma. Anticancer Res. 2020;40(12):6677–84.
76. Filippov-Levy N, Reich R, Davidson B. The Biological and Clinical Role of the Long Non-Coding RNA LOC642852 in Ovarian Carcinoma. Int J Mol Sci. 2020;21(15):5237.
77. Yi L, Li J. CRISPR-Cas9 therapeutics in cancer: promising strategies and present challenges. Biochim Biophys Acta. 2016;1866(2):197–207.
78. Jacinto FV, Link W, Ferreira BI. CRISPR/Cas9-mediated genome editing: From basic research to translational medicine. J Cell Mol Med. 2020;24(7):3766–78.
79. Uddin F, Rudin CM, Sen T. CRISPR Gene Therapy: Applications, Limitations, and Implications for the Future. Front Oncol. 2020;10:1387.
80. Fu Y, Foden JA, Khayter C, Maeder ML, Reyon D, Joung JK, Sander JD. High-frequency off-target mutagenesis induced by CRISPR-Cas nucleases in human cells. Nat Biotechnol. 2013;31(9):822–6.
81. Zhang XH, Tee LY, Wang XG, Huang QS, Yang SH. Off-target Effects in CRISPR/Cas9-mediated Genome Engineering. Mol Ther Nucleic Acids. 2015;4(11):e264.
82. Chen M, Mao A, Xu M, Weng Q, Mao J, Ji J. CRISPR-Cas9 for cancer therapy: Opportunities and challenges. Cancer Lett. 2019;447:48–55.
83. Naeem M, Majeed S, Hoque MZ, Ahmad I. Latest Developed Strategies to Minimize the Off-Target Effects in CRISPR-Cas-Mediated Genome Editing. Cells. 2020;9(7):1608.

84. Mingozzi F, High KA. Therapeutic in vivo gene transfer for genetic disease using AAV: progress and challenges. Nat Rev Genet. 2011;12(5):341–55.
85. Naso MF, Tomkowicz B, Perry WL, 3rd, Strohl WR. Adeno-Associated Virus (AAV) as a Vector for Gene Therapy. BioDrugs. 2017;31(4):317–34.
86. Osborn MJ, Gabriel R, Webber BR, DeFeo AP, McElroy AN, Jarjour J, et al. Fanconi anemia gene editing by the CRISPR/Cas9 system. Hum Gene Ther. 2015;26(2):114–26.
87. Haapaniemi E, Botla S, Persson J, Schmierer B, Taipale J. CRISPR-Cas9 genome editing induces a p53-mediated DNA damage response. Nat Med. 2018;24(7):927–30.
88. Mehta A, Merkel OM. Immunogenicity of Cas9 Protein. J Pharm Sci. 2020;109(1):62–7.
89. Mehravar M, Shirazi A, Nazari M, Banan M. Mosaicism in CRISPR/Cas9-mediated genome editing. Dev Biol. 2019;445(2):156–62.
90. Nelles DA, Fang MY, Aigner S, Yeo GW. Applications of Cas9 as an RNA-programmed RNA-binding protein. Bioessays. 2015;37(7):732–9.

https://doi.org/10.1142/9789819826759_0012

CHAPTER 12

CRISPR/Cas9 in the Treatment of Bone Cancers

Mehrdad Hashemi[1,2], *Alireza Khosravinejad*[1,3], *Mina Alimohammadi*[4], *Reza Mohajer Shirazi*[1,3], *Behdokht Jamali*[5], *Ali Shirazi*[1,3], *Kimia Sadat Esfahani*[1,3], *Rojin Ghannad Zadeh*[1,6], *Faranak Jamshidian*[1,7], *Neda Zali*[3], *Najma Farahani*[1,*], *Afshin Taheriazam*[1,8,*], *Payman Rahimzadeh*[9,*], *Maliheh Entezari*[1,2,*]

[1]Farhikhtegan Medical Convergent Sciences Research Center, Farhikhtegan Hospital, Faculty of Medicine, TeMs. C., Islamic Azad University, Tehran, Iran
[2]Department of Genetics, Faculty of Advanced Sciences and Technology, TeMs. C, Islamic Azad University, Tehran, Iran
[3]Basic and Molecular Epidemiology of Gastrointestinal Disorders Research Center, Research Institute for Gastroenterology and Liver Diseases, Shahid Beheshti University of Medical Sciences, Tehran, Iran
[4]Department of Immunology, School of Medicine, Shahid Beheshti University of Medical Sciences, Tehran, Iran
[5]Department of Microbiology and Genetics, Kherad Institute of Higher Education, Bushehr, Iran

---

* **Corresponding authors:** Najmafarahani@gmail.com (N.F.); a.taheriazam@iautmu.ac.ir (A.T.); P.rahimzadeh76@gmail.com (P.R.); mentezari@iautmu.ac.ir (M.E.)

[6]Department of Art & Sciences, Faculty of Biology, University of North Florida, Jacksonville, Florida, USA
[7]Department of Biology, ET.C., Islamic Azad University, Tehran, Iran
[8]Department of Orthopedics, Faculty of Medicine, TeMs. C, Islamic Azad University, Tehran, Iran
[9]Surgical Research Society (SRS), Students' Scientific Research Center, Tehran University of Medical Sciences, Tehran, Iran

Abstract

In bone cancer research, CRISPR/Cas9 is being used to map oncogenic drivers, resistance mechanisms, and metastatic programs; validate therapeutic targets; and engineer faithful cell and animal models that capture intratumoral heterogeneity and microenvironmental cues. Applications include knockout of oncogenes and drug resistance effectors, restoration or modulation of tumor suppressors, and perturbation of DNA damage response pathways to sensitize tumors to chemotherapy and radiotherapy. These efforts directly address limitations of current standards, multi-agent chemotherapy toxicity, long-term risks of radiotherapy, and high relapse rates, by enabling precision strategies that enhance treatment responsiveness or attenuate malignant circuitry with greater specificity. Ongoing advances in delivery (e.g., tumor-targeted nanoparticles, viral and non-viral vectors, *ex vivo* editing with adoptive transfer) and high-fidelity nucleases (paired nickases, HiFi Cas9, base and prime editors) are reducing off-target risks while expanding the therapeutic toolkit. As these technologies mature, CRISPR/Cas9 is poised to bridge mechanistic discovery and intervention in musculoskeletal malignancies, supporting rational combinations with DNA damage response inhibitors, targeted agents, and immunotherapies, and paving the way for clinically meaningful, genotype- and phenotype-informed gene editing in bone cancers.

Keywords: CRISPR/Cas9; bone cancer; osteosarcoma; gene knockout; homology-directed repair; nonhomologous end joining; functional genomics; translational oncology

12.1 Introduction

Scientists first discovered the CRISPR sequence within *Escherichia coli* [1]. Further research revealed its extensive presence across bacterial and archaeal species. The structure comprises repetitive elements interspersed with spacer segments of comparable length. In conjunction with the nearby Cas9 gene, this sequence forms the CRISPR/Cas9 complex, which serves as a crucial defense mechanism in prokaryotic organisms, enabling them to develop resistance against viral infections and foreign genetic material [2–4].

Through transcription and enzymatic modification, the CRISPR sequence develops into functional CRISPR RNA (crRNA) [5]. This crRNA contains repetitive elements that interact with trans-activated crRNA (tracrRNA) to establish a dual-RNA structure. When bacteria encounter foreign genetic material, the crRNA spacer can incorporate segments of the invading phage genome (prospacer), creating an immunological memory that enhances the organism's defense capabilities [6].

The CAS9 protein utilizes this system to locate and cleave specific DNA sequences, resulting in clean-cut double-strand breaks [7]. In mammalian cell systems, these breaks undergo repair through one of two mechanisms: the precise homology-directed repair (HDR) pathway [8] or the error-prone non-homologous end joining (NHEJ) process [9]. While HDR maintains genetic accuracy during repair, NHEJ often introduces random modifications at the break site through insertions or deletions.

A groundbreaking advancement occurred in 2013 when Mali [10] and Cong [11] independently adapted the CRISPR/Cas9 system for mammalian genome modification. Their innovation involved expressing bacterial CRISPR components in mammalian cells and developing a synthetic crRNA-tracrRNA fusion molecule (gRNA) that guides Cas9 to specific DNA targets for precise genetic alterations. The CRISPR/Cas9 platform rapidly emerged as a leading technology in biomedical research, demonstrating several advantages over previous gene-editing methods like transcription activator-like effector nucleases and zinc finger nucleases: enhanced design simplicity, as targeting new DNA sequences only requires changing the single-guide RNA (sgRNA) while maintaining the same Cas9 enzyme, significantly reducing development time [12, 13]; improved editing capabilities due to the compact nature of sgRNAs, which allows for simultaneous modification of multiple genetic targets [14]; and superior targeting efficiency with reduced experimental costs [13].

These distinctive features have catalyzed significant advances in biomedical applications and therapeutic interventions. A notable clinical success involved treating a patient with dual acute lymphoblastic leukemia and HIV infection using CRISPR-modified CCR5-knockout hematopoietic stem and progenitor cells. This intervention achieved remission without editing-related complications and increased CCR5-ablated CD4+ cell populations following antiretroviral therapy cessation [15]. The technology's therapeutic applications have expanded to numerous clinical trials addressing various conditions [16], including hematological disorders, inherited ocular diseases, viral infections, and multiple cancer types such as malignant glioma, metastatic non-small cell lung cancer, prostate cancer, esophageal cancer, and renal cell carcinoma.

Malignant musculoskeletal neoplasms predominantly affect young populations, with osteosarcoma, Ewing sarcoma, and rhabdomyosarcoma being the most prevalent forms. Current therapeutic protocols integrate surgical intervention, chemotherapeutic agents, and radiation treatments [17]. While this multimodal approach has yielded better outcomes compared to traditional surgical excision alone, several challenges persist: chemotherapy-associated toxicity and adverse effects, risk of tumor recurrence over time, and the potential development of secondary malignancies following radiotherapy. These limitations underscore the urgent need for novel therapeutic strategies offering reduced side effects and enhanced long-term effectiveness.

CRISPR/Cas9 technology has demonstrated promising applications in musculoskeletal tumor research, including the identification and elimination of cancer-promoting genes, neutralization of drug resistance mechanisms, discovery of tumor-suppressing genetic elements, and development of cellular and animal models for cancer research. A comprehensive analysis of CRISPR/Cas9's current applications and implementation challenges in malignant musculoskeletal tumor research could accelerate therapeutic advancements in this field. This section examines recent developments in applying CRISPR/Cas9 technology toward treating these aggressive musculoskeletal malignancies.

12.2 Biology and Molecular Landscape of Bone Cancer

Osteosarcoma, a prevalent form of bone cancer, predominantly emerges during adolescence when long bones undergo rapid growth. The epiphyseal growth plate, particularly in the distal femur and proximal tibia regions, serves as the origin point for over 50% of cases. These areas are crucial for skeletal development and height increase during teenage years [18].

The pathogenesis of osteosarcoma involves several mechanisms, including disruptions in mesenchymal stem cell (MSC) differentiation into mature osteoblasts [19]. The malignant transformation process is facilitated by irregular oncogene expression and tumor suppressor gene function, which results from both genetic and epigenetic modifications that disrupt essential cellular signaling pathways [20, 21]. The heightened bone remodeling activity during growth periods increases the likelihood of irregularities in differentiation and signaling processes [18].

Bone marrow stromal MSCs possess unique characteristics, including self-renewal capabilities and the ability to differentiate into various tissues such as bone, muscle, tendon, and adipose tissue [22]. The transformation of MSCs into osteoblasts through osteogenesis relies on multiple internal and external factors. When these factors become dysregulated or encounter unusual stimuli like inflammatory or tumorigenic cytokines, it can disrupt the balance between cellular differentiation and multiplication, potentially leading to malignancy [23, 24]. Within the tumor microenvironment, MSCs play a significant role in facilitating cancer cell proliferation, metastatic spread, and treatment resistance in osteosarcoma [25].

Research has revealed that osteosarcoma is characterized by diverse alterations at genetic, epigenetic, and molecular levels. These modifications include chromosomal abnormalities, suppressor gene deactivation, and disrupted signaling pathways [26]. These mechanisms will be explored in greater depth in subsequent sections.

12.3 CRISPR/Cas9 in Osteosarcoma Management and Treatment

Osteosarcoma represents the most prevalent skeletal tumor in young populations, ranking as the third most common childhood cancer after lymphoma and brain tumors, while constituting about 1% of adult malignancies [27, 28]. Despite its relatively low occurrence rate, with only 800 new diagnoses yearly in the United States, patient outcomes remain concerning [28]. The ten-year survival rate hovers around 50% [29, 30].

The disease presents significant challenges: 30–40% of patients experience local recurrence post-treatment [27], over 80% of localized tumors may develop metastases, and approximately 20% of cases already show metastatic spread at initial diagnosis [28]. For patients with metastatic disease or recurrence, the five-year survival rate falls below 30% [27].

Current treatment protocols involve neoadjuvant chemotherapy, surgical intervention, and post-operative chemotherapy extending 6–8 months. The standard MAP regimen combines cisplatin, high-dose methotrexate, and adriamycin [28, 29, 31]. While combination chemotherapy has improved survival rates, serious concerns exist regarding toxic side effects, including doxorubicin's cardiotoxicity [32], cisplatin's otorenal toxicity and carcinogenic potential [33–35], and methotrexate's adverse effects on bone marrow, liver, kidneys, and ocular mucosa [34, 35]. Additionally, chemotherapy resistance often leads to recurrence and decreased survival rates.

Understanding osteosarcoma's genetic basis is crucial for addressing these clinical challenges. While its exact etiology remains unclear, certain hereditary conditions are associated with increased risk, including retinoblastoma, Li-Fraumeni syndrome, Rothmund-Thomson syndrome, and Werner syndrome, involving mutations in RB1, TP53, RECQL4, and WRN genes respectively [28, 36].

Treatment outcomes are significantly influenced by germline genes and pharmacogenetics, particularly those involved in drug transport (ABCC3, ABCB1, RFC1, GST family) and DNA repair (ERCC1, ERCC2, XPC). The latter group specifically affects cisplatin-induced DNA damage repair. Research has shown that mutations in these genes impact drug sensitivity and often correlate with poor prognosis in osteosarcoma patients [37–43]. The precision targeting capability of CRISPR/Cas9 technology shows promise for future therapeutic applications in osteosarcoma treatment.

The pioneering application of CRISPR/Cas9 technology in osteosarcoma research was initiated by Feng et al. Their study demonstrated that CD11K gene deletion in KHOS and U-2OS osteosarcoma cell lines significantly reduced cell migration, invasion, and proliferation [44].

Subsequent research has extensively utilized CRISPR/Cas9 for targeting various oncogenes in osteosarcoma. Research revealed that Saos osteosarcoma cells became non-viable following GLT25D1 and GLT25D2 gene elimination [45]. In highly invasive osteosarcoma cell lines (143B and MNNG/HOS), CD44 deletion resulted in decreased cell mobility and significantly reduced spheroid formation and growth [46].

The effectiveness of CRISPR/Cas9 gene editing has also been validated through *in vivo* studies. CD81-deleted 143B cells, when introduced into nude mice, showed markedly reduced pulmonary metastases compared to controls [47]. Similarly, FGF5-knockout in MG63 and U2OS cells, followed by tibia transplantation in nude mice, demonstrated significant tumor growth suppression [48].

CRISPR/Cas9 technology has shown particular promise in enhancing chemotherapy effectiveness. In the multidrug-resistant KHOSR2 cell line, mutant TP53 deletion increased sensitivity to adriamycin [49]. PD-L1 elimination in KHOS and MNNG/HOS cells enhanced their response to paclitaxel and doxorubicin treatments [50]. In KHOSR2 and U-2OSR2 cells, CD44 knockout led to decreased expression of the drug efflux protein p-gp (encoded by ABCB1), resulting in improved doxorubicin absorption and sensitivity [51]. Direct ABCB1 gene knockout in KHOSR2 and U-2OS cells effectively reversed their adriamycin resistance [52].

These experimental findings suggest that targeted oncogene elimination through CRISPR/Cas9 technology shows promising potential for both inhibiting osteosarcoma progression and addressing chemotherapy resistance issues.

12.4 CRISPR/Cas9 and Gene Targeting in Osteosarcoma

CRISPR/Cas9 technology has proven valuable in studying tumor suppressor genes through targeted deletion experiments. Research showed that eliminating CNE9, CNE10, or STAG2 genes in U2OS cells reduced apoptotic activity. While CNE9 or CNE10 deletion resulted in decreased cell proliferation, confirming their tumor-suppressive nature, STAG2 knockout produced different effects. STAG2-deficient cells showed enhanced epithelial-mesenchymal transition (EMT), increased invasiveness, and elevated PD-L1 expression. These cells also exhibited altered immune-related gene expression and increased cisplatin resistance, suggesting that STAG2 loss might protect tumor cells from immune responses through PD-L1 mediation. This finding indicates STAG2's potential as a biomarker for PD-1-PD-L1 inhibitor therapy in STAG2-deficient osteosarcoma [53, 54].

Studies with decitabine (DAC), a DNA methylation inhibitor, demonstrated its ability to suppress various cancer cell behaviors including proliferation, mobility, anchorage-independent growth, and spheroid formation. DAC also reduced xenograft tumor growth, metastasis, and expression of stem cell markers (SOX2, OCT4, NANOG). Notably, CRISPR/Cas9-mediated ESR1 gene knockout nullified these DAC effects, indicating ESR1's crucial role in DAC's anti-tumor activity [55].

CRISPR/Cas9 research also revealed SENP2's potential as a therapeutic target, as it shows reduced expression in primary osteosarcoma tissues and cell lines. Experimental SENP2 overexpression significantly inhibited cancer cell activities, while CRISPR/Cas9-mediated SENP2 knockout reversed these effects [56].

Beyond gene knockout applications, CRISPR/Cas9 has been used to create stable gene overexpression cell lines. For instance, RECQL5, typically downregulated in osteosarcoma, was inserted into the human AAVS1 safe harbor using CRISPR/Cas9. The resulting stable RECQL5-overexpressing MG63 cell line showed reduced proliferation, cell cycle arrest, and increased apoptosis, establishing RECQL5's role as a tumor suppressor in osteosarcoma [57].

CRISPR/Cas9 technology has been instrumental in developing animal and cellular models for studying human osteosarcoma. In one significant study [58], researchers demonstrated that when TP53 was knocked out in pig zygotes using CRISPR/Cas9, approximately 50% of the surviving piglets developed various tumors, including osteosarcoma, after being transplanted *in vivo*. This innovative combination of CRISPR/Cas9 and *in vitro* fertilization technologies offers a cost-effective approach to generating genetically modified pigs, providing a physiologically and anatomically relevant model for preclinical osteosarcoma studies.

Research utilizing CRISPR/Cas9 to create a RAD52-deficient U2OS cell model [59] revealed RAD52's crucial role in repairing collapsed DNA replication forks damaged by chemicals or oncogenes. The study showed that RAD52 deletion impaired fork recovery and triggered DNA damage.

Another investigation [60] employed CRISPR/Cas9 to generate PAWS1 and CD2AP knockout U2OS cell models. This research highlighted the vital functions of these proteins in maintaining proper actin organization and focal adhesion formation. Their absence led to disrupted actin networks, diminished cell motility, and impaired focal adhesion development. These findings contribute significantly to understanding cytoskeletal regulation, embryonic development, blood vessel formation, EMT, and cancer cell migration.

Additional cell models created through CRISPR/Cas9 include NRF-2-deficient U2OS cells for exploring sulforaphane's mTOR inhibition mechanisms [61], CNN3 knockout cells for studying stress fiber formation [62], G3BP-deficient cells for viral interaction studies [63], and CRY1/CRY2 knockout models for circadian rhythm research [64].

CRISPR/Cas9 technology shows promising potential in identifying and analyzing genes associated with cancer development. A notable study by Marko and colleagues [65] employed forward genetic screening using a cancer gene database to identify SRGAP2, a genetic locus potentially linked to osteosarcoma progression. Their research, utilizing CRISPR/Cas9-mediated knockout and doxycycline-induced overexpression in mouse osteosarcoma cells, revealed SRGAP2's role as a migration suppressor. The findings showed that eliminating SRGAP2 enhanced cell migration, while increasing its expression had the opposite effect.

Various research approaches, including candidate gene analysis, pathway-based investigations, and GWAS, have identified crucial genes involved in MAP therapy pharmacokinetics (**Table 12.1**) [35]. These include genes encoding drug metabolism enzymes (GSTT1, GSTM1, GSTM3*B, and GSTP1) and transport proteins (ABCB1, ABCB3, and RFC1). Additionally, genes involved in DNA repair (REV1, REV3, ERCC1, ERCC2, ERCC5, and XPC) were identified as significant in cisplatin treatment response. Implementing CRISPR/Cas9 to modify these genes could potentially reveal new therapeutic targets for osteosarcoma treatment and enhance our understanding of how these genes influence the disease's development and progression.

Given osteosarcoma's challenging characteristics — high metastatic potential and frequent chemotherapy resistance — and the lack of significant treatment advances in recent decades, CRISPR/Cas9 technology presents a promising avenue for addressing these persistent clinical challenges in the foreseeable future.

12.5 CRISPR/Cas9 and Ewing Sarcoma

Ewing sarcoma ranks as the second most prevalent skeletal malignancy after osteosarcoma, with an incidence rate of 2.93 per million in the United States over three decades. Statistics from 2000–2005 indicate approximately 208 new diagnoses annually, with over 25%

Table 12.1 CRISPR/Cas9 applications in osteosarcoma research and therapy.

Target Gene	Biological Function	CRISPR/Cas9 Effects	Therapeutic or Research Implications	Experimental Models	Reference
CNE9/ CNE10	Putative tumor suppressors	Knockout decreased apoptosis; inhibited cell proliferation	Identification of novel tumor suppressor genes; potential therapeutic targets	U2OS osteosarcoma cells	[54]
STAG2	Tumor suppressor; cohesin complex component	Knockout promoted EMT, cell invasion, PD-L1 expression; increased cisplatin resistance; immune-related gene changes	Potential biomarker for PD-1/PD-L1 inhibitor therapy in STAG2-deficient tumors	U2OS osteosarcoma cells	[53]
ESR1	Estrogen receptor; tumor regulation	Knockout eliminated DAC inhibitory effects on tumor growth, metastasis, and stem cell markers	Demonstrates DAC mechanism of action; ESR1-dependent therapy	Osteosarcoma models	[55]
SENP2	Potential tumor suppressor; SUMO protease	Knockout reversed anti-proliferative, anti-migration, anti-invasion effects of SENP2 overexpression	Potential therapeutic target for osteosarcoma treatment	Primary human osteosarcoma tissue and cell lines	[56]
RECQL5	DNA helicase; tumor suppressor	Stable overexpression inhibited proliferation; caused cell cycle arrest; promoted apoptosis	Tumor suppressor role confirmation; potential gene therapy approach	MG63 osteosarcoma cells with AAVS1 safe **harbor insertion**	[57]

(Continued)

Table 12.1 (*Continued*)

Target Gene	Biological Function	CRISPR/Cas9 Effects	Therapeutic or Research Implications	Experimental Models	Reference
TP53	Tumor suppressor; cell cycle regulation	Knockout in pig zygotes led to osteosarcoma development in half of piglets	Large animal model for preclinical osteosarcoma research	Pig models (*in vitro* zygotes)	[58]
RAD52	DNA repair; replication fork restart	Knockout compromised restart of collapsed forks; led to DNA damage	Understanding DNA repair mechanisms; potential synthetic lethality targets	U2OS osteosarcoma cells	[59]
PAWS1/ CD2AP	Cytoskeleton regulation; cell adhesion	Knockout caused disorganized actin mesh; reduced migration; impaired focal adhesion formation	Insights into cell migration mechanisms; cancer metastasis research	U2OS osteosarcoma cells	[60]
SRGAP2	Cell migration regulator	Knockout increased cell migration; overexpression reduced migration	Identification of migration inhibitor; potential metastasis target	Murine osteosarcoma cell lines	[65]

of patients presenting with metastatic disease at initial diagnosis [66]. Survival rates vary significantly between non-metastatic and metastatic cases, with 10-year survival rates of 66.8% and 28.1%, respectively [67].

Unlike osteosarcoma, Ewing sarcoma has a distinct genetic signature characterized by chromosomal translocation between the EWSR gene on chromosome 22 and various ETS family genes (FL1, ERG, ETV1, ETV4, and FEV) on chromosome 11. The EWSR-FL1 fusion occurs in approximately 85% of cases. These fusion products create potent transcriptional activators that trigger Ewing sarcoma development [68, 69]. Additional genes implicated in Ewing sarcoma progression include telomerase reverse transcriptase, VEGF, IGF-1, CAV1, EZH2, BMI1, NKX2.2, NROB1, GLI1, RB, and p53 [69].

Current treatment protocols combine surgery, radiation therapy, and chemotherapy using vincristine, doxorubicin, cyclophosphamide, ifosphamide, and etoposide [68]. The nuclear localization of EWSR1-FLI1 fusion protein presents a significant therapeutic challenge, often rendering traditional chemotherapeutic approaches ineffective [70, 71]. Despite improved survival rates through multimodal treatment, significant challenges persist, including poor long-term survival, metastasis, recurrence, drug resistance, and increased risk of secondary cancers [69, 72, 73].

A Swedish national study of long-term Ewing sarcoma survivors revealed elevated risks of secondary malignancies: breast cancer risk increased 4.7-fold and soft tissue sarcoma risk increased 67-fold compared to the general population [74]. Analysis of 23,603 childhood cancer survivors in North America identified radiotherapy as a significant factor in secondary malignancy development [73].

Given the suboptimal long-term outcomes in Ewing sarcoma patients, there is an urgent need for novel therapeutic approaches. Recent years have witnessed significant progress in applying CRISPR/Cas9 technology to Ewing sarcoma research. The first breakthrough came in 2014 [75], when researchers successfully used CRISPR/Cas9 to create an Ewing sarcoma cell model featuring EWSR1-FLI1 translocation mutations in both HEK293 cells and human adult MSCs, the latter being a potential cell of origin for Ewing sarcoma. The model demonstrated EWSR1-FLI1 fusion protein expression and increased expression of six target genes, validating CRISPR/Cas9's potential for Ewing sarcoma modeling.

To enhance CRISPR/Cas9's efficiency, Torres-Ruiz and colleagues [76] developed an improved method called ssODN-RNP CRISPR/Cas9 coupling [11,22] translocations in hMSCs and human induced pluripotent stem cells, advancing Ewing sarcoma modeling through the integration of stem cell and CRISPR/Cas9 technologies.

A significant advancement came from Spraggon et al. [77], who developed an innovative approach combining CRISPR/Cas9 with HDR to engineer and regulate chromosomal translocation products. This method enabled temporal control over EWSR1-FLI1 fusion gene expression, addressing a crucial limitation: the challenge of precisely studying target gene expression changes caused by permanent EWSR1-FLI1 fusion gene generation. This strategic improvement has enhanced the ability of researchers to investigate genetic and pathogenic mechanisms of Ewing sarcoma.

CRISPR/Cas9 has proven valuable in elucidating Ewing sarcoma gene functions. Research by Stolte et al. [78] revealed important insights through knockout studies of MDM2, MDM4, PPM1D, and USP7 in Ewing sarcoma cell lines with different TP53 status. Their findings showed significant viability reduction only in cells with wild-type TP53, suggesting its necessity for these oncogenes' function. Furthermore, their CRISPR/Cas9-based gene screening identified enhanced antitumor effects with MDM2/MDM4 double knockout. When combining the MDM2/MDM4 dual inhibitor ATSP-7041 with conventional chemotherapy drugs (doxorubicin, etoposide, and vincristine), they observed superior tumor growth inhibition in xenograft models, supporting the potential clinical application of this combination therapy.

Another significant study [79] demonstrated that PHF19 deletion via CRISPR/Cas9 in SK-N-MC Ewing sarcoma cells decreased proliferation, colony formation, and invasion while enhancing sensitivity to JQ1, a BET bromodomain protein inhibitor known for its anti-proliferative and pro-apoptotic effects. These findings highlighted JQ-1's therapeutic potential in Ewing sarcoma treatment.

Research using CRISPR/Cas9 to knockout TNC in A673 and SKNMC cells [80] showed significant reduction in cell proliferation, migration, and angiogenesis. *In vivo* studies using nude mice demonstrated decreased metastatic and colonization capabilities of TNC-knockout cells compared to controls.

A recent innovative study [81] used CRISPR/Cas9 to create a defective DNA mismatch repair phenotype by knocking out MSH2 in A673 cells. This increased mutation rates and served as a forward genetics system for identifying compound targets. The approach revealed resistance alleles to three cellular toxins (PSMB5, CD437, and MLN4924). This methodology offers valuable insights into both compound mechanisms of action and the genetic basis of chemotherapy resistance.

The application of CRISPR/Cas9 technology in Ewing sarcoma research is still in its early stages. While significant progress has been made in developing cellular models, there remains a notable gap in establishing effective animal models. Future research efforts should focus on advancing animal model development and expanding the exploration of Ewing sarcoma-related genetic modifications, particularly targeting EWS/ETS-regulated genes using CRISPR/Cas9 technology. These advancements are crucial as they hold the potential to expand the range of therapeutic options available for Ewing sarcoma patients in clinical settings.

Overall and in the context of osteosarcoma and Ewing sarcoma, **Figure 12.1** illustrates CRISPR/Cas9-mediated approaches for understanding tumor biology, identifying therapeutic targets, and enhancing chemotherapy responses in these two subtypes of sarcoma.

12.6 CRISPR/Cas9 and Rhabdomyosarcoma

Rhabdomyosarcoma represents the most common soft tissue sarcoma in humans, constituting 4–5% of pediatric malignancies. It comprises two main histological subtypes: embryonal sarcomas

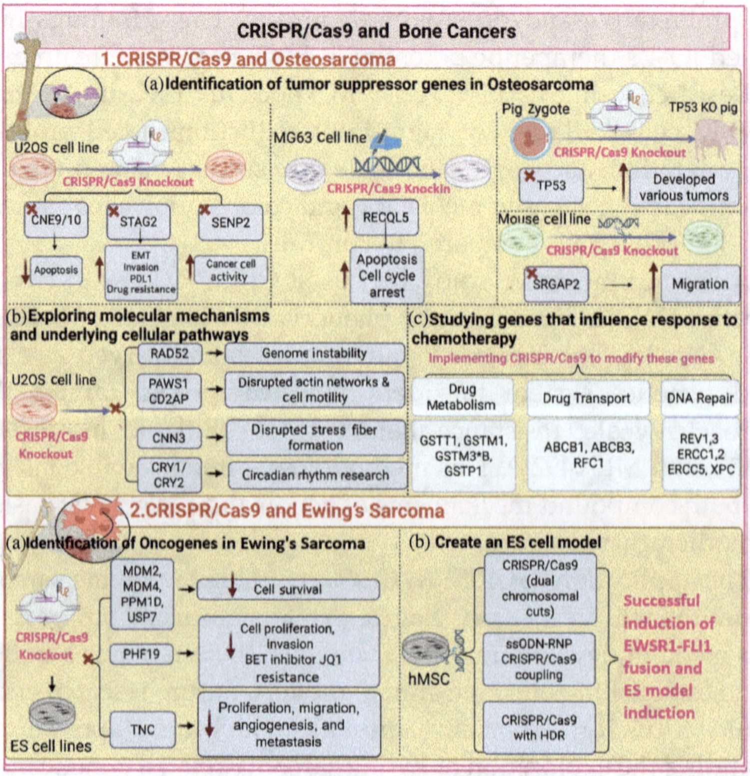

Figure 12.1 CRISPR/Cas9 applications in bone cancers: osteosarcoma and Ewing sarcoma. (1) CRISPR/Cas9 and osteosarcoma: (1a) Identification of tumor suppressor genes: CNE9/CNE10 knockout: CRISPR/Cas9-mediated knockout of CNE9 or CNE10 (conserved non-coding elements regulating SHOX gene expression) in U2OS osteosarcoma cells significantly decreases apoptosis and increases cell growth. Sanger sequencing confirmed successful knockout, with CNE9/CNE10 disruption resulting in reduced SHOX mRNA and protein expression. These knockout cells exhibited enhanced proliferation and reduced apoptotic rates compared to controls, establishing CNE9/CNE10 as regulatory elements with tumor-suppressive functions. STAG2 knockout: CRISPR/Cas9-mediated STAG2 gene disruption in U2OS cells reduces apoptosis and promotes EMT, invasion, and drug resistance. STAG2, a cohesin complex component, functions as a tumor suppressor, and its loss induces PD-L1 expression in osteosarcoma cells, contributing to immune evasion mechanisms. STAG2 mutations in Ewing sarcoma also alter enhancer-promoter interactions and promote metastatic phenotypes. SENP2 knockout: CRISPR/Cas9-mediated knockout of SENP2 (SUMO-specific protease 2) in U2OS cells decreases apoptosis and increases cancer cell activity. SENP2

Figure 12.1 (*Continued on facing page*) disruption promotes osteosarcoma progression through altered post-translational modifications of key regulatory proteins. RECQL5 knockin: CRISPR/Cas9 technology was used to insert the RECQL5 gene into the AAVS1 safe harbor locus in MG-63 osteosarcoma cells, establishing stable overexpression. RECQL5 overexpression induced cell cycle arrest in G0/G1 phase, promoted apoptosis, and inhibited cell proliferation. Immunohistochemical analysis of patient tissues revealed that RECQL5 expression was downregulated in osteosarcoma and correlated with advanced tumor stage and low histologic grade. These findings establish RECQL5 as a tumor suppressor and potential therapeutic target in osteosarcoma. TP53 knockout in pigs: CRISPR/Cas9-mediated TP53 knockout in pig zygotes via electroporation of Cas9 protein generated large animal models of osteosarcoma that closely recapitulate human disease. TP53^-/-^ pigs developed mandibular osteosarcoma and other tumors, with heterozygous knockout animals exhibiting spontaneous osteosarcoma in older animals, while homozygous knockouts developed multiple large osteosarcomas by 7–8 months of age. Unlike Trp53 mutant mice, these porcine models develop osteosarcomas in long bones and skulls—the characteristic anatomical sites of human disease—providing superior translational models for juvenile osteosarcoma research. SRGAP2 knockout in mice: CRISPR/Cas9-mediated SRGAP2 (SLIT-ROBO Rho GTPase-activating protein 2) knockout in mouse osteosarcoma cell lines increases cell migration. SRGAP2 functions as a negative regulator of cell motility, and its disruption promotes metastatic behavior in osteosarcoma models. **(1b) Molecular mechanisms and cellular pathways:** CRISPR/Cas9 knockout in U2OS cells reveals critical molecular mechanisms underlying osteosarcoma biology. RAD52: Knockout disrupts genome stability and DNA repair pathways, revealing RAD52's role in maintaining chromosomal integrity in osteosarcoma cells. PAWS1/CD2AP: Disruption of these actin cytoskeleton-associated proteins impairs actin network formation and cell motility, demonstrating their importance in osteosarcoma cell migration and invasion. CNN3 (Calponin 3): Knockout disrupts stress fiber formation and cytoskeletal organization, compromising mechanical properties and migratory capacity of osteosarcoma cells. CRY1/CRY2 (Cryptochrome 1/2): Disruption of circadian rhythm regulatory genes provides insights into temporal regulation of osteosarcoma cell proliferation and metabolism. **(1c) Genes influencing chemotherapy response:** CRISPR/Cas9-mediated modification of genes involved in drug metabolism, transport, and DNA repair pathways reveals mechanisms of chemotherapy resistance and sensitivity in osteosarcoma. Drug metabolism: GSTT1, GSTM1, GSTM3B, and GSTP1 (glutathione S-transferases) modulate cellular detoxification of chemotherapeutic agents and oxidative stress responses. Drug transport: ABCB1, ABCB3, and RFC1 (ATP-binding cassette transporters and reduced folate carrier) regulate intracellular drug accumulation and efflux, directly impacting chemotherapy efficacy. DNA repair: REV1, REV3, ERCC1, ERCC2, ERCC5, and XRCC1 participate in nucleotide

Figure 12.1 (*Continued*) excision repair and translesion DNA synthesis pathways that counteract platinum-based chemotherapy damage. **(2) CRISPR/Cas9 and Ewing sarcoma: (2a) Identification of oncogene dependencies:** Genome-scale CRISPR-Cas9 screens in Ewing sarcoma cell lines identified critical dependencies for tumor cell survival. MDM2/MDM4/PPM1D/USP7: These genes emerged as selective dependencies in TP53 wild-type Ewing sarcoma cell lines. CRISPR/Cas9-mediated knockout of MDM2 and MDM4 (negative regulators of p53) dramatically reduced cell survival specifically in TP53 wild-type cells. USP7 (ubiquitin-specific protease 7) disruption and PPM1D (Wip1 phosphatase) knockout similarly demonstrated selective cytotoxicity in TP53 wild-type Ewing sarcoma lines, validating these genes as druggable targets for p53 pathway activation. Pharmacologic validation using MDM2/MDM4 inhibitor ATSP-7041, USP7 inhibitors P5091 and XL-188, and PPM1D inhibitor GSK2830371 confirmed antitumor efficacy, with effects rescued by concurrent TP53 knockout, demonstrating p53 pathway dependence. PHF19: CRISPR-Cas9-mediated deletion of PHF19 (PRC2-associated factor) reduced cell proliferation, invasion, and BET inhibitor JQ1 resistance in Ewing sarcoma. PHF19 is transcriptionally activated by EWS-FLI1 through direct binding to distal regulatory elements, and its deletion decreased tumorigenic phenotype while increasing sensitivity to BET bromodomain inhibition. PHF19 expression correlates with poor prognosis in Ewing sarcoma patients, establishing it as both a biomarker and therapeutic target. TNC (Tenascin-C): CRISPR/Cas9-mediated TNC knockout in Ewing sarcoma cell lines reduces proliferation, migration, angiogenesis, and metastatic capacity both *in vitro* and *in vivo*. The EWS-FLI1 oncoprotein directly binds the TNC promoter to drive overexpression, and TNC promotes tumor progression through integrin $\alpha 5\beta 1$-mediated YAP activation and subsequent MALAT1 upregulation. Immunohistochemical analysis demonstrated that TNC overexpression in Ewing sarcoma tissues associates with poor patient survival, validating TNC as a prognostic marker and therapeutic target. **(2b) Creating Ewing sarcoma cell models:** CRISPR/Cas9 enables generation of human Ewing sarcoma models through engineering chromosomal translocations and fusion oncogenes. Dual chromosomal cuts: CRISPR/Cas9 with dual-guide RNAs targeting chromosomes 11 and 22 generates EWSR1-FLI1 fusion oncogenes in human MSCs, successfully inducing transformation and Ewing sarcoma-like phenotypes. ssODN-RNP CRISPR/Cas9 coupling: Single-stranded oligodeoxynucleotide (ssODN) template-mediated HDR combined with CRISPR/Cas9 ribonucleoprotein delivery enables precise generation of EWSR1-FLI1 fusion sequences at defined chromosomal breakpoints. CRISPR/Cas9 with HDR: HDR templates facilitate precise engineering of patient-specific EWS-ETS fusion variants for mechanistic studies and drug screening applications. These approaches enable successful induction of EWSR1-FLI1 fusion oncogenes in primary cells, creating authentic cellular models that recapitulate the molecular and phenotypic features of Ewing sarcoma for translational research.

(ERSMs, ~80%) and alveolar sarcomas (ARSMs, 15–20%) [82]. Despite current multimodal treatments including chemotherapy, surgery, and radiation successfully treating about two-thirds of non-metastatic cases, patients with metastatic or recurrent disease face poor outcomes, with three-year overall survival rates of only 34–56% [83, 84].

Rhabdomyosarcoma originates from skeletal myoblasts and shows distinct genetic characteristics: ERSM typically displays chromosome 11 allelic deletions, while ARSM features chromosomal translocations (1,13 and 2,13) producing PAX7-FOXO1 or PAX3-FOXO1 fusion genes. These fusion genes disrupt normal transcription and differentiation processes, making ARSM generally more aggressive than ERSM [17, 85, 86]. Additional genes implicated in rhabdomyosarcoma development include NRAS, KRAS, HRAS, PIK3CA, FBXW7, BCOR, FGFR4, and CTNNB1 [87].

CRISPR/Cas9 technology has advanced rhabdomyosarcoma research significantly. The first breakthrough came in 2015 when Lagutina et al. [88] created a human ARSM-like chromosomal translocation t [1,3] model in mouse myoblasts. Subsequent studies developed DMD-KO [89, 90] and Dysf-KO TE671 [91] cells from WT-TE671 human ERMS cells for muscle disease research.

Using iExCN analysis tools with CRISPR/Cas9, researchers identified numerous rhabdomyosarcoma-related genes [86]. These include oncogenes (CDCA2, HAS2, SNAI2, WAR, EZH2, SCARA3, ARL4A, CDK6, ETV1, RAD54B, RIPK2, ZFHX4) and tumor suppressor genes (PTEN, ZRSR2, TJP2), many influencing rhabdomyosarcoma growth and differentiation.

Further functional studies using CRISPR/Cas9 revealed that HDAC3 knockout in 381T ERSM cells significantly reduced proliferation *in vitro* and tumor growth *in vivo*, while promoting extensive tumor differentiation in xenograft models. These findings suggest CRISPR/Cas9's potential role in differentiation-induction therapy for rhabdomyosarcoma [92].

Research into the PAX3-FOXO1 fusion gene's role in rhabdomyosarcoma utilized immortalized human myoblasts with doxycycline-inducible PAX3-FOXO1 and constitutive MYCN expression. When injected into nude mice, cells expressing both constructs rapidly formed tumors, while those expressing only PAX3-FOXO1 showed delayed tumor development. Although stopping doxycycline administration led to initial tumor regression, most tumors eventually recurred without doxycycline induction. CRISPR/Cas9-mediated PAX3-FOXO1 knockout in primary tumor-derived cells eliminated their oncogenic potential and promoted differentiation after doxycycline withdrawal. However, cells derived from recurrent tumors maintained resistance to differentiation despite PAX3-FOXO1 knockout. These findings demonstrate that PAX3-FOXO1 collaborates with MYCN to promote rhabdomyosarcoma development by inhibiting myogenic differentiation and cell death, while recurrent tumors develop independently of PAX3-FOXO1 [85].

Another promising therapeutic target emerged in the RAS gene. CRISPR/Cas9-mediated RAS elimination significantly reduced xenograft tumor growth while increasing tumor cell death, myogenic differentiation, and survival in tumor-bearing mice. Notably, this study introduced an innovative CRISPR/Cas9 MYXV vector delivery system that effectively achieved targeted RAS knockout in ERSM tumors in transplanted mice [93]. This breakthrough offers a potential solution to the challenge of *in vivo* CRISPR/Cas9 delivery.

The application of CRISPR/Cas9 technology in rhabdomyosarcoma research has shown considerable promise, particularly in tumor differentiation-induction therapy. However, additional research is necessary to facilitate its translation into clinical applications.

12.7 Future Perspectives

Future developments in CRISPR/Cas9 therapy for bone cancers should concentrate on delivery and editing strategies specifically tailored to the unique characteristics of these malignancies. Key priorities include the development of targeted delivery systems such as ligand-directed nanoparticles, polymeric carriers, engineered extracellular vesicles, and optimized viral or hybrid vectors. These platforms must be capable of reaching both primary bone lesions and pulmonary metastases while minimizing exposure to healthy tissues, and should support both local and systemic delivery approaches.

Technical optimization efforts should focus on the use of transient editing formats like ribonucleoproteins or mRNA, integration of high-fidelity Cas variants to enhance precision, and the design of multiplex guide RNAs to improve targeting efficiency while reducing off-target effects. Therapeutic strategies should incorporate combination approaches that disable resistance mechanisms to boost chemotherapy effectiveness, modulate DNA repair pathways to increase radiation sensitivity, and reprogram immune checkpoints to enhance T cell therapy within immunosuppressive tumor microenvironments.

Monitoring and assessment protocols must include robust pharmacodynamic tracking, quantification of editing efficiency, and analysis of pathway modifications and circulating tumor DNA. The integration of single-cell and spatial profiling will enable adaptive treatment strategies that respond to tumor evolution. Clinical implementation should involve biomarker-driven early-phase trials focused on patient-centered outcomes, along with comprehensive long-term safety monitoring. Ethical and regulatory frameworks must address treatment durability, off-target risks, and equitable access to emerging therapies.

Looking ahead, technological expansion will involve the integration of advanced editing tools such as base editors, prime editors, and CRISPR interference/activation systems. The development of epigenome editing capabilities, establishment of scalable GMP-compliant manufacturing processes, and creation of modular guide RNA libraries will be essential to accelerating clinical translation and broadening therapeutic impact.

12.8 Conclusion

With its precision, modularity, and scalability, CRISPR/Cas9 offers a coherent path to close the gap between biological understanding and therapeutic control in bone cancers. By enabling systematic target validation, restoration or ablation of pathogenic gene functions, and synergy with existing modalities, gene editing can move beyond discovery to deliver clinically meaningful benefits in malignancies historically constrained by toxicity and recurrence. Translational success will hinge on selective delivery, rigorous safety engineering, and biomarker-guided patient selection, but the trajectory of progress across human gene-editing applications indicates that CRISPR/Cas9 can become a cornerstone technology in the development of durable, mechanism-based treatments for osteosarcoma, Ewing sarcoma, and rhabdomyosarcoma.

References

1. Ishino Y, Shinagawa H, Makino K, Amemura M, Nakata A. Nucleotide sequence of the iap gene, responsible for alkaline phosphatase isozyme conversion in Escherichia coli, and identification of the gene product. J Bacteriol. 1987;169(12):5429–33.
2. Marraffini LA. CRISPR-Cas immunity against phages: its effects on the evolution and survival of bacterial pathogens. PLoS Pathog. 2013;9(12):e1003765.
3. Marraffini LA. CRISPR-Cas immunity in prokaryotes. Nature. 2015;526(7571):55–61.
4. Sorek R, Kunin V, Hugenholtz P. CRISPR--a widespread system that provides acquired resistance against phages in bacteria and archaea. Nat Rev Microbiol. 2008;6(3):181–6.
5. Brouns SJ, Jore MM, Lundgren M, Westra ER, Slijkhuis RJ, Snijders AP, et al. Small CRISPR RNAs guide antiviral defense in prokaryotes. Science. 2008;321(5891):960–4.
6. Deveau H, Barrangou R, Garneau JE, Labonté J, Fremaux C, Boyaval P, et al. Phage response to CRISPR-encoded resistance in Streptococcus thermophilus. J Bacteriol. 2008;190(4):1390–400.
7. Jinek M, Chylinski K, Fonfara I, Hauer M, Doudna JA, Charpentier E. A programmable dual-RNA-guided DNA endonuclease in adaptive bacterial immunity. Science. 2012;337(6096):816–21.
8. San Filippo J, Sung P, Klein H. Mechanism of eukaryotic homologous recombination. Annu Rev Biochem. 2008;77:229–57.
9. Lieber MR. The mechanism of double-strand DNA break repair by the nonhomologous DNA end-joining pathway. Annu Rev Biochem. 2010;79:181–211.

10. Mali P, Yang L, Esvelt KM, Aach J, Guell M, DiCarlo JE, et al. RNA-guided human genome engineering via Cas9. Science. 2013;339(6121): 823–6.
11. Cong L, Ran FA, Cox D, Lin S, Barretto R, Habib N, et al. Multiplex genome engineering using CRISPR/Cas systems. Science. 2013;339(6121):819–23.
12. Chandrasegaran S, Carroll D. Origins of Programmable Nucleases for Genome Engineering. J Mol Biol. 2016;428(5 Pt B):963–89.
13. Ran FA, Hsu PD, Wright J, Agarwala V, Scott DA, Zhang F. Genome engineering using the CRISPR-Cas9 system. Nat Protoc. 2013;8(11):2281–308.
14. Wang H, Yang H, Shivalila CS, Dawlaty MM, Cheng AW, Zhang F, Jaenisch R. One-step generation of mice carrying mutations in multiple genes by CRISPR/Cas-mediated genome engineering. Cell. 2013;153(4):910–8.
15. Xu L, Wang J, Liu Y, Xie L, Su B, Mou D, et al. CRISPR-Edited Stem Cells in a Patient with HIV and Acute Lymphocytic Leukemia. N Engl J Med. 2019;381(13):1240–7.
16. Li H, Yang Y, Hong W, Huang M, Wu M, Zhao X. Applications of genome editing technology in the targeted therapy of human diseases: mechanisms, advances and prospects. Signal Transduct Target Ther. 2020;5(1):1.
17. Arndt CA, Rose PS, Folpe AL, Laack NN. Common musculoskeletal tumors of childhood and adolescence. Mayo Clin Proc. 2012;87(5):475–87.
18. Ottaviani G, Jaffe N. The epidemiology of osteosarcoma. Cancer Treat Res. 2009;152:3–13.
19. Yang Y, Yang R, Roth M, Piperdi S, Zhang W, Dorfman H, et al. Genetically transforming human osteoblasts to sarcoma: development of an osteosarcoma model. Genes Cancer. 2017;8(1–2):484–94.
20. Broadhead ML, Clark JC, Myers DE, Dass CR, Choong PF. The molecular pathogenesis of osteosarcoma: a review. Sarcoma. 2011;2011:959248.
21. Denduluri SK, Wang Z, Yan Z, Wang J, Wei Q, Mohammed MK, et al. Molecular pathogenesis and therapeutic strategies of human osteosarcoma. J Biomed Res. 2016;30(1):5–18.
22. Deng ZL, Sharff KA, Tang N, Song WX, Luo J, Luo X, et al. Regulation of osteogenic differentiation during skeletal development. Front Biosci. 2008;13:2001–21.
23. Mori T, Sato Y, Miyamoto K, Kobayashi T, Shimizu T, Kanagawa H, et al. TNF α promotes osteosarcoma progression by maintaining tumor cells in an undifferentiated state. Oncogene. 2014;33(33):4236–41.

24. Tu B, Peng ZX, Fan QM, Du L, Yan W, Tang TT. Osteosarcoma cells promote the production of pro-tumor cytokines in mesenchymal stem cells by inhibiting their osteogenic differentiation through the TGF-β/Smad2/3 pathway. Exp Cell Res. 2014;320(1):164–73.
25. Zheng Y, Wang G, Chen R, Hua Y, Cai Z. Mesenchymal stem cells in the osteosarcoma microenvironment: their biological properties, influence on tumor growth, and therapeutic implications. Stem Cell Res Ther. 2018;9(1):22.
26. Tang N, Song WX, Luo J, Haydon RC, He TC. Osteosarcoma development and stem cell differentiation. Clin Orthop Relat Res. 2008; 466(9):2114–30.
27. Luetke A, Meyers PA, Lewis I, Juergens H. Osteosarcoma treatment — where do we stand? A state of the art review. Cancer Treat Rev. 2014;40(4):523–32.
28. Simpson E, Brown HL. Understanding osteosarcomas. Jaapa. 2018;31(8):15–9.
29. Anninga JK, Gelderblom H, Fiocco M, Kroep JR, Taminiau AH, Hogendoorn PC, Egeler RM. Chemotherapeutic adjuvant treatment for osteosarcoma: where do we stand? Eur J Cancer. 2011;47(16): 2431–45.
30. Berner K, Johannesen TB, Berner A, Haugland HK, Bjerkehagen B, Bøhler PJ, Bruland Ø S. Time-trends on incidence and survival in a nationwide and unselected cohort of patients with skeletal osteosarcoma. Acta Oncol. 2015;54(1):25–33.
31. Ritter J, Bielack SS. Osteosarcoma. Ann Oncol. 2010;21 Suppl 7: vii320–5.
32. Lipshultz SE, Lipsitz SR, Mone SM, Goorin AM, Sallan SE, Sanders SP, et al. Female sex and higher drug dose as risk factors for late cardiotoxic effects of doxorubicin therapy for childhood cancer. N Engl J Med. 1995;332(26):1738–43.
33. Aung L, Gorlick RG, Shi W, Thaler H, Shorter NA, Healey JH, et al. Second malignant neoplasms in long-term survivors of osteosarcoma: Memorial Sloan-Kettering Cancer Center Experience. Cancer. 2002;95(8):1728–34.
34. Daw NC, Neel MD, Rao BN, Billups CA, Wu J, Jenkins JJ, et al. Frontline treatment of localized osteosarcoma without methotrexate: results of the St. Jude Children's Research Hospital OS99 trial. Cancer. 2011;117(12):2770–8.

35. Vos HI, Coenen MJ, Guchelaar HJ, Te Loo DM. The role of pharmacogenetics in the treatment of osteosarcoma. Drug Discov Today. 2016;21(11):1775–86.
36. Gorlick R. Current concepts on the molecular biology of osteosarcoma. Cancer Treat Res. 2009;152:467–78.
37. Caronia D, Patiño-García A, Milne RL, Zalacain-Díez M, Pita G, Alonso MR, et al. Common variations in ERCC2 are associated with response to cisplatin chemotherapy and clinical outcome in osteosarcoma patients. Pharmacogenomics J. 2009;9(5):347–53.
38. Caronia D, Patiño-Garcia A, Peréz-Martínez A, Pita G, Moreno LT, Zalacain-Díez M, et al. Effect of ABCB1 and ABCC3 polymorphisms on osteosarcoma survival after chemotherapy: a pharmacogenetic study. PLoS One. 2011;6(10):e26091.
39. Hao T, Feng W, Zhang J, Sun YJ, Wang G. Association of four ERCC1 and ERCC2 SNPs with survival of bone tumour patients. Asian Pac J Cancer Prev. 2012;13(8):3821–4.
40. Jabeen S, Holmboe L, Alnæs GI, Andersen AM, Hall KS, Kristensen VN. Impact of genetic variants of RFC1, DHFR and MTHFR in osteosarcoma patients treated with high-dose methotrexate. Pharmacogenomics J. 2015;15(5):385–90.
41. Liu S, Yi Z, Ling M, Shi J, Qiu Y, Yang S. Predictive potential of ABCB1, ABCC3, and GSTP1 gene polymorphisms on osteosarcoma survival after chemotherapy. Tumour Biol. 2014;35(10):9897–904.
42. Teng JW, Yang ZM, Li J, Xu B. Predictive role of Glutathione S-transferases (GSTs) on the prognosis of osteosarcoma patients treated with chemotherapy. Pak J Med Sci. 2013;29(5):1182–6.
43. Wang MJ, Zhu Y, Guo XJ, Tian ZZ. Genetic variability of genes involved in DNA repair influence treatment outcome in osteosarcoma. Genet Mol Res. 2015;14(3):11652–7.
44. Feng Y, Sassi S, Shen JK, Yang X, Gao Y, Osaka E, et al. Targeting CDK11 in osteosarcoma cells using the CRISPR-Cas9 system. J Orthop Res. 2015;33(2):199–207.
45. Baumann S, Hennet T. Collagen Accumulation in Osteosarcoma Cells lacking GLT25D1 Collagen Galactosyltransferase. J Biol Chem. 2016;291(35):18514–24.
46. Liu T, Yan Z, Liu Y, Choy E, Hornicek FJ, Mankin H, Duan Z. CRISPR-Cas9-Mediated Silencing of CD44 in Human Highly Metastatic Osteosarcoma Cells. Cell Physiol Biochem. 2018;46(3):1218–30.

47. Mizoshiri N, Shirai T, Terauchi R, Tsuchida S, Mori Y, Hayashi D, et al. The tetraspanin CD81 mediates the growth and metastases of human osteosarcoma. Cell Oncol (Dordr). 2019;42(6):861–71.
48. Han D, Wang M, Yu Z, Yin L, Liu C, Wang J, et al. FGF5 promotes osteosarcoma cells proliferation via activating MAPK signaling pathway. Cancer Manag Res. 2019;11:6457–66.
49. Tang F, Min L, Seebacher NA, Li X, Zhou Y, Hornicek FJ, et al. Targeting mutant TP53 as a potential therapeutic strategy for the treatment of osteosarcoma. J Orthop Res. 2019;37(3):789–98.
50. Liao Y, Chen L, Feng Y, Shen J, Gao Y, Cote G, et al. Targeting programmed cell death ligand 1 by CRISPR/Cas9 in osteosarcoma cells. Oncotarget. 2017;8(18):30276–87.
51. Xiao Z, Wan J, Nur AA, Dou P, Mankin H, Liu T, Ouyang Z. Targeting CD44 by CRISPR-Cas9 in Multi-Drug Resistant Osteosarcoma Cells. Cell Physiol Biochem. 2018;51(4):1879–93.
52. Liu T, Li Z, Zhang Q, De Amorim Bernstein K, Lozano-Calderon S, Choy E, et al. Targeting ABCB1 (MDR1) in multi-drug resistant osteosarcoma cells using the CRISPR-Cas9 system to reverse drug resistance. Oncotarget. 2016;7(50):83502–13.
53. Nie Z, Gao W, Zhang Y, Hou Y, Liu J, Li Z, et al. STAG2 loss-of-function mutation induces PD-L1 expression in U2OS cells. Ann Transl Med. 2019;7(7):127.
54. Xu XJ, Xin SJ, Mao HY, Zhang HJ, Chen LN, Li L, et al. SHOX CNE9/10 Knockout in U2OS Osteosarcoma Cells and Its Effects on Cell Growth and Apoptosis. Med Sci Monit. 2020;26:e921233.
55. Lillo Osuna MA, Garcia-Lopez J, El Ayachi I, Fatima I, Khalid AB, Kumpati J, et al. Activation of Estrogen Receptor Alpha by Decitabine Inhibits Osteosarcoma Growth and Metastasis. Cancer Res. 2019;79(6):1054–68.
56. Pei H, Chen L, Liao QM, Wang KJ, Chen SG, Liu ZJ, Zhang ZC. SUMO-specific protease 2 (SENP2) functions as a tumor suppressor in osteosarcoma via SOX9 degradation. Exp Ther Med. 2018;16(6):5359–65.
57. Wu J, Zhi L, Dai X, Cai Q, Ma W. Decreased RECQL5 correlated with disease progression of osteosarcoma. Biochem Biophys Res Commun. 2015;467(4):617–22.
58. Tanihara F, Hirata M, Nguyen NT, Le QA, Hirano T, Takemoto T, et al. Generation of a TP53-modified porcine cancer model by CRISPR/Cas9-mediated gene modification in porcine zygotes via electroporation. PLoS One. 2018;13(10):e0206360.

59. Sotiriou SK, Kamileri I, Lugli N, Evangelou K, Da-Ré C, Huber F, et al. Mammalian RAD52 Functions in Break-Induced Replication Repair of Collapsed DNA Replication Forks. Mol Cell. 2016;64(6):1127–34.
60. Cummins TD, Wu KZL, Bozatzi P, Dingwell KS, Macartney TJ, Wood NT, et al. PAWS1 controls cytoskeletal dynamics and cell migration through association with the SH3 adaptor CD2AP. J Cell Sci. 2018;131(1):jcs202390.
61. Zhang Y, Gilmour A, Ahn YH, de la Vega L, Dinkova-Kostova AT. The isothiocyanate sulforaphane inhibits mTOR in an NRF2-independent manner. Phytomedicine. 2021;86:153062.
62. Ciuba K, Hawkes W, Tojkander S, Kogan K, Engel U, Iskratsch T, Lappalainen P. Calponin-3 is critical for coordinated contractility of actin stress fibers. Sci Rep. 2018;8(1):17670.
63. Götte B, Panas MD, Hellström K, Liu L, Samreen B, Larsson O, et al. Separate domains of G3BP promote efficient clustering of alphavirus replication complexes and recruitment of the translation initiation machinery. PLoS Pathog. 2019;15(6):e1007842.
64. Börding T, Abdo AN, Maier B, Gabriel C, Kramer A. Generation of Human CRY1 and CRY2 Knockout Cells Using Duplex CRISPR/Cas9 Technology. Front Physiol. 2019;10:577.
65. Marko TA, Shamsan GA, Edwards EN, Hazelton PE, Rathe SK, Cornax I, et al. Slit-Robo GTPase-Activating Protein 2 as a metastasis suppressor in osteosarcoma. Sci Rep. 2016;6:39059.
66. Esiashvili N, Goodman M, Marcus RB, Jr. Changes in incidence and survival of Ewing sarcoma patients over the past 3 decades: Surveillance Epidemiology and End Results data. J Pediatr Hematol Oncol. 2008;30(6):425–30.
67. Duchman KR, Gao Y, Miller BJ. Prognostic factors for survival in patients with Ewing's sarcoma using the surveillance, epidemiology, and end results (SEER) program database. Cancer Epidemiol. 2015;39(2):189–95.
68. Haybaeck J, Roessner A. [Malignant round cell tumors : The Ewing sarcoma and beyond]. Pathologe. 2020;41(2):116–22.
69. Toomey EC, Schiffman JD, Lessnick SL. Recent advances in the molecular pathogenesis of Ewing's sarcoma. Oncogene. 2010;29(32): 4504–16.
70. Balamuth NJ, Womer RB. Ewing's sarcoma. Lancet Oncol. 2010; 11(2):184–92.

71. Gaspar N, Hawkins DS, Dirksen U, Lewis IJ, Ferrari S, Le Deley MC, et al. Ewing Sarcoma: Current Management and Future Approaches Through Collaboration. J Clin Oncol. 2015;33(27):3036–46.
72. Chin M, Yokoyama R, Sumi M, Okita H, Kawai A, Hosono A, et al. Multimodal treatment including standard chemotherapy with vincristine, doxorubicin, cyclophosphamide, ifosfamide, and etoposide for the Ewing sarcoma family of tumors in Japan: Results of the Japan Ewing Sarcoma Study 04. Pediatr Blood Cancer. 2020;67(5):e28194.
73. Turcotte LM, Liu Q, Yasui Y, Arnold MA, Hammond S, Howell RM, et al. Temporal Trends in Treatment and Subsequent Neoplasm Risk Among 5-Year Survivors of Childhood Cancer, 1970–2015. Jama. 2017;317(8):814–24.
74. Hesla AC, Discacciati A, Tsagkozis P, Smedby KE. Subsequent primary neoplasms among bone sarcoma survivors; increased risks remain after 30 years of follow-up and in the latest treatment era, a nationwide population-based study. Br J Cancer. 2020;122(8):1242–9.
75. Torres R, Martin MC, Garcia A, Cigudosa JC, Ramirez JC, Rodriguez-Perales S. Engineering human tumour-associated chromosomal translocations with the RNA-guided CRISPR-Cas9 system. Nat Commun. 2014;5:3964.
76. Torres-Ruiz R, Martinez-Lage M, Martin MC, Garcia A, Bueno C, Castaño J, et al. Efficient Recreation of t(11;22) EWSR1-FLI1(+) in Human Stem Cells Using CRISPR/Cas9. Stem Cell Reports. 2017;8(5):1408–20.
77. Spraggon L, Martelotto LG, Hmeljak J, Hitchman TD, Wang J, Wang L, et al. Generation of conditional oncogenic chromosomal translocations using CRISPR-Cas9 genomic editing and homology-directed repair. J Pathol. 2017;242(1):102–12.
78. Stolte B, Iniguez AB, Dharia NV, Robichaud AL, Conway AS, Morgan AM, et al. Genome-scale CRISPR-Cas9 screen identifies druggable dependencies in TP53 wild-type Ewing sarcoma. J Exp Med. 2018;215(8):2137–55.
79. Gollavilli PN, Pawar A, Wilder-Romans K, Natesan R, Engelke CG, Dommeti VL, et al. EWS/ETS-Driven Ewing Sarcoma Requires BET Bromodomain Proteins. Cancer Res. 2018;78(16):4760–73.
80. He S, Huang Q, Hu J, Li L, Xiao Y, Yu H, et al. EWS-FLI1-mediated tenascin-C expression promotes tumour progression by targeting MALAT1 through integrin α5β1-mediated YAP activation in Ewing sarcoma. Br J Cancer. 2019;121(11):922–33.

81. Povedano JM, Liou J, Wei D, Srivatsav A, Kim J, Xie Y, et al. Engineering Forward Genetics into Cultured Cancer Cells for Chemical Target Identification. Cell Chem Biol. 2019;26(9):1315–21.e3.
82. Bisogno G, Jenney M, Bergeron C, Gallego Melcón S, Ferrari A, Oberlin O, et al. Addition of dose-intensified doxorubicin to standard chemotherapy for rhabdomyosarcoma (EpSSG RMS 2005): a multicentre, open-label, randomised controlled, phase 3 trial. Lancet Oncol. 2018;19(8):1061–71.
83. Meza JL, Anderson J, Pappo AS, Meyer WH. Analysis of prognostic factors in patients with nonmetastatic rhabdomyosarcoma treated on intergroup rhabdomyosarcoma studies III and IV: the Children's Oncology Group. J Clin Oncol. 2006;24(24):3844–51.
84. Vaarwerk B, Bisogno G, McHugh K, Brisse HJ, Morosi C, Corradini N, et al. Indeterminate Pulmonary Nodules at Diagnosis in Rhabdomyosarcoma: Are They Clinically Significant? A Report From the European Paediatric Soft Tissue Sarcoma Study Group. J Clin Oncol. 2019;37(9):723–30.
85. Pandey PR, Chatterjee B, Olanich ME, Khan J, Miettinen MM, Hewitt SM, Barr FG. PAX3-FOXO1 is essential for tumour initiation and maintenance but not recurrence in a human myoblast model of rhabdomyosarcoma. J Pathol. 2017;241(5):626–37.
86. Xu L, Zheng Y, Liu J, Rakheja D, Singleterry S, Laetsch TW, et al. Integrative Bayesian Analysis Identifies Rhabdomyosarcoma Disease Genes. Cell Rep. 2018;24(1):238–51.
87. Shern JF, Chen L, Chmielecki J, Wei JS, Patidar R, Rosenberg M, et al. Comprehensive genomic analysis of rhabdomyosarcoma reveals a landscape of alterations affecting a common genetic axis in fusion-positive and fusion-negative tumors. Cancer Discov. 2014;4(2):216–31.
88. Lagutina IV, Valentine V, Picchione F, Harwood F, Valentine MB, Villarejo-Balcells B, et al. Modeling of the human alveolar rhabdomyosarcoma Pax3-Foxo1 chromosome translocation in mouse myoblasts using CRISPR-Cas9 nuclease. PLoS Genet. 2015;11(2):e1004951.
89. Maruyama R, Yokota T. Creation of DMD Muscle Cell Model Using CRISPR-Cas9 Genome Editing to Test the Efficacy of Antisense-Mediated Exon Skipping. Methods Mol Biol. 2018;1828:165–71.
90. Shimo T, Hosoki K, Nakatsuji Y, Yokota T, Obika S. A novel human muscle cell model of Duchenne muscular dystrophy created by CRISPR/Cas9 and evaluation of antisense-mediated exon skipping. J Hum Genet. 2018;63(3):365–75.

91. De Luna N, Suarez-Calvet X, Garicano M, Fernandez-Simon E, Rojas-García R, Diaz-Manera J, et al. Effect of MAPK Inhibition on the Differentiation of a Rhabdomyosarcoma Cell Line Combined With CRISPR/Cas9 Technology: An In Vitro Model of Human Muscle Diseases. J Neuropathol Exp Neurol. 2018;77(10):964–72.
92. Phelps MP, Bailey JN, Vleeshouwer-Neumann T, Chen EY. CRISPR screen identifies the NCOR/HDAC3 complex as a major suppressor of differentiation in rhabdomyosarcoma. Proc Natl Acad Sci U S A. 2016;113(52):15090–5.
93. Phelps MP, Yang H, Patel S, Rahman MM, McFadden G, Chen E. Oncolytic Virus-Mediated RAS Targeting in Rhabdomyosarcoma. Mol Ther Oncolytics. 2018;11:52–61.
94. Moon SB, Kim DY, Ko JH, Kim JS, Kim YS. Improving CRISPR Genome Editing by Engineering Guide RNAs. Trends Biotechnol. 2019;37(8):870–81.
95. Kleinstiver BP, Pattanayak V, Prew MS, Tsai SQ, Nguyen NT, Zheng Z, Joung JK. High-fidelity CRISPR-Cas9 nucleases with no detectable genome-wide off-target effects. Nature. 2016;529(7587):490–5.
96. Lee JK, Jeong E, Lee J, Jung M, Shin E, Kim YH, et al. Directed evolution of CRISPR-Cas9 to increase its specificity. Nat Commun. 2018;9(1):3048.
97. Liang C, Li F, Wang L, Zhang ZK, Wang C, He B, et al. Tumor cell-targeted delivery of CRISPR/Cas9 by aptamer-functionalized lipopolymer for therapeutic genome editing of VEGFA in osteosarcoma. Biomaterials. 2017;147:68–85.

https://doi.org/10.1142/9789819826759_0013

CHAPTER 13

CRISPR/Cas9 in the Study and Reversal of Cancer Drug Resistance

Mehrdad Hashemi[1,2], *Alireza Khosravinejad*[1,3], *Mina Alimohammadi*[4], *Behdokht Jamali*[5], *Reza Mohajer Shirazi*[1,3], *Kimia Sadat Esfahani*[1,3], *Ali Shirazi*[1,3], *Rojin Ghannad Zadeh*[1,6], *Faranak Jamshidian*[1,7], *Neda Zali*[3], *Najma Farahani*[1,*], *Afshin Taheriazam*[1,8,*], *Payman Rahimzadeh*[9,*], *Maliheh Entezari*[1,2,*]

[1]Farhikhtegan Medical Convergent Sciences Research Center, Farhikhtegan Hospital, Faculty of Medicine, TeMs. C., Islamic Azad University, Tehran, Iran
[2]Department of Genetics, Faculty of Advanced Sciences and Technology, TeMs. C, Islamic Azad University, Tehran, Iran
[3]Basic and Molecular Epidemiology of Gastrointestinal Disorders Research Center, Research Institute for Gastroenterology and Liver Diseases, Shahid Beheshti University of Medical Sciences, Tehran, Iran
[4]Department of Immunology, School of Medicine, Shahid Beheshti University of Medical Sciences, Tehran, Iran
[5]Department of Microbiology and Genetics, Kherad Institute of Higher Education, Bushehr, Iran

* **Corresponding authors:** Najmafarahani@gmail.com (N.F.); a.taheriazam@iautmu.ac.ir (A.T.); P.rahimzadeh76@gmail.com (P.R.); mentezari@iautmu.ac.ir (M.E.)

[6]Department of Art & Sciences, Faculty of Biology, University of North Florida, Jacksonville, Florida, USA
[7]Department of Biology, ET.C., Islamic Azad University, Tehran, Iran
[8]Department of Orthopedics, Faculty of Medicine, TeMs. C, Islamic Azad University, Tehran, Iran
[9]Surgical Research Society (SRS), Students' Scientific Research Center, Tehran University of Medical Sciences, Tehran, Iran

Abstract

CRISPR/Cas9 has emerged as a versatile platform to dissect and therapeutically counteract cancer drug resistance by enabling precise, programmable edits across the core pathways that govern drug efflux, DNA repair, apoptosis, and adaptive signaling. By modeling resistance-causing mutations, executing focused loss- or gain-of-function screens, and functionally validating candidate drivers, CRISPR/Cas9 bridges mechanistic insight with translational action. In cellular and animal studies, targeted knockout or correction of resistance mediators, including ABC transporters, KRAS and downstream effectors, PI3K/AKT nodes, apoptosis regulators, and lineage-plasticity factors, has restored chemosensitivity and enhanced responses to targeted agents, supporting the concept that editing the determinants of resistance can convert refractory disease into a treatable state. Beyond single-gene interventions, pooled CRISPR screens have mapped context-dependent vulnerabilities and resistance trajectories under therapeutic pressure, informing rational drug combinations and sequence strategies. As early clinical studies of CRISPR-based therapies advance and safety engineering improves, the framework is set to move from discovery to intervention: pairing molecularly guided edits with standard regimens to delay resistance onset, reverse established resistance, and improve durability of response. At the same time, delivery constraints, off-target risks, tumor heterogeneity, and the potential for compensatory rewiring necessitate careful design, favoring transient, high-fidelity editors; robust off-target profiling; and longitudinal biomarker monitoring, to ensure that precision at the genome level translates into meaningful clinical benefit.

Keywords: CRISPR/Cas9; cancer drug resistance; functional genomics; efflux transporters; DNA repair; apoptosis; genome-wide screens; chemosensitization

13.1 Introduction

Addressing cancer remains one of the most critical medical challenges in healthcare. Clinical treatment protocols typically include combinations of surgical intervention, chemotherapeutic agents, precision-targeted treatments, and radiation therapy, with specific approaches tailored to individual cases [1, 2]. Despite these interventions, cancer persists as a major cause of mortality, ranking second only to heart disease in the United States, with 598,932 fatalities recorded in 2020 [3]. These concerning statistics underscore the urgency for continued research in cancer therapeutics.

Contemporary research efforts focus on two primary objectives: discovering novel therapeutic strategies and enhancing existing treatment modalities. Among emerging therapeutic innovations, genetic modification through CRISPR/Cas9 technology has emerged as a promising approach. This gene-editing platform enables precise genomic alterations in cancerous cells, with both laboratory and animal studies demonstrating encouraging outcomes. Currently, multiple clinical trials are evaluating the therapeutic potential of CRISPR/Cas9 in cancer treatment [4, 5].

Drug resistance presents a significant obstacle in cancer therapy, contributing to approximately 90% of cancer-related deaths [6]. While the complete mechanisms of drug resistance remain partially understood, research has identified multiple contributing factors, including genes associated with drug transport, DNA repair mechanisms, programmed cell death, and various cellular signaling cascades [7]. The application of CRISPR/Cas9 technology to target these resistance-related genes has shown promising results in diminishing drug resistance and improving therapeutic efficacy.

The scope of this discussion encompasses key drug resistance mechanisms, investigated countermeasures, and the potential applications of CRISPR/Cas9 in overcoming treatment resistance in cancer therapy. Additionally, the text examines the current limitations and challenges associated with CRISPR/Cas9 implementation.

13.2 Molecular Mechanisms of Drug Resistance in Cancer

Chemotherapy resistance in cancer is driven by a network of fundamental molecular mechanisms, including drug efflux, enhanced DNA damage repair, apoptosis evasion, epigenetic modifications, cancer stem cell dynamics, and alterations in intracellular drug metabolism. These mechanisms are highly interconnected and mutually influential, forming a complex landscape that remains only partially understood. This section systematically describes these molecular pathways, highlighting their roles in the development of chemotherapy resistance.

13.2.1 *Efflux of Chemotherapeutics*

Chemotherapy resistance frequently develops due to enhanced drug expulsion from cancer cells, which reduces the effectiveness of therapeutic agents. This process is primarily orchestrated by ATP-binding cassette (ABC) transport proteins, specifically ABCB1, ABCG2, and ABCC1, which are naturally present in organs including the liver, intestinal tissue, kidneys, and brain tissue [8–10]. These molecular pumps harness ATP energy to actively transport various substances, including chemotherapeutic compounds, out of cells.

P-glycoprotein (P-gp), which is encoded by the ABCB1 (MDR1) gene and positioned on epithelial cell surfaces, represents one of the most extensively researched drug transporters [11]. Its primary function involves chemotherapeutic agent removal from malignant cells, thereby limiting drug effectiveness. Studies have demonstrated increased MDR1 expression in gallbladder cancer, correlating with enhanced resistance to treatments such as gemcitabine and 5-fluorouracil (5-FU) [12]. Similar elevated MDR1 levels have been documented across various malignancies, including colorectal, breast, bone, and pancreatic cancers, contributing to broad drug resistance patterns [13].

The multidrug resistance-associated protein 1 (MRP1), another member of the ABCC family, also significantly influences drug resistance through its export capabilities [14]. Research has shown that targeting MRP1, particularly through miR-145 regulation, may help overcome chemotherapy resistance [15]. In gallbladder cancer specifically, MRP1 facilitates the removal of glutathione-bound cisplatin complexes from cells. Research indicates that strategies reducing MRP1 activity or glutathione levels can enhance cisplatin's therapeutic efficacy, suggesting promising treatment approaches [16].

The ABCG2 gene produces breast cancer resistance protein (BCRP), another key transport protein that influences drug resistance. This protein serves a protective function by removing harmful substances, including chemotherapeutic agents, and is naturally present in various body tissues such as intestinal walls, bile ducts, placental tissue, and protective barriers in the testes and brain [17]. Research has demonstrated that elevated BCRP levels correlate with increased resistance to chemotherapy treatments [18]. Of particular concern is the observation that metastatic cancer cells often show high BCRP expression, resulting in inherent drug resistance even before chemotherapy exposure [19].

Beyond the ABC transporter family, copper-regulating ATPases ATP7A and ATP7B play dual roles: while they maintain cellular copper homeostasis, they can also bind and compartmentalize platinum-based chemotherapy drugs like cisplatin. This binding action diminishes the therapeutic effectiveness of these drugs, contributing to treatment resistance [20]. Understanding how ATP7A and ATP7B function in gallbladder cancer could potentially reveal new strategies for combating resistance to platinum-based treatments.

Despite considerable advances in understanding cellular drug elimination mechanisms, additional research remains essential to fully comprehend the complex pathways involved in chemotherapy resistance, especially in specific cancers such as gallbladder cancer. The development of therapeutic approaches targeting these transport mechanisms represents a promising direction for enhancing treatment efficacy and overcoming drug resistance.

13.2.2 *DNA Damage Repair*

Cancer cells activate sophisticated DNA damage response mechanisms when confronted with chemotherapeutic agents like topoisomerase inhibitors, alkylating compounds, or DNA cross-linking medications such as cisplatin and cyclophosphamide. These pathways form an intricate network that preserves genomic stability [21]. Several DNA repair systems operate within cells, including direct damage reversal, base excision repair (BER), nucleotide excision repair, and mismatch repair. For more severe damage involving double-strand breaks, cells employ either homologous recombination or non-homologous end joining (NHEJ) [22].

The effectiveness of DNA repair mechanisms influences both cancer progression and therapeutic response. For instance, cancer cells with hyperactive RAS and PI3K pathways generate increased reactive oxygen species, leading to oxidative DNA damage. While these cells upregulate BER to address oxidative injuries, this enhanced repair capability can unexpectedly increase resistance to chemotherapeutic agents like temozolomide and cisplatin [23]. Research has also revealed that DNA damage triggers increased production of Dicer, an RNA-processing enzyme, which enhances DNA repair through NHEJ pathways, contributing to chemotherapy resistance in colorectal cancers [24].

Enhanced DNA repair capabilities enable cancer cells to survive chemotherapy by quickly remedying treatment-induced DNA damage. This understanding of repair pathways suggests potential therapeutic targets for addressing drug resistance. For example, PARP inhibitors have demonstrated promise in making resistant cancer cells more susceptible to chemotherapy by interfering with their DNA repair capabilities.

13.2.3 *Escape from Apoptosis*

Programmed cell death, or apoptosis, represents a precisely controlled mechanism for eliminating compromised cells. While chemotherapy typically works by triggering apoptosis [25], cancer cells often develop resistance by acquiring various mechanisms to circumvent this process [26]. These evasion strategies include modifications to apoptotic pathways, activation of protective autophagy, and increased production of proteins that inhibit cell death.

Protective autophagy represents a significant mechanism through which cancer cells resist apoptosis. This self-degradation process activates under stressful conditions, helping tumor cells survive [27]. When exposed to chemotherapy, cancer cells often initiate autophagy, which suppresses apoptotic processes and reduces treatment effectiveness [28]. For example, cervical cancer cells resistant to cisplatin employ autophagy to minimize endoplasmic reticulum stress, thereby preventing mitochondria-mediated cell death [29]. In gallbladder cancer, nutrient-poor conditions activate autophagy through the IL-6/STAT3 pathway, enhancing gemcitabine resistance [30]. Similarly, pancreatic cancer cells utilize Girdin-mediated autophagy through interaction with p62/SQSTM1 to suppress apoptosis and develop drug resistance [31]. Research suggests that autophagy inhibition could enhance chemotherapy efficacy [32, 33], with compounds like chloroquine showing promise in restoring drug sensitivity.

The disruption of apoptotic signaling pathways also significantly influences chemotherapy resistance. The B-cell lymphoma 2 (Bcl-2) protein family controls mitochondrial membrane permeability, crucial for apoptosis initiation. Enhanced expression of antiapoptotic Bcl-2 proteins, particularly myeloid cell leukemia-1 (Mcl-1) and Bcl-2, correlates with chemotherapy resistance in various cancers including leukemia [34]. Studies of ovarian cancer demonstrate that cells expressing high levels of Bcl-2 exhibit increased chemotherapy resistance [35], while reducing Mcl-1 expression can restore drug sensitivity [36].

The development of chemotherapy resistance is also influenced by alterations in pro-apoptotic proteins, either through mutations or decreased expression. For example, alterations in the proapoptotic BAX gene have been linked to treatment resistance in colorectal cancer [37]. In acute myeloid leukemia, reduced levels of pro-apoptotic proteins including BAX and NOXA contribute to therapeutic resistance [38–40].

The inhibitor of apoptosis proteins (IAPs) represent another crucial group of proteins that regulate cell death. These proteins promote cancer cell survival by preventing caspase activation. Enhanced expression of various IAP family proteins, including XIAP, Survivin, and cIAP, correlates with resistance to cisplatin and other chemotherapeutic drugs [41]. New therapeutic approaches, such as SMAC mimetics, are being developed to counteract IAP-mediated apoptosis resistance [42].

Dysregulation of the NF-κB signaling pathway also plays a significant role in treatment resistance across various cancers, such as breast cancer. Abnormal NF-κB activation has been shown to reduce the effectiveness of several chemotherapy agents, including doxorubicin, cisplatin, and paclitaxel [43]. Research in gallbladder cancer has demonstrated that combining NF-κB inhibitors with chemotherapy can enhance the tumor cells' response to gemcitabine [44].

The ability of cancer cells to evade apoptosis involves multiple interconnected mechanisms that collectively contribute to chemotherapy resistance. Therapeutic strategies targeting proteins involved in autophagy regulation, anti-apoptotic signaling, and cell death pathways show promise in enhancing chemotherapy effectiveness and overcoming drug resistance.

13.2.4 *Epigenetic Alterations*

Epigenetic modifications represent heritable but reversible changes in gene expression that occur without altering DNA sequences. These modifications, which include DNA methylation, histone modifications, and non-coding RNA regulation, significantly influence cancer development and treatment resistance [45].

DNA methylation, involving methyl group addition to CpG sites, represents a fundamental epigenetic mechanism [46]. Cancer cells typically exhibit widespread hypomethylation alongside specific hypermethylation of tumor suppressors [47]. Studies have shown that BRCA1 gene hypermethylation in ovarian cancer correlates with increased platinum-based therapy effectiveness [48]. However, TGF-βRI hypermethylation in gastric cancer reduces TGF-β signaling response [49]. Modifying these methylation patterns could potentially overcome treatment resistance.

Chromatin structure and gene expression are also regulated by histone modifications, including acetylation, methylation, ubiquitination, and phosphorylation. Histone acetylation, controlled by HATs and HDACs, particularly influences treatment resistance [50]. While acetylation typically promotes gene expression through chromatin relaxation, deacetylation suppresses gene activity through chromatin condensation [51]. For instance, elevated p300 (a HAT) levels correlate with gemcitabine resistance in pancreatic cancer [52], while increased HDAC expression links to resistance in melanoma and ovarian cancers [53, 54]. HDAC inhibitors like belinostat show promise in reversing resistance [55]. Histone methylation also affects drug response, with EZH2 methyltransferase overexpression contributing to cisplatin resistance in ovarian cancer. Reducing EZH2-mediated H3K27 trimethylation enhances cisplatin effectiveness [56]. Similar mechanisms influence lung cancer resistance through effects on cancer stem cells, epithelial-mesenchymal transition (EMT), and cell migration [57].

Non-coding RNAs, including miRNAs and lncRNAs, represent another layer of epigenetic regulation in chemoresistance [58]. miRNAs, which post-transcriptionally regulate gene expression, can function as either tumor suppressors or promoters [59]. In gallbladder cancer, they influence drug resistance gene expression [60]. lncRNAs affect drug resistance through various signaling pathway interactions [61, 62]. For example, GBCDRlnc1 promotes resistance in gallbladder cancer by enhancing autophagy [63], while HOTTIP modulates chemotherapy sensitivity in cholangiocarcinoma through the HOTTIP/miR-637/LASP1 pathway [64]. Epigenetic mechanisms offer potential therapeutic targets, as their reversible nature provides opportunities for intervention. By targeting specific epigenetic alterations, such as using DNA demethylating agents or histone deacetylase inhibitors, chemotherapy resistance may be mitigated.

13.2.5 *Changes in Drug Metabolism*

The metabolic processing of chemotherapy drugs within cancer cells significantly influences treatment effectiveness. Drug metabolism occurs in two distinct phases: Phase I, involving oxidation, reduction, or hydrolysis processes mediated by enzymes like cytochrome P450 (CYP), and Phase II, where drugs undergo conjugation by enzymes such as glutathione S-transferases (GSTs) [65].

CYP enzymes serve as crucial mediators of drug biotransformation. Changes in CYP enzyme expression can dramatically affect drug metabolism and treatment response. Research has shown that elevated levels of CYP1B1, CYP2E1, and CYP3A4 in non-rhabdomyosarcoma soft tissue sarcomas contribute to chemotherapy resistance [66, 67]. Interestingly, reduced CYP expression in medulloblastoma cells also correlates with increased drug resistance [67].

The glutathione (GSH) system represents another major factor in drug resistance. High cellular GSH levels enable cancer cells to detoxify chemotherapy drugs through conjugation, leading to their elimination [68]. This mechanism is particularly relevant in cisplatin resistance, where GSH binding neutralizes the drug's therapeutic effects [69]. Enhanced expression of gamma-glutamyl transferase, an enzyme involved in GSH metabolism, further promotes resistance by protecting cancer cells from oxidative stress and chemotherapy-induced damage [70].

Additional metabolic enzymes also influence treatment resistance. For instance, deoxycytidine kinase (dCK), which activates gemcitabine, often shows reduced expression in resistant cancer cells. Studies of gallbladder cancer have demonstrated that dCK mutations or decreased expression correlate with resistance, while restoring dCK activity can re-establish drug sensitivity [71, 72].

The intricate nature of drug metabolism pathways, encompassing both Phase I and II processes, highlights its fundamental role in chemotherapy resistance. Therapeutic approaches targeting specific metabolic enzymes like CYPs, GSTs, or dCK may offer promising strategies for overcoming drug resistance and enhancing treatment outcomes.

13.2.6 *Cancer Stem Cells*

Cancer stem cells [CSCs] represent a distinct tumor cell subset with unique capabilities for self-renewal, differentiation, and tumor initiation. These cells demonstrate remarkable resistance to traditional chemotherapy treatments, which typically target rapidly proliferating cells. Consequently, surviving CSCs often lead to cancer recurrence and spread [73, 74]. These cells can be identified through specific markers including CD133, CD44, and aldehyde dehydrogenase [75].

CSCs employ several resistance mechanisms, with drug efflux being particularly significant. This process involves ABC transporters, especially ABCG2, which actively remove chemotherapy drugs from cells [76]. For example, gallbladder cancer cells expressing CD133 show high ABCG2 levels, conferring resistance to treatments like gemcitabine and 5-FU [77]. Similarly, CD133-positive lung cancer cells resist DNA-damaging agents through enhanced DNA repair capabilities [78].

Advanced DNA repair mechanisms further protect CSCs from chemotherapy effects. These cells typically express elevated levels of DNA repair proteins, enabling rapid recovery from treatment-induced damage. This is exemplified by high XRCC1 expression in CD133-positive gallbladder cancer cells, contributing to 5-FU resistance [79]. CSCs also maintain low reactive oxygen species levels through increased antioxidant enzyme production, protecting them from oxidative damage-based therapies [80–82].

Cell dormancy provides another protective mechanism for CSCs. By entering a quiescent state (G0 phase), these cells avoid the effects of chemotherapy drugs targeting actively dividing cells. These dormant CSCs can later reactivate, causing tumor recurrence [83, 84]. Additionally, high aldehyde dehydrogenase expression in quiescent CSCs helps neutralize harmful aldehydes and reduce oxidative stress, enhancing their survival [85, 86]. Understanding these resistance mechanisms has become crucial in cancer research, with potential therapeutic strategies focusing on targeting CSC-specific pathways including drug transporters, DNA repair mechanisms, and reactive oxygen species metabolism [87].

In this section, the molecular mechanisms underlying chemotherapy resistance in cancer are comprehensively described. These intricately connected pathways play a pivotal role in the failure of chemotherapeutic interventions, posing substantial challenges in clinical oncology. By gaining a deeper understanding of how these mechanisms contribute to resistance, researchers can more effectively identify novel therapeutic targets, paving the way for advanced treatment strategies and improved outcomes for cancer patients.

13.3 Developments in Research on Chemoresistance Inhibition to Increase Chemosensitivity

Recent years have witnessed an acceleration in research aimed at addressing drug resistance in cancer, with numerous strategies being developed [88]. Researchers have extensively investigated various chemical and natural compounds, targeting specific mechanisms, signaling pathways, and RNA molecules (including lncRNAs and miRNAs) in drug-resistant cancer cells.

Understanding cellular and animal models of drug resistance is essential before examining key research findings. Scientists employ three primary protocols to establish resistant cell lines, each varying in dosage and timing. The initial approach involves gradually increasing drug concentrations on sensitive cell lines. The second method maintains constant drug exposure over an extended period, while the third protocol implements cyclical treatment patterns — typically alternating between 3-day drug treatments and 7-day control medium periods [88].

Since ABC family transporters significantly contribute to multidrug resistance (MDR) in cancer cells [17], researchers also develop resistant cells by transfecting cancer cells with mdr1-expressing vectors, such as plasmids containing mdr1 cDNA [89]. Animal models provide another avenue for studying resistance mechanisms. These models are created by injecting drug-resistant cancer cells subcutaneously into mice, monitoring tumor growth, administering chemotherapy, and analyzing tumor tissue post-treatment [90].

Many contemporary studies concentrate on counteracting the function of ABC family transporters in MDR. Several inhibitory compounds have shown promise, including NSC23925, NSC77037, and curcumin. For instance, YS-7a, derived from NSC23925, effectively reduces p-gp transport function and helps reverse MDR [91]. Research on osteosarcoma demonstrated NSC-77037's ability to counter ABCB1/ABCC1-dependent resistance and enhance doxorubicin effectiveness [92].

Curcumin, a natural compound notable for its low toxicity even at high doses, has been extensively researched. Studies on colorectal cancer cells reveal its capacity to inhibit p-gp transport and increase intracellular doxorubicin levels in resistant cells, ultimately enhancing doxorubicin's cytotoxic and apoptotic effects [93].

Recent attention has also turned to metformin, an antidiabetic medication, for its potential in combating cancer drug resistance. Research indicates it can reduce p-gp activity in doxorubicin-resistant cells dose-dependently while amplifying doxorubicin's apoptotic effects [94]. This suggests that repurposing existing medications might offer viable strategies for overcoming MDR in cancer treatment.

DNA damage response and repair mechanisms play crucial roles in cancer cell resistance to many chemotherapeutic agents that function by inducing DNA damage [95]. Recent research has focused on addressing drug resistance by developing compounds that target these DNA damage response pathways and reduce DNA repair capabilities. Research has demonstrated that in cisplatin-resistant gastric cancer, PARP1 inhibitors (specifically AG14361 and BYK204165) can enhance cisplatin's effectiveness by promoting DNA damage and cell death. This occurs through the inhibitors' ability to decrease DNA-PKcs stability and impair the NHEJ repair mechanism [96].

Nevertheless, resistance to PARP inhibitors themselves presents a significant challenge. One potential solution involves using miR-200c to target neuropilin 1, which has shown promise in reducing olaparib resistance in ovarian cancer cells [97]. PARP1's significance stems from its role as a DNA damage detector and its essential function in DNA repair processes [98].

Another promising approach involves melatonin, which can diminish cancer drug resistance by interfering with DNA repair mechanisms. The combination of melatonin with conventional chemotherapy agents represents a promising strategy that warrants further investigation [99]. Studies on hepatocellular carcinoma have revealed that melatonin induces lncRNA RAD51-AS1, which inhibits RAD51 translation (a crucial DNA repair protein), thereby reducing DNA repair capacity and enhancing chemotherapy effectiveness [100].

Various pathway inhibitors have shown positive results in combating cancer cell drug resistance. For instance, trigonelline, an alkaloid that inhibits Nrf2, shows promise in addressing oxaliplatin resistance in colorectal cancer [101]. Similarly, targeting the PI3K/AKT pathway has demonstrated potential in improving chemotherapy sensitivity [102]. Additionally, reducing CSC characteristics through compounds like bufalin, a traditional medicine, has proven effective in decreasing cisplatin resistance in colorectal cancer cells [103].

Recent research has shown significant promise in utilizing nanoparticle technology to deliver anticancer compounds and combat drug resistance. A notable example is the combined delivery of metformin and doxorubicin using PLGA-TPGS nanoparticles, which improves cellular drug uptake while reducing drug efflux in doxorubicin-resistant breast cancer cells, ultimately leading to increased cell death and reduced drug resistance [104]. More comprehensive information about nanotechnology's role in addressing cancer drug resistance can be found in specialized reviews [105].

Targeting inflammation through conventional medications and antibodies presents another strategy for reducing cancer cell drug resistance. Research has demonstrated that aspirin, a common anti-inflammatory medication, can enhance cisplatin's ability to induce cell death in resistant lung cancer cells [106]. Additionally, the anti-IL6 antibody MEDI5117 has demonstrated effectiveness in improving chemotherapy response across various cancer types [107].

Among the most promising approaches to addressing cancer drug resistance is the targeting of non-coding RNAs, particularly miRNAs and lncRNAs. lncRNAs, defined as non-coding RNA molecules exceeding 200 nucleotides in length [108], have been linked to key drug resistance mechanisms in cancer cells. For instance, lncRNA H19 has been shown to reduce p-gp expression in doxorubicin-resistant liver cancer cells [109]. Research has also revealed that lncRNA-MALAT1 increases ABCC1 and ABCB1 expression in cisplatin-resistant lung cancer cells, potentially through STAT3 activation [110]. This same lncRNA has been found to enhance doxorubicin resistance in breast cancer by targeting miR-570-3p, while increased miR-570-3p levels can improve chemotherapy effectiveness [111].

lncRNA NEAT1 appears to play a role in enhancing DNA repair, with its inhibition leading to decreased expression of homologous recombination pathway genes. Suppressing this lncRNA can improve the effectiveness of various anticancer drugs, including bortezomib, carfilzomib, and melphalan in multiple myeloma [112]. Similarly, reducing LINC00963 expression has shown promise in decreasing stemness and drug resistance in head and neck carcinomas [113]. These findings suggest that modulating lncRNA levels through antisense oligonucleotides or expression enhancement could be valuable strategies for overcoming cancer drug resistance.

miRNAs function by targeting mRNA, leading to its degradation, destabilization, and translation inhibition, thereby regulating post-transcriptional processes [114, 115]. The development of cancer therapeutics based on miRNA mimics and antagomiRs has gained significant attention, with some candidates advancing to clinical trials. For instance, cobomarsen, an antagomiR-155, is currently undergoing phase I trials for cutaneous T cell lymphoma treatment [116].

Research has revealed promising results regarding miRNAs as therapeutic targets for cancer drug resistance. Studies have shown that miR-221 inhibition can significantly decrease p-gp and bcl-2 expression in doxorubicin-resistant osteosarcoma, reducing drug resistance [117]. Additionally, miR-21 has been found to increase p-gp expression and contribute to cisplatin resistance in ovarian cancer [118]. As a well-documented oncomiR, miR-21's role in drug resistance spans multiple cancer types [119], making its inhibition a focal point in resistance research.

Enhanced miR-506 expression has shown potential in reducing MDR1/p-gp levels and improving chemotherapy response in oxaliplatin-resistant colorectal cancer [120], suggesting miR-506 mimics as promising candidates for further investigation. miR-140 has demonstrated ability to reduce DNA repair by inhibiting FEN1, thereby enhancing breast cancer chemosensitivity [121]. In gastric cancer, miR-200c can reverse drug resistance by reducing ERCC3 and ERCC4 expression, which are involved in nucleotide excision repair [122].

miR-451a has shown effectiveness in reducing EMT and increasing doxorubicin sensitivity in lung cancer by downregulating c-Myc, with promising results both *in vitro* and *in vivo* [123]. Conversely, miR-372 and miR-373 promote stemness and 5-FU resistance in colorectal cancer [124], suggesting their inhibition as a potential therapeutic strategy. miR-144 mimics have shown potential in enhancing 5-FU's effects in liver cancer by promoting Nrf2 degradation [125], while miR-29c improves cisplatin sensitivity in lung cancer through PI3K/AKT pathway regulation [126]. The broader relationship between miRNAs and signaling pathways is extensively documented elsewhere [127].

Recent advances in genome editing, particularly CRISPR/Cas9 technology, offer new possibilities for addressing cancer drug resistance by targeting key resistance mechanisms and improving treatment efficacy. The following sections will explore CRISPR/Cas9 applications in overcoming cancer drug resistance.

13.4 CRISPR/Cas9 Technology to Combat Cancer Chemoresistance

The CRISPR/Cas9 system, which functions as an RNA-based immune system in bacteria, can be adapted for editing genes in eukaryotic cells, including those associated with multiple drug resistance. This system employs single-guide RNA (sgRNA) designed to complement specific sequences, working in conjunction with Cas9 endonuclease. When introduced into target cells, the sgRNA directs Cas9 to create double-strand breaks at specific DNA sequences, enabling targeted gene deletion or insertion [128].

Recent studies applying CRISPR/Cas9 technology to cancer drug resistance have yielded promising results. Research has particularly focused on ABC family transporters, which play a crucial role in drug resistance through enhanced drug efflux. A study using KBV200 and HCT-8/V cancer cells demonstrated that CRISPR/Cas9-mediated ABCB1 gene knockout significantly increased intracellular doxorubicin accumulation and chemotherapy sensitivity [129].

In doxorubicin-resistant breast cancer cells, MDR1 gene targeting using CRISPR/Cas9 substantially increased doxorubicin cytotoxicity. Flow cytometry analysis revealed a fourfold increase in drug uptake compared to untreated cells [130]. Similarly, research on ovarian cancer cells using three sgRNAs targeting ABCB1 gene's fourth and fifth exons showed significant reduction in ABCB1 expression and increased doxorubicin sensitivity, as confirmed by MTT assays [131]. A meta-analysis further supported these findings, showing that CRISPR/Cas9-mediated ABCB1 targeting effectively reduced doxorubicin resistance in resistant osteosarcoma cells [132].

The system has also shown promise in targeting other resistance mechanisms. GST and glutathione, which contribute to drug resistance through chemotherapy drug detoxification and apoptosis suppression [133], have been successfully targeted. Research demonstrated that CRISPR/Cas9-mediated knockout of glutathione S-transferase omega 1 in colorectal cancer cells enhanced the effectiveness of cisplatin and oxaliplatin.

DNA repair enhancement represents another significant resistance mechanism. Cyclin-dependent kinases (CDKs), which regulate cell cycle, proliferation, and DNA repair [134, 135], play a crucial role in this process. These kinase enzymes have been confirmed as important factors in cancer drug resistance.

Research has demonstrated elevated expression of CDK enzymes in cancers, with CDK inhibitors showing promising therapeutic results. Palbociclib, a CDK4/6 inhibitor, has received the U.S. Food and Drug Administration (FDA) approval for breast cancer treatment [136]. However, resistance to palbociclib has emerged, potentially linked to increased CDK6 expression. Studies on palbociclib-resistant breast cancer cells have shown that CRISPR/Cas9-mediated CDK6 knockout can restore drug sensitivity and reduce cancer cell survival [137].

CDK11 has also been implicated in cancer drug resistance. Research on ovarian cancer cells has revealed CDK11's role in enhancing proliferation while reducing apoptosis and paclitaxel sensitivity [138]. In osteosarcoma cells, CRISPR/Cas9-mediated CDK11 knockout using specific sgRNA (sequence: TCCGAGA CATTTGCTGGGTGG) significantly increased cell death and reduced cancer cell invasiveness [139].

BRCA1, a crucial tumor suppressor involved in DNA repair [140], shows mutation rates of 1–7% in breast and ovarian cancers, regardless of age or family history [141]. This protein can reduce chemotherapy effectiveness by enhancing DNA repair pathways [142], with high BRCA1 expression correlating with chemoresistance in lung cancer [143]. While heterogeneous BRCA1 mutations are challenging to target directly, targeting its synthetic lethality partner PARP1 offers an alternative approach. Research on triple-negative breast cancer cells with mBRCA1 demonstrated that CRISPR/Cas9-mediated PARP1 targeting increased sensitivity to various chemotherapy drugs, including doxorubicin, gemcitabine, and docetaxel, allowing for reduced dosage requirements [144].

Another study focused on breast cancer cells used CRISPR/Cas9 to target HER2 exon 12, showing that combining this approach with PARP inhibitors significantly inhibited cancer cell growth [145]. The combination of CRISPR/Cas9 technology with DNA repair inhibitors represents a promising direction for future cancer treatment research.

RECQL4 helicase, a protein involved in DNA repair and drug resistance, has been shown to enhance MDR1 expression [146, 147].

Recent research on glioma cells demonstrated that CRISPR/Cas9-mediated RECQL4 knockout increased temozolomide effectiveness, as evidenced by elevated levels of DNA damage and apoptosis markers, including phospho-H2AX, PARP-1, and cleaved caspases 3 and 7 [146]. This suggests RECQL4 targeting via CRISPR/Cas9 as a potential strategy for addressing cancer drug resistance.

Multiple proteins and signaling pathways contribute to cancer drug resistance. Research has shown that mutations in oncogenes and tumor suppressors, particularly K-Ras and P53, significantly impact drug resistance through various mechanisms, including reduced apoptosis, increased ABC transporter expression, and enhanced DNA repair [148–150]. Additionally, mutations in growth-related receptors, their associated signaling pathways, and proteins involved in proliferation and apoptosis can lead to increased proliferation and drug resistance.

K-Ras mutations particularly stand out as crucial factors in cancer development, progression, and treatment resistance, especially in colorectal cancer [151, 152]. A notable study on colorectal cancer cells employed CRISPR/Cas9 technology, delivered via nanoparticles, to edit the KRAS gene. The results demonstrated that K-Ras targeting significantly enhanced cetuximab-induced apoptosis. In mouse models with KRAS-mutated colorectal cancer, this approach led to substantial tumor size reduction and improved cetuximab effectiveness. This is particularly significant as cetuximab, an EGFR inhibitor, is typically used for treating colorectal cancer with wild-type K-Ras [153].

The CRISPR/Cas9 findings suggest potential for expanding cetuximab use to K-Ras-mutated colorectal cancer cases, though extensive additional research is needed. P53 mutations, another factor in cancer drug resistance [154], have been successfully addressed using CRISPR/Cas9 technology in osteosarcoma cells, resulting in increased doxorubicin sensitivity and reduced anti-apoptotic protein expression, including Bcl-2 and survivin [155].

The epidermal growth factor receptor (EGFR), a receptor tyrosine kinase that responds to EGF family proteins, normally regulates epithelial tissue development and homeostasis. However, mutation-induced overexpression can promote tumorigenesis and drug resistance, particularly in lung cancer and glioblastoma [156, 157]. While EGFR inhibitors show promise in treating EGFR-mutant non-small-cell lung cancer, drug resistance remains problematic [158].

A breakthrough study on non-small-cell lung cancer employed CRISPR/Cas9 to specifically target EGFR containing a single-nucleotide missense mutation (CTG > CGG). Using adenoviral vectors to deliver sgRNA-EGFR and Cas9, researchers achieved successful disruption of mutated EGFR, leading to enhanced cell death. *In vivo* studies demonstrated significant tumor reduction and improved survival rates in mouse models [159].

Additional research on renal cancer cells utilized two sgRNAs with homology-directed repair templates to target EGFR's exon 2. The combination of CRISPR/Cas9-mediated EGFR knockout with sunitinib showed enhanced anti-proliferative effects compared to sunitinib alone in wild-type EGFR cells [160]. Sunitinib, an FDA-approved renal cell carcinoma treatment, targets VEGFR and PDGF-R receptors [161].

The urokinase plasminogen activator receptor (uPAR), a GPI-linked membrane receptor, represents another significant target. This protein, which regulates urokinase's proteolytic activity in extracellular matrix breakdown, is frequently overexpressed in various cancers. uPAR contributes to enhanced EMT, stemness, invasion, metastasis, and drug resistance [162, 163].

Research on MDR cancer cells (HCT8/T and KBV200) demonstrated that CRISPR/Cas9-mediated uPAR knockout significantly reduced IC50 values for various chemotherapy drugs, including 5-FU, cisplatin, docetaxel, and doxorubicin, indicating enhanced drug sensitivity [164].

Mucin glycoproteins, particularly MUC4, show elevated expression in various cancers and correlate with drug resistance [165]. Studies have linked MUC4 to gemcitabine resistance in pancreatic cancer [166]. Recent research has shown that CRISPR/Cas9-mediated MUC4 knockout significantly improves gemcitabine sensitivity in pancreatic ductal adenocarcinoma cells [167]. Given this cancer's high mortality rate, further research into CRISPR/Cas9-based resistance reduction strategies is warranted.

Topoisomerase 2 (TOP2), an enzyme crucial for managing DNA topological issues during chromosome processes [168], exists in two isoforms in etoposide-resistant leukemia cells: TOP2α/170 and TOP2α/90. While TOP2α/170 serves as a drug target, resistant cells show decreased TOP2α/170 and increased TOP2α/90 expression [169]. A recent study used CRISPR/Cas9 to modify the exon 19/intron 19 5′ splice site (GAG//GTAA AC → GAG//GTAA GT), successfully reducing TOP2α/90 expression while increasing TOP2α/170, thereby enhancing etoposide sensitivity [169].

Additional research on chronic myeloid leukemia has shown that CRISPR/Cas9-mediated disruption of the BCR/ABL oncogene can reduce proliferation and increase apoptosis in imatinib-resistant cells [170], suggesting potential applications in overcoming leukemia drug resistance.

RUNX1 has also emerged as a significant factor in cancer drug resistance. Studies of ovarian cancer cells have revealed its role, along with FOXO3a and hyperactive IGF1R, in driving drug resistance [171].

Recent research has demonstrated that CRISPR/Cas9-mediated RUNX1 knockout can enhance cisplatin's apoptotic effects in ovarian cancer cells [172]. The technology has also shown promise in targeting various signaling pathways involved in cancer drug resistance. The PI3K/AKT pathway, crucial for cell proliferation, apoptosis resistance, and drug resistance [173], has been successfully targeted through CRISPR/Cas9 knockout of PI3K-110α and PI3K-110β genes (Pik3ca and Pik3cb). This intervention reduced ABCB1(p-gp) and ABCG2 (BCRP) expression, improving sensitivity to colchicine and paclitaxel in epidermoid carcinoma and lung cancer cells [174].

The interaction between PI3K/AKT signaling and programmed cell death ligand 1 (PD-L1) presents another interesting aspect of drug resistance. PD-L1, frequently upregulated in resistant cancer cells, influences drug resistance through PI3K/AKT pathway enhancement and immune suppression [175, 176]. Research has shown that CRISPR/Cas9-mediated PD-L1 knockout reduces doxorubicin and paclitaxel IC50 values in osteosarcoma cells [175].

The NFE2L2 gene, encoding NRF2, has also been successfully targeted using CRISPR/Cas9, resulting in increased sensitivity to cisplatin, vinorelbine, and carboplatin in lung cancer cells [177].

CSCs, a major contributor to treatment resistance and disease recurrence, have been addressed through CRISPR/Cas9 targeting of stem cell markers. A study on prostate cancer cells demonstrated that CRISPR/Cas9-mediated knockout of NANOG1 and NANOGP8 significantly enhanced docetaxel sensitivity [178]. This approach of targeting stemness characteristics shows promise in addressing cancer drug resistance.

Research has demonstrated significant findings regarding CD44's role in cancer treatment. As a glycoprotein that functions as a hyaluronic acid receptor in the extracellular matrix, CD44 serves as an indicator of both drug resistance and CSCs [179]. Research on ovarian cancer has revealed elevated CD44 levels in drug-resistant cells, particularly noting its significance in paclitaxel resistance [180].

CD44 contributes to cancer cell drug resistance through several pathways, including reducing ABCB1 ubiquitination and breakdown, boosting anti-apoptotic protein expression like Bcl-xL, and influencing glucose metabolism by enhancing glycolysis and the pentose phosphate pathway [179, 181, 182]. In drug-resistant osteosarcoma research, CRISPR/Cas9-mediated CD44 targeting led to decreased ABCB1 expression and enhanced doxorubicin effectiveness [181]. Similarly, CD44 knockout in hepatocellular carcinoma cells via CRISPR/Cas9 improved responsiveness to both sorafenib and 5-FU treatments [183]. Meta-analysis results indicated that CRISPR/Cas9-based CD44 knockout inhibited osteosarcoma cell invasion, metastasis, and spheroid development [184].

Non-coding RNAs, including miRNAs and lncRNAs, have emerged as potential therapeutic targets due to their connection to cancer drug resistance. The miR-371/372/373 cluster, known for its oncogenic characteristics, was successfully eliminated using CRISPR/Cas9 in oral carcinoma cells, resulting in enhanced cisplatin-induced apoptosis after 48-hour exposure to 15 μM cisplatin [185]. Another investigation employed CRISPR/Cas9 and lentiviral vectors to suppress miR-21 (an established oncomiR) in ovarian cancer cells, leading to increased paclitaxel-induced apoptosis and reduced EMT [186]. Regarding lncRNA MALAT1's role in breast cancer doxorubicin resistance, researchers found that CRISPR/Cas9-mediated deletion of the lncRNA promoter in triple-negative breast cancer cells improved sensitivity to both doxorubicin and paclitaxel [187].

Research indicates that employing CRISPR/Cas9 technology to target drug resistance-associated miRNAs and lncRNAs could be a promising strategy for combating cancer drug resistance, warranting further investigation. The applications of CRISPR/Cas9 gene editing extend beyond human protein targeting to include viral oncoproteins. papillomavirus (HPV), particularly HPV16 and HPV18, stands out as a crucial oncogenic virus, accounting for approximately 70% of cervical cancer cases and pre-cancerous lesions [188]. Research has demonstrated that viral proteins E6 and E7 contribute to both metastasis and drug resistance in cervical cancer [188, 189]. Scientists have successfully shown that CRISPR/Cas9 can effectively disrupt these E6 and E7 genes.

In HPV16-positive cervical cancer cells, E7 gene disruption via CRISPR/Cas9 resulted in enhanced apoptosis, growth inhibition, and increased pRb expression [190]. Additional research revealed that CRISPR/Cas9-mediated disruption of HPV16 E6/E7 enhanced cisplatin's effectiveness in both cellular and xenograft mouse models, improving growth inhibition and apoptosis induction [191]. Similarly, HPV18 E6 knockout using CRISPR/Cas9 strengthened cisplatin's anti-proliferative and pro-apoptotic effects in cervical cancer cells [**Table 13.1**] [192].

The collective evidence suggests that CRISPR/Cas9 gene editing holds significant potential for addressing drug resistance across various cancer types by targeting different resistance mechanisms. With numerous ongoing studies, researchers are optimistic that overcoming the current limitations of CRISPR/Cas9 technology will pave the way for its clinical application in treating drug-resistant cancers.

Table 13.1 CRISPR/Cas9 applications in overcoming cancer drug resistance.

Target Gene or Protein	Cancer Type	Drug Resistance Mechanism	CRISPR/Cas9 Intervention	Outcome	Reference
ABCB1	KBV200 and HCT-8/V cancer cells	Enhanced drug efflux	Gene knockout	Increased doxorubicin accumulation and chemosensitivity	[129]
MDR1	Doxorubicin-resistant breast cancer	Enhanced drug efflux	Gene downregulation	4 × increased drug uptake, enhanced cytotoxicity	[130]
ABCB1	Ovarian cancer	Enhanced drug efflux	Targeted exons 4–5	Reduced gene expression, increased doxorubicin susceptibility	[131]
ABCB1	Osteosarcoma	Enhanced drug efflux	Gene targeting	Attenuated doxorubicin resistance (meta-analysis)	[132]
CDK6	Breast cancer	Enhanced DNA repair	Gene knockout	Increased palbociclib sensitivity, reduced cell survival	[137]
CDK11	Osteosarcoma	Enhanced proliferation, attenuated apoptosis	Gene knockout	Increased cell death, reduced invasiveness	[139]
PARP1	Triple-negative breast cancer (mBRCA1)	Enhanced DNA repair	Gene targeting	Increased sensitivity to multiple chemotherapy drugs	[144]
RECQL4	Glioma	Enhanced DNA repair, MDR1 expression	Gene knockout	Enhanced temozolomide toxicity, increased DNA damage markers	[146]

K-Ras	Colorectal cancer	Enhanced proliferation, drug resistance	Gene editing	Enhanced cetuximab apoptotic effects, reduced tumor size	[193]
Mutant TP53	Osteosarcoma	Attenuated apoptosis	Gene knockout	Increased doxorubicin sensitivity, reduced anti-apoptotic proteins	[155]
EGFR	Non-small-cell lung cancer	Enhanced tumorigenesis	Selective mutation targeting	Enhanced cell death, reduced tumor size, increased survival	[159]
uPAR	MDR cancer cells	Enhanced EMT, stemness, invasion	Gene knockout	Reduced IC50 of multiple chemotherapy drugs	[164]
MUC4	Pancreatic cancer	Gemcitabine resistance	Gene knockout	Increased gemcitabine sensitivity in pancreatic ductal adenocarcinoma	[167]
TOP2α/90	Etoposide-resistant leukemia	Alternative RNA processing	Splice site targeting	Reduced TOP2α/90 expression, increased etoposide sensitivity	[169]
BCR/ABL	Chronic myeloid leukemia	Enhanced proliferation	Gene disruption	Attenuated proliferation, enhanced apoptosis in imatinib-resistant cells	[170]
RUNX1	Ovarian cancer	Drug resistance with FOXO3a/IGF1R	Gene knockout	Potentiated cisplatin apoptotic effects	[172]
PI3K-110α/β	Epidermoid carcinoma, lung cancer	Enhanced drug resistance	Gene knockout	Reduced ABCB1/ABCG2 expression, enhanced drug sensitivity	[174]
PD-L1	Osteosarcoma	Enhanced PI3K/AKT signaling	Gene knockout	Reduced IC50 of doxorubicin and paclitaxel	[175]

(Continued)

Table 13.1 (*Continued*)

Target Gene or Protein	Cancer Type	Drug Resistance Mechanism	CRISPR/Cas9 Intervention	Outcome	Reference
NFE2L2 (NRF2)	Lung cancer	Enhanced detoxification	Function disruption	Increased sensitivity to multiple chemotherapy drugs	[177]
NANOG1/ NANOGP8	Prostate cancer	CSC resistance	Gene knockout	Increased docetaxel sensitivity	[178]
CD44	Osteosarcoma	Enhanced drug resistance, stemness	Gene targeting	Reduced ABCB1 expression, increased doxorubicin sensitivity	[194]
miR-371/ 372/373	Oral carcinoma	Drug resistance	Cluster removal	Enhanced cisplatin apoptotic effects	[185]
miR-21	Ovarian cancer	Enhanced EMT, drug resistance	Expression inhibition	Potentiated paclitaxel apoptotic effects, attenuated EMT	[186]
lncRNA MALAT1	Triple-negative breast cancer	Doxorubicin resistance	Promoter deletion	Enhanced doxorubicin and paclitaxel sensitivity	[187]

13.5 CRISPR/Cas9-mediated Identification and Targeting of Chemoresistance-related Genes

CRISPR/Cas9 technology has emerged as a valuable tool for investigating cancer drug resistance mechanisms, helping researchers identify crucial genes involved in this process. Recent studies have highlighted several significant genes, including SLFN11, APE1, RSF1, and CDK5, in their contribution to cancer drug resistance [195].

Schlafen 11 (SLFN11), functioning as a DNA/RNA helicase, plays a dual role in replication blocking and cell death promotion [196]. This protein enhances cancer cell sensitivity to various anticancer treatments, including platinum derivatives, gemcitabine (DNA synthesis inhibitor), and irinotecan (topoisomerase inhibitor) [197]. CRISPR/Cas9-mediated SLFN11 knockout studies in small-cell lung cancer cells demonstrated increased resistance to the PARP inhibitor talazoparib, suggesting SLFN11 expression could serve as a predictive marker for PARP inhibitor response [198].

Further CRISPR/Cas9 research revealed SLFN11's mechanism in PARP inhibitor sensitivity. Studies using SLFN11-deleted cells showed reduced replication inhibition at 24 hours post-talazoparib treatment, G2 phase progression at 48 hours, and minimal increase in apoptotic cells. These findings suggest SLFN11 enhances cancer cell sensitivity to PARP inhibitors through S-phase arrest promotion [199].

APE1 (apurinic/apyrimidyl endonuclease 1), a key enzyme in BER DNA repair, was investigated using CRISPR/Cas9 in triple-negative breast cancer. Research showed that APE1 gene knockout significantly increased olaparib's IC50, indicating that APE1 deletion may contribute to olaparib resistance [200].

Remodeling and spacing factor 1 (RSF-1), a protein crucial for chromosome stabilization, oncogene transcription reduction, and DNA repair enhancement, has been linked to cancer drug resistance when overexpressed [201].

Research on lung cancer cells demonstrated that RSF-1 silencing through CRISPR/Cas9 enhanced paclitaxel's antitumor and apoptotic effects. The study revealed reduced tumor volume and weight in xenograft mice following RSF-1 knockout, suggesting RSF-1's role in drug resistance through NFKB signaling enhancement [202].

CDK5, unlike typical cell cycle-regulating CDKs, is an atypical CDK primarily known for its central nervous system functions [203]. It plays vital roles in neuronal migration during central nervous system development, drug addiction, and synaptic plasticity [204]. Studies have linked CDK5 to both tumorigenesis and drug resistance across various cancers [203].

CRISPR/Cas9-mediated CDK5 silencing research demonstrated enhanced sorafenib effectiveness in hepatocellular carcinoma cells by reducing proliferation and survival. The study revealed that CDK5 knockdown reduced EGFR and AKT phosphorylation post-sorafenib treatment and prevented increased cell surface EGFR levels. These mechanisms, particularly EGFR signaling activation, are crucial in sorafenib resistance [205, 206].

Additional genes implicated in cancer drug resistance include ARID1A, Aurora-B, ATRX, and BIRC5, with their mechanisms clarified through CRISPR/Cas9 technology. In endometrial cancer, where progesterone resistance challenges medroxyprogesterone (MPA) treatment, CRISPR/Cas9 studies revealed that ARID1A (a tumor suppressor) knockout led to progesterone receptor B downregulation, increased AKT phosphorylation, and reduced MPA sensitivity [207].

Studies revealed Aurora-B's role in mitotic division regulation, with its overexpression linked to increased cisplatin and paclitaxel resistance in non-small-cell lung cancer and reduced patient survival. CRISPR/Cas9-mediated Aurora-B knockout enhanced chemosensitivity and p53 expression, suggesting Aurora-B reduces drug sensitivity by suppressing p53-dependent DNA damage responses [208].

ATRX serves multiple cellular functions, including telomere structure maintenance and DNA replication/repair [209, 210]. CRISPR/Cas9 knockout studies in glioma cells showed ATRX deletion enhanced temozolomide-induced apoptosis by reducing histone H3K9me3 availability and weakening ATM-dependent DNA repair, indicating ATRX's role in drug resistance through DNA repair enhancement [209].

The BIRC5 gene, encoding the anti-apoptotic protein survivin [211], was studied in ovarian cancer using CRISPR/Cas9. Gene disruption increased cytokeratin-7 (epithelial marker) expression while decreasing mesenchymal markers (vimentin, snai2, β-catenin), enhancing paclitaxel sensitivity. These findings suggest BIRC5 contributes to drug resistance through EMT promotion [212].

The identification of drug resistance genes and their mechanisms through CRISPR/Cas9 technology opens new avenues for therapeutic targeting. Genome-wide CRISPR/Cas9 screening has emerged as a powerful tool for identifying drug resistance genes in cancer cells. This technique employs commercially available sgRNA libraries delivered via lentiviral vectors alongside Cas9. The process involves designing sgRNA pools, infecting cell populations with lentiviral vectors containing sgRNAs and Cas9, administering drug treatment, selecting clones based on phenotype, and using next-generation sequencing to identify genes present in drug-sensitive versus resistant cells [213, 214].

Genome-wide CRISPR knockout screening can be conducted using an arrayed screen method, where individual wells contain specific sgRNAs, eliminating the need for next-generation sequencing [213]. This technique enables simultaneous examination of numerous genes, yielding significant findings regarding drug resistance mechanisms.

Research utilizing CRISPR screens has revealed the roles of PBRM1 and SGOL1 in cancer drug resistance. PBRM1, a SWI/SNF complex component involved in nucleosome positioning and chromatin accessibility, exhibits tumor-suppressive characteristics [215, 216]. CRISPR screening of lung cancer cells demonstrated that PBRM1 mutations might reduce EGFR inhibitor effectiveness by maintaining AKT signaling [216].

SGOL1, which protects centromeric cohesion during meiosis, has been linked to chromosomal stability [217]. A comprehensive CRISPR screen using 123,411 sgRNAs identified SGOL1 as a prognostic marker in sorafenib-treated patients. CRISPR/Cas9-mediated

SGOL1 silencing induced sorafenib resistance in hepatocellular carcinoma cells, with *in vivo* studies confirming reduced sorafenib cytotoxicity following SGOL1 loss [218].

Recent CRISPR/Cas9 screening studies have identified additional drug resistance genes. In prostate cancer research, 17 genes were found crucial for docetaxel resistance, with transcription elongation factor A-like 1 (Tceal1) emerging as particularly significant. Tceal1 suppression enhanced docetaxel's effects on subG1 cell death and polyploidy [219]. Similarly, cervical cancer studies identified 374 paclitaxel resistance-related genes, including ABCC9 and IL37 [220].

Genome-wide CRISPR/Cas9 screening in bladder cancer cells identified MSH2's significance in cisplatin resistance, showing that its downregulation decreased cisplatin-induced apoptosis [221]. In gallbladder cancer research, the technique revealed elongator complex subunit 5 (ELP5)'s role in gemcitabine sensitivity, with reduced ELP5 expression correlating with poor survival outcomes following gemcitabine treatment [222].

Studies in renal cell carcinoma using genome-wide CRISPR/Cas9 screening identified farnesyltransferase as a key factor in sunitinib resistance. Further investigation using siRNA-mediated knockdown demonstrated enhanced sunitinib-induced apoptosis, while the farnesyltransferase inhibitor lonafarnib increased sunitinib's antitumor effects [223].

In NRAS-mutant melanoma, the screening technique identified FBXO42 (an E3 ubiquitin ligase) as crucial in trametinib resistance, revealing its involvement in TAK1 signaling. This finding suggested potential effectiveness of combined TAK1 inhibitor and trametinib therapy [224].

Acute myeloid leukemia studies revealed that negative regulators of MAPK and mTORC1 pathways (LZTR1, NF1, TSC1/TSC2) contributed to sorafenib resistance [225]. Additional acute myeloid leukemia research identified BEND3's role in TAK-243 (UBA1 inhibitor) effectiveness. BEND3 knockout reduced TAK-243's impact on DNA repair response and proteotoxic stress, while increasing ABCG2 expression and decreasing intracellular TAK-243 levels, potentially causing drug resistance [226].

Research using genome-wide CRISPR/Cas9 screens in k-ras mutated colorectal cancer cells revealed the Wnt/B-catenin signaling pathway's involvement in ABT-263 (BCL-XL inhibitor) resistance. The study showed depletion of sgRNAs targeting WNT signaling's positive regulators and enrichment of those targeting negative regulators in resistant cells [227].

Glioblastoma cell studies identified MSH2, CLCA2, and PTCH2 as key genes in temozolomide resistance. These genes regulate mismatch repair, Wnt signaling inhibition, and Sonic Hedgehog pathway inhibition, respectively. siRNA-mediated silencing of these genes increased cell survival after temozolomide treatment, demonstrating how Wnt and Sonic Hedgehog pathway activation contributes to glioblastoma drug resistance [228].

The genome-wide CRISPR/Cas9 screen technology has transformed our understanding of cancer drug resistance mechanisms. Recent studies have identified crucial resistance-related genes that warrant investigation as therapeutic targets. These discoveries suggest potential breakthroughs in cancer treatment through overcoming drug resistance barriers. The technology's continued application is expected to reveal. **Figure 13.1** comprehensively demonstrates how CRISPR/Cas9 knockout systems and genome-wide screens systematically identify chemoresistance mechanisms across cancer types, providing theoretical guidance for clinical combination therapies and personalized treatment strategies.

13.6 Challenges and Limitations in Utilizing CRISPR/Cas9 System in Overcoming Chemoresistance

Despite CRISPR/Cas9's extensive applications, several limitations must be addressed before clinical implementation. Off-target mutagenesis represents a primary concern, where sgRNA may affect unintended DNA regions similar to the target sequence, potentially disrupting gene function and causing genomic

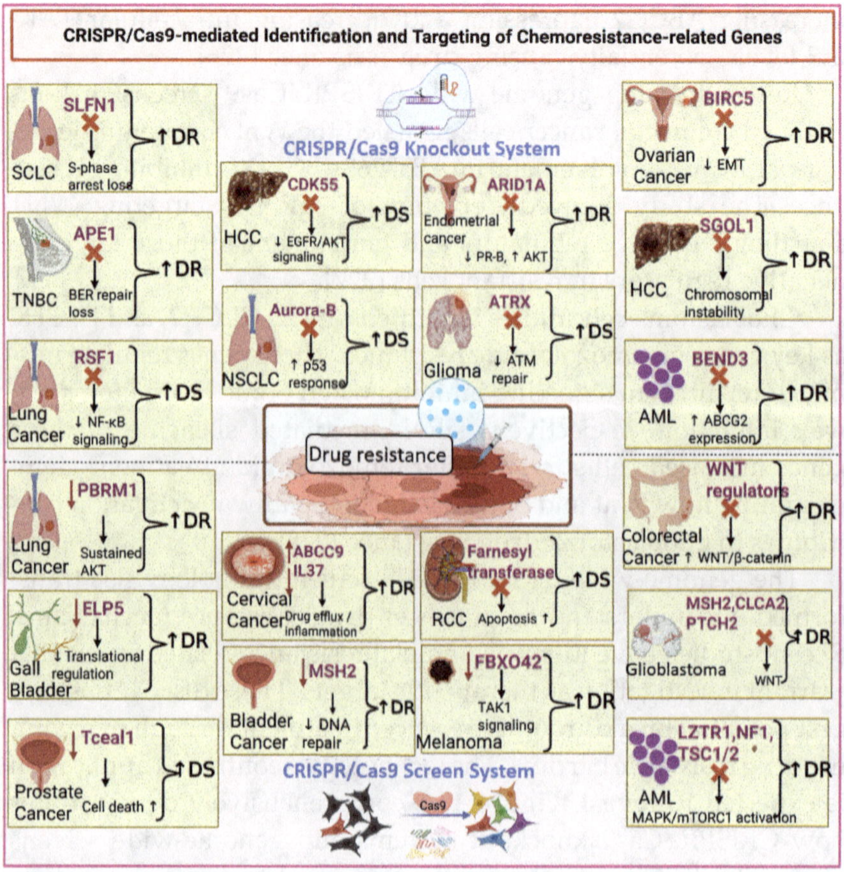

Figure 13.1 CRISPR/Cas9-mediated identification and targeting of chemoresistance-related genes across multiple cancer types. CRISPR/Cas9 knockout and screening approaches to identify and target chemoresistance-related genes across diverse cancer types, revealing mechanisms of drug resistance and potential therapeutic targets. **Small cell lung cancer:** SLFN11 knockout confers drug resistance through loss of S-phase arrest following DNA damage. SLFN11 is the strongest predictor of sensitivity to DNA-damaging agents including PARP inhibitors and platinum chemotherapy, with its loss occurring in approximately 50% of cancer cells. CRISPR/Cas9-mediated SLFN11 knockout demonstrates that this protein promotes CDT1 degradation through CUL4-DDB1 E3 ubiquitin ligase, irreversibly arresting DNA replication and inducing cell death in response to topoisomerase inhibitors, platinum agents, and PARP inhibitors. SLFN11-deficient cells can reactivate replication under DNA damage conditions, enabling chemoresistance. Clinical validation shows SLFN11 expression strongly correlates with

Figure 13.1 (*Conitnued on facing page*) prolonged progression-free survival and overall survival in patients receiving chemotherapy. **Triple-negative breast cancer:** APE1 is significantly overexpressed in 85.6% of tissues compared to 14.4% in adjacent normal tissues. CRISPR/Cas9-based studies targeting the BER pathway reveal that high APE1 expression associates with larger tumor size, poor prognosis, and reduced overall survival. APE1 and PARP1 compete for the same site in the BER pathway, and elevated APE1 expression is a key factor affecting sensitivity to PARP inhibitors. The median survival time for low APE1 expression is 82.0 months compared to 66.9 months for high expression groups. **Lung cancer:** RSF1 influences sensitivity to paclitaxel through regulation of the NF-κB pathway. CRISPR/Cas9-mediated knockout of RSF1 in NCI-H1299 and NCI-H460 lung cancer cells reduces migration and proliferation while increasing apoptosis and paclitaxel sensitivity. RSF1 knockout decreases NF-κB signaling by reducing phosphorylated p65 levels and downregulating downstream antiapoptotic genes including BCL2, CFLAR, and XIAP. Xenograft studies confirm that RSF1 knockout enhances paclitaxel-mediated tumor volume and weight reduction. PBRM1 (polybromo 1) loss sustains AKT survival signaling in lung cancer cells despite gefitinib treatment, conferring EGFR inhibitor resistance. CRISPR studies demonstrate that PBRM1 deficiency maintains activated AKT phosphorylation, enabling cancer cells to evade apoptosis under targeted therapy pressure. **Hepatocellular carcinoma:** CRISPR screening libraries identify genes regulating drug sensitivity, with particular focus on resistance to sorafenib and lenvatinib. CDK55 knockout studies reveal decreased drug sensitivity through dysregulation of EGFR/AKT signaling pathways. CRISPR screening discovered that feedback activation of the EGFR-PAK2-ERK5 pathway after lenvatinib treatment contributes to resistance, leading to clinical trials combining lenvatinib with EGFR inhibitor gefitinib. SGOL1 (shugoshin 1) is highly expressed in hepatocellular carcinoma tissues and promotes chromosomal instability. CRISPR knockout library screening identifies SGOL1 as a druggable target for sorafenib-treated hepatocellular carcinoma. SGOL1 expression positively correlates with disease stage, tumor grade, and tumor size, representing an independent prognostic factor. *In vitro* experiments demonstrate that SGOL1 silencing alters cell cycle markers and decreases proliferation, invasion, and migration of hepatocellular carcinoma cells. **Endometrial cancer:** ARID1A mutations occur in 26–40% of endometrial cancers. CRISPR/Cas9-mediated ARID1A knockout promotes primary progesterone resistance by downregulating progesterone receptor B expression and increasing AKT phosphorylation. ARID1A-deficient cells show insensitivity to [MPA, and AKT inhibition cannot rescue progesterone receptor B expression or resensitize cells to MPA in ARID1A knockout cells. These findings establish ARID1A as a reliable biomarker to predict response to combination AKT inhibitor and MPA treatment. **Non-small cell lung cancer:** Aurora-B overexpression correlates with significantly

Figure 13.1 (*Conitnued*) reduced overall survival, disease-free survival, and chemoresistance in patients. CRISPR/Cas9-mediated Aurora-B knockout resensitizes cells to cisplatin and paclitaxel by ensuring correct chromosome segregation, restoring p53 expression, and activating p53-related DNA damage response and apoptotic pathways. Aurora-B knockout increases apoptotic rates from 1.29% to 12.01% in paclitaxel-treated cells. Aurora-B impairs drug response by disturbing cell proliferation and inhibiting p53-mediated mechanisms. **Glioma:** ATRX (alpha thalassemia/mental retardation syndrome X-linked) mutations are highly prevalent in gliomas. CRISPR/Cas9-mediated ATRX knockout suppresses ATM-dependent DNA damage repair by reducing H3K9me3 histone marks, enhancing temozolomide sensitivity. ATRX knockout induces greater DNA damage, increased apoptosis, and decreased cell proliferation and invasion following temozolomide treatment. ATRX-deficient cells show selective sensitivity to PARP inhibitors due to increased replication stress and defective homologous recombination repair. Patients with low ATRX expression exhibit preferable overall survival and benefit more from temozolomide treatment. **Acute myeloid leukemia:** BEND3 (BEN domain containing 3) emerged as the top hit from genome-wide CRISPR/Cas9 knockout screens, with BEND3 knockout conferring resistance to UBA1 inhibitor TAK-243. BEND3 functions as a transcriptional repressor interacting with chromatin-modifying complexes. While BEND3 knockout confers drug resistance *in vitro* and *in vivo*, it does not alter basal cell proliferation. ABCG2 knockout increases drug sensitivity by reducing efflux transporter activity. ShRNA-mediated knockdown of ABCG2 sensitizes cells to TAK-243 and reduces IC50 by 7–9 fold across multiple cell lines. LZTR1/NF1/TSC1/TSC2: CRISPR screens identify these genes as regulators of MAPK/mTORC1 activation pathways that modulate drug resistance. Loss of TSC1, TSC2, or PTEN hyperactivates PI3K-AKT-mTOR signaling, reducing MAPK pathway inhibitor activity. **Colorectal cancer:** WNT regulators including components of the WNT/β-catenin signaling pathway contribute to chemoresistance in colorectal cancer. CRISPR/Cas9-mediated disruption of WNT pathway genes increases drug resistance by maintaining stem cell properties and promoting tumor survival. **Cervical cancer:** CRISPR studies reveal that increased ABCC9 and IL37 expression contributes to drug resistance through enhanced drug efflux and inflammatory responses. ABCC9 upregulation promotes chemoresistance by reducing intracellular drug accumulation. **Renal cell carcinoma:** Farnesyl transferase knockout using CRISPR/Cas9 decreases apoptosis and increases drug sensitivity. Farnesyl transferase inhibition disrupts post-translational modification of key signaling proteins, sensitizing cells to therapeutic intervention. **Bladder cancer:** MSH2 (mutS homolog 2) knockout reduces cisplatin-mediated apoptosis, diminishes DNA damage response signaling, and increases drug resistance in bladder cancer. Low MSH2 protein levels in bladder tumors predict poor survival with

Figure 13.1 (*Conitnued*) platinum-based chemotherapy. **Melanoma:** FBXO42 knockout disrupts TAK1 signaling, increasing drug resistance in melanoma cells. FBXO42 functions in ubiquitin-mediated protein degradation pathways that regulate therapeutic response. **Glioblastoma:** MSH2/CLCA2/PTCH2 knockout studies in glioblastoma reveal contributions to drug resistance through disruption of DNA repair (MSH2), altered chloride channel activity (CLCA2), and dysregulated WNT signaling (PTCH2). These genes represent potential therapeutic targets for overcoming chemoresistance in glioblastoma. **Gallbladder cancer:** ELP5 is identified through genome-wide CRISPR screens as a determinant of gemcitabine sensitivity. ELP5 loss reduces gemcitabine-induced apoptosis in a P53-dependent manner through impaired translational regulation. ELP5 knockout disrupts wobble U34 tRNA modification, impeding translation of hnRNPQ mRNA, which is required for P53 IRES-dependent translation. Gallbladder cancer patients with lower ELP5, hnRNPQ, or P53 expression have poor survival outcomes after gemcitabine chemotherapy. **Prostate Cancer:** Tceal1 represents the top candidate from *in vivo* genome-wide CRISPR screens under docetaxel treatment pressure. TCEAL1 suppression enhances docetaxel efficacy by increasing subG1 cell death and polyploidy. This represents the first *in vivo* genome-wide treatment sensitization CRISPR screen in prostate cancer.

instability. With off-target mutation rates exceeding 50%, addressing this limitation is crucial for clinical application [229].

Several strategies exist to minimize off-target effects. Computational platforms like CHOPCHOP, E-CRISP, and CRISPR-ERA enable design of specific sgRNAs. The D10A-mutated Cas9 variant, which creates single-strand breaks rather than double-strand breaks, can significantly reduce off-target effects when used with paired sgRNAs, as off-target single-strand breaks can be repaired by local enzymes [230]. Additional Cas9 variants, including SpCas9-HF1 and eSpCas9 [1.1], have demonstrated reduced off-target effects [230].

The requirement for PAM sequence recognition near target sites by Cas9 presents another limitation. The commonly used SpCas9 requires a specific 5′NGG3′ PAM sequence (where N represents any nucleotide). To expand targeting capabilities, new Cas9 variants like SpCas9-NG and xCas9 have been developed [231].

CRISPR/Cas9-induced double-strand breaks can trigger p53 activation and cellular apoptosis. To address this, researchers suggest using Cas9 variants capable of creating single-strand breaks instead [231].

A major obstacle to CRISPR/Cas9's clinical implementation is the potential presence of anti-SpCas9 antibodies, as reported in several studies [231, 232]. Research on alternative systems, such as Campylobacter jejuni Cas9 [CjCas9], may offer solutions to this challenge [231].

The delivery system for CRISPR/Cas9 requires further investigation. While AAV vectors are currently the standard delivery method, they present limitations including immune response stimulation and increased off-target mutations due to prolonged component expression. Researchers suggest non-viral vectors, such as nanoparticles, as alternatives to reduce immune response activation. *In vivo* delivery faces additional challenges, including enzymatic degradation and immune cell interference [231, 233].

Before CRISPR/Cas9 can be clinically applied to address cancer drug resistance, extensive research is needed to overcome these limitations. Successfully addressing these challenges could enable the future clinical application of CRISPR/Cas9 gene-editing technology.

13.7 Conclusion

Drug resistance remains the principal barrier to durable cancer control, yet the programmability of CRISPR/Cas9 now allows direct interrogation and reversal of its genetic and epigenetic drivers. By combining mechanistic mapping (via genome-scale screens and isogenic modeling) with targeted editing of validated resistance nodes, CRISPR/Cas9 provides a coherent route to resensitize tumors, rationalize combinations, and personalize therapy. Real-world impact will depend on delivery solutions suited to solid tumors, minimization of off-target effects, and adaptive, biomarker-driven trial designs that track edit efficiency and evolving clonal architecture. With these guardrails in place, CRISPR/Cas9 can shift the paradigm from reacting to resistance after clinical failure to proactively engineering tumor susceptibility, enhancing the durability and depth of response across chemotherapy, targeted therapy, and immunotherapy.

References

1. Padma VV. An overview of targeted cancer therapy. Biomedicine (Taipei). 2015;5(4):19.
2. Yan J, Yao Y, Yan S, Gao R, Lu W, He W. Chiral Protein Supraparticles for Tumor Suppression and Synergistic Immunotherapy: An Enabling Strategy for Bioactive Supramolecular Chirality Construction. Nano Lett. 2020;20(8):5844–52.
3. Ahmad FB, Anderson RN. The Leading Causes of Death in the US for 2020. Jama. 2021;325(18):1829–30.
4. Khalaf K, Janowicz K, Dyszkiewicz-Konwińska M, Hutchings G, Dompe C, Moncrieff L, et al. CRISPR/Cas9 in Cancer Immunotherapy: Animal Models and Human Clinical Trials. Genes (Basel). 2020;11(8):921.
5. Zhan T, Rindtorff N, Betge J, Ebert MP, Boutros M. CRISPR/Cas9 for cancer research and therapy. Semin Cancer Biol. 2019;55:106–19.
6. Bukowski K, Kciuk M, Kontek R. Mechanisms of Multidrug Resistance in Cancer Chemotherapy. Int J Mol Sci. 2020;21(9):3233.
7. Haider T, Pandey V, Banjare N, Gupta PN, Soni V. Drug resistance in cancer: mechanisms and tackling strategies. Pharmacol Rep. 2020;72(5):1125–51.
8. Liu X. ABC Family Transporters. Adv Exp Med Biol. 2019;1141: 13–100.
9. Lusvarghi S, Robey RW, Gottesman MM, Ambudkar SV. Multidrug transporters: recent insights from cryo-electron microscopy-derived atomic structures and animal models. F1000Res. 2020;9.
10. Robey RW, Pluchino KM, Hall MD, Fojo AT, Bates SE, Gottesman MM. Revisiting the role of ABC transporters in multidrug-resistant cancer. Nat Rev Cancer. 2018;18(7):452–64.
11. Morau MV, Seguin CS, Visacri MB, Pincinato EC, Moriel P. Genetic Variants in the ABCB1 and ABCG2 Gene Drug Transporters Involved in Gefitinib-Associated Adverse Reaction: A Systematic Review and Meta-Analysis. Genes (Basel). 2024;15(5):591.
12. Li Q, Mou LJ, Tao L, Chen W, Sun XT, Xia XF, et al. Inhibition of mTOR suppresses human gallbladder carcinoma cell proliferation and enhances the cytotoxicity of 5-fluorouracil by downregulating

MDR1 expression. Eur Rev Med Pharmacol Sci. 2016;20(9): 1699–706.

13. Zhan M, Wang H, Chen T, Chen W, Yang L, He M, et al. NOX1 mediates chemoresistance via HIF1α/MDR1 pathway in gallbladder cancer. Biochem Biophys Res Commun. 2015;468(1–2):79–85.
14. Dong Q, Zhou C, Ren H, Zhang Z, Cheng F, Xiong Z, et al. Lactate-induced MRP1 expression contributes to metabolism-based etoposide resistance in non-small cell lung cancer cells. Cell Commun Signal. 2020;18(1):167.
15. Zhan M, Zhao X, Wang H, Chen W, Xu S, Wang W, et al. miR-145 sensitizes gallbladder cancer to cisplatin by regulating multidrug resistance associated protein 1. Tumour Biol. 2016;37(8):10553–62.
16. Wang H, Li X, Chen T, Wang W, Liu Q, Li H, et al. Mechanisms of verapamil-enhanced chemosensitivity of gallbladder cancer cells to platinum drugs: glutathione reduction and MRP1 downregulation. Oncol Rep. 2013;29(2):676–84.
17. Pote MS, Gacche RN. ATP-binding cassette efflux transporters and MDR in cancer. Drug Discov Today. 2023;28(5):103537.
18. Zhao CC, Sun X, Chen J, Geng BD. NAT10-mediated mRNA N4-acetylcytidine modification of MDR1 and BCRP promotes breast cancer progression. Thorac Cancer. 2024;15(10):820–9.
19. Uceda-Castro R, Margarido AS, Song JY, de Gooijer MC, Messal HA, Chambers CR, et al. BCRP drives intrinsic chemoresistance in chemotherapy-naïve breast cancer brain metastasis. Sci Adv. 2023;9(42):eabp9530.
20. Kalayda GV, Wagner CH, Buss I, Reedijk J, Jaehde U. Altered localisation of the copper efflux transporters ATP7A and ATP7B associated with cisplatin resistance in human ovarian carcinoma cells. BMC Cancer. 2008;8:175.
21. Federica G, Michela C, Giovanna D. Targeting the DNA damage response in cancer. MedComm (2020). 2024;5(11):e788.
22. Jeppesen DK, Bohr VA, Stevnsner T. DNA repair deficiency in neurodegeneration. Prog Neurobiol. 2011;94(2):166–200.
23. Vickridge E, Faraco CCF, Nepveu A. Base excision repair accessory factors in senescence avoidance and resistance to treatments. Cancer Drug Resist. 2022;5(3):703–20.
24. Chen X, Li WF, Wu X, Zhang HC, Chen L, Zhang PY, et al. Dicer regulates non-homologous end joining and is associated with

chemosensitivity in colon cancer patients. Carcinogenesis. 2017;38(9):873–82.
25. Wei S, Han C, Mo S, Huang H, Luo X. Advancements in programmed cell death research in antitumor therapy: a comprehensive overview. Apoptosis. 2025;30(1–2):401–21.
26. Hanahan D, Weinberg RA. Hallmarks of cancer: the next generation. Cell. 2011;144(5):646–74.
27. Yamamoto K, Iwadate D, Naito E, Tateishi K, Fujishiro M. Autophagy as a critical driver of metabolic adaptation, therapeutic resistance, and immune evasion of cancer. Curr Opin Biotechnol. 2023;84:103012.
28. Pimentel JM, Zhou JY, Wu GS. Autophagy and cancer therapy. Cancer Lett. 2024;605:217285.
29. Xu Y, Yu H, Qin H, Kang J, Yu C, Zhong J, et al. Inhibition of autophagy enhances cisplatin cytotoxicity through endoplasmic reticulum stress in human cervical cancer cells. Cancer Lett. 2012;314(2):232–43.
30. Yang B, Li Y, Zhang R, Liu L, Miao H, Li Y, et al. MOB1A regulates glucose deprivation-induced autophagy via IL6-STAT3 pathway in gallbladder carcinoma. Am J Cancer Res. 2020;10(11):3896–910.
31. Wang S, Feng W, Wang W, Ye X, Chen H, Yu C. Girdin Knockdown Increases Gemcitabine Chemosensitivity to Pancreatic Cancer by Modulating Autophagy. Front Oncol. 2021;11:618764.
32. Chen N, Qi Y, Ma X, Xiao X, Liu Q, Xia T, et al. Rediscovery of Traditional Plant Medicine: An Underestimated Anticancer Drug of Chelerythrine. Front Pharmacol. 2022;13:906301.
33. Wang FT, Wang H, Wang QW, Pan MS, Li XP, Sun W, Fan YZ. Inhibition of autophagy by chloroquine enhances the antitumor activity of gemcitabine for gallbladder cancer. Cancer Chemother Pharmacol. 2020;86(2):221–32.
34. Urrutia S, Takahashi K. Precision medicine in AML: overcoming resistance. Int J Hematol. 2024;120(4):439–54.
35. Yuan J, Lan H, Jiang X, Zeng D, Xiao S. Bcl-2 family: Novel insight into individualized therapy for ovarian cancer (Review). Int J Mol Med. 2020;46(4):1255–65.
36. Zhang J, Wang Y, Yin C, Gong P, Zhang Z, Zhao L, et al. Artesunate improves venetoclax plus cytarabine AML cell targeting by regulating the Noxa/Bim/Mcl-1/p-Chk1 axis. Cell Death Dis. 2022;13(4):379.

37. Miquel C, Borrini F, Grandjouan S, Aupérin A, Viguier J, Velasco V, et al. Role of bax mutations in apoptosis in colorectal cancers with microsatellite instability. Am J Clin Pathol. 2005;123(4):562–70.
38. Carter BZ, Mak PY, Tao W, Zhang Q, Ruvolo V, Kuruvilla VM, et al. Maximal Activation of Apoptosis Signaling by Cotargeting Antiapoptotic Proteins in BH3 Mimetic-Resistant AML and AML Stem Cells. Mol Cancer Ther. 2022;21(6):879–89.
39. Carter JL, Su Y, Qiao X, Zhao J, Wang G, Howard M, et al. Acquired resistance to venetoclax plus azacitidine in acute myeloid leukemia: In vitro models and mechanisms. Biochem Pharmacol. 2023;216: 115759.
40. Oakes SA, Scorrano L, Opferman JT, Bassik MC, Nishino M, Pozzan T, Korsmeyer SJ. Proapoptotic BAX and BAK regulate the type 1 inositol trisphosphate receptor and calcium leak from the endoplasmic reticulum. Proc Natl Acad Sci U S A. 2005;102(1):105–10.
41. Cetraro P, Plaza-Diaz J, MacKenzie A, Abadía-Molina F. A Review of the Current Impact of Inhibitors of Apoptosis Proteins and Their Repression in Cancer. Cancers (Basel). 2022;14(7):1671.
42. Rathore R, McCallum JE, Varghese E, Florea AM, Büsselberg D. Overcoming chemotherapy drug resistance by targeting inhibitors of apoptosis proteins (IAPs). Apoptosis. 2017;22(7):898–919.
43. Guo Q, Jin Y, Lin M, Zeng C, Zhang J. NF-κB signaling in therapy resistance of breast cancer: Mechanisms, approaches, and challenges. Life Sci. 2024;348:122684.
44. Yang MH, Lee KT, Yang S, Lee JK, Lee KH, Moon IH, Rhee JC. Guggulsterone enhances antitumor activity of gemcitabine in gallbladder cancer cells through suppression of NF-κB. J Cancer Res Clin Oncol. 2012;138(10):1743–51.
45. Nwabo Kamdje AH, Dongmo Fogang HP, Mimche PN. Role of epigenetic in cancer biology, in hematologic malignancies and in anticancer therapy. Front Mol Med. 2024;4:1426454.
46. Panda R, Mohan S, Vellapandian C. Harnessing Epigenetic Mechanisms to Overcome Immune Evasion in Cancer: The Current Strategies and Future Directions. Cureus. 2024;16(10):e70631.
47. Urban T, Pokorná P, Slabý O. Significance of aberrant DNA methylation for cancer diagnostics and therapy. Klin Onkol. 2024;38(2): 88–94.
48. Yang D, Khan S, Sun Y, Hess K, Shmulevich I, Sood AK, Zhang W. Association of BRCA1 and BRCA2 mutations with survival,

chemotherapy sensitivity, and gene mutator phenotype in patients with ovarian cancer. Jama. 2011;306(14):1557–65.
49. Kang SH, Bang YJ, Im YH, Yang HK, Lee DA, Lee HY, et al. Transcriptional repression of the transforming growth factor-beta type I receptor gene by DNA methylation results in the development of TGF-beta resistance in human gastric cancer. Oncogene. 1999;18(51):7280–6.
50. Skouras P, Markouli M, Papadatou I, Piperi C. Targeting epigenetic mechanisms of resistance to chemotherapy in gliomas. Crit Rev Oncol Hematol. 2024;204:104532.
51. Seto E, Yoshida M. Erasers of histone acetylation: the histone deacetylase enzymes. Cold Spring Harb Perspect Biol. 2014;6(4):a018713.
52. Ono H, Basson MD, Ito H. P300 inhibition enhances gemcitabine-induced apoptosis of pancreatic cancer. Oncotarget. 2016;7(32):51301–10.
53. Emmons MF, Faião-Flores F, Sharma R, Thapa R, Messina JL, Becker JC, et al. HDAC8 Regulates a Stress Response Pathway in Melanoma to Mediate Escape from BRAF Inhibitor Therapy. Cancer Res. 2019;79(11):2947–61.
54. Kim MG, Pak JH, Choi WH, Park JY, Nam JH, Kim JH. The relationship between cisplatin resistance and histone deacetylase isoform overexpression in epithelial ovarian cancer cell lines. J Gynecol Oncol. 2012;23(3):182–9.
55. Vagapova E, Kozlov M, Lebedev T, Ivanenko K, Leonova O, Popenko V, et al. Selective Inhibition of HDAC Class I Sensitizes Leukemia and Neuroblastoma Cells to Anticancer Drugs. Biomedicines. 2021;9(12):1846.
56. Hu S, Yu L, Li Z, Shen Y, Wang J, Cai J, et al. Overexpression of EZH2 contributes to acquired cisplatin resistance in ovarian cancer cells in vitro and in vivo. Cancer Biol Ther. 2010;10(8):788–95.
57. Zhang L, Zhang X, Shi Y, Ni Y, Fei J, Jin Z, et al. Role and potential therapeutic value of histone methyltransferases in drug resistance mechanisms in lung cancer. Front Oncol. 2024;14:1376916.
58. Yan H, Bu P. Non-coding RNA in cancer. Essays Biochem. 2021;65(4):625–39.
59. Rahdan F, Saberi A, Saraygord-Afshari N, Hadizadeh M, Fayeghi T, Ghanbari E, et al. Deciphering the multifaceted role of microRNAs in hepatocellular carcinoma: Integrating literature review and bioinformatics analysis for therapeutic insights. Heliyon. 2024;10(20):e39489.

60. Shahin RK, Elkady MA, Abulsoud AI, Abdelmaksoud NM, Abdel Mageed SS, El-Dakroury WA, et al. miRNAs orchestration of gallbladder cancer — Particular emphasis on diagnosis, progression and drug resistance. Pathol Res Pract. 2023;248:154684.
61. Chen LL. Linking Long Noncoding RNA Localization and Function. Trends Biochem Sci. 2016;41(9):761–72.
62. Quinn JJ, Chang HY. Unique features of long non-coding RNA biogenesis and function. Nat Rev Genet. 2016;17(1):47–62.
63. Cai Q, Wang S, Jin L, Weng M, Zhou D, Wang J, et al. Long noncoding RNA GBCDRlnc1 induces chemoresistance of gallbladder cancer cells by activating autophagy. Mol Cancer. 2019;18(1):82.
64. Gao K, Chen S, Yang X. HOTTIP Enhances Gemcitabine and Cisplatin Resistance Through Sponging miR-637 in Cholangiocarcinoma. Front Oncol. 2021;11:664916.
65. Kaur G, Gupta SK, Singh P, Ali V, Kumar V, Verma M. Drug-metabolizing enzymes: role in drug resistance in cancer. Clin Transl Oncol. 2020;22(10):1667–80.
66. Torres-Zárate C, Vences-Mejía A, Espinosa-Aguirre JJ, Díaz-Díaz E, Palacios-Acosta JM, Cárdenas-Cardós R, et al. Expression of Cytochrome P450 Enzymes in Pediatric Non-Rhabdomyosarcoma Soft Tissue Sarcomas: Possible Role in Carcinogenesis and Treatment Response. Int J Toxicol. 2022;41(3):234–42.
67. Valencia-Cervantes J, Huerta-Yepez S, Aquino-Jarquín G, Rodríguez-Enríquez S, Martínez-Fong D, Arias-Montaño JA, Dávila-Borja VM. Hypoxia increases chemoresistance in human medulloblastoma DAOY cells via hypoxia-inducible factor 1α-mediated downregulation of the CYP2B6, CYP3A4 and CYP3A5 enzymes and inhibition of cell proliferation. Oncol Rep. 2019;41(1):178–90.
68. Marengo B, Pulliero A, Izzotti A, Domenicotti C. miRNA Regulation of Glutathione Homeostasis in Cancer Initiation, Progression and Therapy Resistance. Microrna. 2020;9(3):187–97.
69. Niu B, Liao K, Zhou Y, Wen T, Quan G, Pan X, Wu C. Application of glutathione depletion in cancer therapy: Enhanced ROS-based therapy, ferroptosis, and chemotherapy. Biomaterials. 2021;277:121110.
70. Zhang T, Yao C, Zhou X, Liu S, Qi L, Zhu S, et al. Glutathione-degrading enzymes in the complex landscape of tumors (Review). Int J Oncol. 2024;65(1):72.

71. Nakano T, Saiki Y, Kudo C, Hirayama A, Mizuguchi Y, Fujiwara S, et al. Acquisition of chemoresistance to gemcitabine is induced by a loss-of-function missense mutation of DCK. Biochem Biophys Res Commun. 2015;464(4):1084–9.
72. Ueno H, Kiyosawa K, Kaniwa N. Pharmacogenomics of gemcitabine: can genetic studies lead to tailor-made therapy? Br J Cancer. 2007;97(2):145–51.
73. Aponte PM, Caicedo A. Stemness in Cancer: Stem Cells, Cancer Stem Cells, and Their Microenvironment. Stem Cells Int. 2017;2017:5619472.
74. Batlle E, Clevers H. Cancer stem cells revisited. Nat Med. 2017;23(10):1124–34.
75. Gires O. Lessons from common markers of tumor-initiating cells in solid cancers. Cell Mol Life Sci. 2011;68(24):4009–22.
76. Najafi M, Mortezaee K, Majidpoor J. Cancer stem cell (CSC) resistance drivers. Life Sci. 2019;234:116781.
77. Shi C, Tian R, Wang M, Wang X, Jiang J, Zhang Z, et al. CD44+ CD133+ population exhibits cancer stem cell-like characteristics in human gallbladder carcinoma. Cancer Biol Ther. 2010;10(11):1182–90.
78. Desai A, Webb B, Gerson SL. CD133+ cells contribute to radioresistance via altered regulation of DNA repair genes in human lung cancer cells. Radiother Oncol. 2014;110(3):538–45.
79. Wu Z, Miao X, Zhang Y, Li D, Zou Q, Yuan Y, et al. XRCC1 Is a Promising Predictive Biomarker and Facilitates Chemo-Resistance in Gallbladder Cancer. Front Mol Biosci. 2020;7:70.
80. Donadelli M, Dando I, Zaniboni T, Costanzo C, Dalla Pozza E, Scupoli MT, et al. Gemcitabine/cannabinoid combination triggers autophagy in pancreatic cancer cells through a ROS-mediated mechanism. Cell Death Dis. 2011;2(4):e152.
81. Sosa V, Moliné T, Somoza R, Paciucci R, Kondoh H, ME LL. Oxidative stress and cancer: an overview. Ageing Res Rev. 2013;12(1):376–90.
82. Wang Y, Qi H, Liu Y, Duan C, Liu X, Xia T, et al. The double-edged roles of ROS in cancer prevention and therapy. Theranostics. 2021;11(10):4839–57.
83. De Angelis ML, Francescangeli F, La Torre F, Zeuner A. Stem Cell Plasticity and Dormancy in the Development of Cancer Therapy Resistance. Front Oncol. 2019;9:626.

84. Sosa MS, Bragado P, Aguirre-Ghiso JA. Mechanisms of disseminated cancer cell dormancy: an awakening field. Nat Rev Cancer. 2014;14(9):611–22.
85. Pors K, Moreb JS. Aldehyde dehydrogenases in cancer: an opportunity for biomarker and drug development? Drug Discov Today. 2014;19(12):1953–63.
86. Vassalli G. Aldehyde Dehydrogenases: Not Just Markers, but Functional Regulators of Stem Cells. Stem Cells Int. 2019;2019:3904645.
87. Ma S, Lee TK, Zheng BJ, Chan KW, Guan XY. CD133+ HCC cancer stem cells confer chemoresistance by preferential expression of the Akt/PKB survival pathway. Oncogene. 2008;27(12):1749–58.
88. Wang J, Seebacher N, Shi H, Kan Q, Duan Z. Novel strategies to prevent the development of multidrug resistance (MDR) in cancer. Oncotarget. 2017;8(48):84559–71.
89. Chen YB, Yan ML, Gong JP, Xia RP, Liu LX, Li N, et al. Establishment of hepatocellular carcinoma multidrug resistant monoclone cell line HepG2/mdr1. Chin Med J (Engl). 2007;120(8):703–7.
90. Chen SY, Hu SS, Dong Q, Cai JX, Zhang WP, Sun JY, et al. Establishment of paclitaxel-resistant breast cancer cell line and nude mice models, and underlying multidrug resistance mechanisms in vitro and in vivo. Asian Pac J Cancer Prev. 2013;14(10):6135–40.
91. Quan X, Du H, Xu J, Hou X, Gong X, Wu Y, et al. Novel Quinoline Compound Derivatives of NSC23925 as Potent Reversal Agents Against P-Glycoprotein-Mediated Multidrug Resistance. Front Chem. 2019;7:820.
92. Fanelli M, Hattinger CM, Vella S, Tavanti E, Michelacci F, Gudeman B, et al. Targeting ABCB1 and ABCC1 with their Specific Inhibitor CBT-1® can Overcome Drug Resistance in Osteosarcoma. Curr Cancer Drug Targets. 2016;16(3):261–74.
93. Zhang N, Gao M, Wang Z, Zhang J, Cui W, Li J, et al. Curcumin reverses doxorubicin resistance in colon cancer cells at the metabolic level. J Pharm Biomed Anal. 2021;201:114129.
94. Shafiei-Irannejad V, Samadi N, Yousefi B, Salehi R, Velaei K, Zarghami N. Metformin enhances doxorubicin sensitivity via inhibition of doxorubicin efflux in P-gp-overexpressing MCF-7 cells. Chem Biol Drug Des. 2018;91(1):269–76.
95. Sadoughi F, Hallajzadeh J, Asemi Z, Mansournia MA, Alemi F, Yousefi B. Signaling pathways involved in cell cycle arrest during the DNA breaks. DNA Repair (Amst). 2021;98:103047.

96. Wang Q, Xiong J, Qiu D, Zhao X, Yan D, Xu W, et al. Inhibition of PARP1 activity enhances chemotherapeutic efficiency in cisplatin-resistant gastric cancer cells. Int J Biochem Cell Biol. 2017;92: 164–72.
97. Vescarelli E, Gerini G, Megiorni F, Anastasiadou E, Pontecorvi P, Solito L, et al. MiR-200c sensitizes Olaparib-resistant ovarian cancer cells by targeting Neuropilin 1. J Exp Clin Cancer Res. 2020;39(1):3.
98. Ray Chaudhuri A, Nussenzweig A. The multifaceted roles of PARP1 in DNA repair and chromatin remodelling. Nat Rev Mol Cell Biol. 2017;18(10):610–21.
99. Shafabakhsh R, Reiter RJ, Mirzaei H, Teymoordash SN, Asemi Z. Melatonin: A new inhibitor agent for cervical cancer treatment. J Cell Physiol. 2019;234(12):21670–82.
100. Chen CC, Chen CY, Wang SH, Yeh CT, Su SC, Ueng SH, et al. Melatonin Sensitizes Hepatocellular Carcinoma Cells to Chemotherapy Through Long Non-Coding RNA RAD51-AS1-Mediated Suppression of DNA Repair. Cancers (Basel). 2018;10(9):320.
101. Pirpour Tazehkand A, Salehi R, Velaei K, Samadi N. The potential impact of trigonelline loaded micelles on Nrf2 suppression to overcome oxaliplatin resistance in colon cancer cells. Mol Biol Rep. 2020;47(8):5817–29.
102. Wang Z, Huang Y, Zhang J. Molecularly targeting the PI3K-Akt-mTOR pathway can sensitize cancer cells to radiotherapy and chemotherapy. Cell Mol Biol Lett. 2014;19(2):233–42.
103. Sun J, Xu K, Qiu Y, Gao H, Xu J, Tang Q, Yin P. Bufalin reverses acquired drug resistance by inhibiting stemness in colorectal cancer cells. Oncol Rep. 2017;38(3):1420–30.
104. Shafiei-Irannejad V, Samadi N, Salehi R, Yousefi B, Rahimi M, Akbarzadeh A, Zarghami N. Reversion of Multidrug Resistance by Co-Encapsulation of Doxorubicin and Metformin in Poly(lactide-co-glycolide)-d-α-tocopheryl Polyethylene Glycol 1000 Succinate Nanoparticles. Pharm Res. 2018;35(6):119.
105. Majidinia M, Mirza-Aghazadeh-Attari M, Rahimi M, Mihanfar A, Karimian A, Safa A, Yousefi B. Overcoming multidrug resistance in cancer: Recent progress in nanotechnology and new horizons. IUBMB Life. 2020;72(5):855–71.
106. Zhao M, Wang T, Hui Z. Aspirin overcomes cisplatin resistance in lung cancer by inhibiting cancer cell stemness. Thorac Cancer. 2020;11(11):3117–25.

107. Zhong H, Davis A, Ouzounova M, Carrasco RA, Chen C, Breen S, et al. A Novel IL6 Antibody Sensitizes Multiple Tumor Types to Chemotherapy Including Trastuzumab-Resistant Tumors. Cancer Res. 2016;76(2):480–90.
108. Liu K, Gao L, Ma X, Huang JJ, Chen J, Zeng L, et al. Long non-coding RNAs regulate drug resistance in cancer. Mol Cancer. 2020;19(1):54.
109. Tsang WP, Kwok TT. Riboregulator H19 induction of MDR1-associated drug resistance in human hepatocellular carcinoma cells. Oncogene. 2007;26(33):4877–81.
110. Fang Z, Chen W, Yuan Z, Liu X, Jiang H. LncRNA-MALAT1 contributes to the cisplatin-resistance of lung cancer by upregulating MRP1 and MDR1 via STAT3 activation. Biomed Pharmacother. 2018;101:536–42.
111. Yue X, Wu WY, Dong M, Guo M. LncRNA MALAT1 promotes breast cancer progression and doxorubicin resistance via regulating miR-570–3p. Biomed J. 2021;44(6 Suppl 2):S296–S304.
112. Taiana E, Favasuli V, Ronchetti D, Todoerti K, Pelizzoni F, Manzoni M, et al. Long non-coding RNA NEAT1 targeting impairs the DNA repair machinery and triggers anti-tumor activity in multiple myeloma. Leukemia. 2020;34(1):234–44.
113. Lee SP, Hsieh PL, Fang CY, Chu PM, Liao YW, Yu CH, et al. LINC00963 Promotes Cancer Stemness, Metastasis, and Drug Resistance in Head and Neck Carcinomas via ABCB5 Regulation. Cancers (Basel). 2020;12(5):1073.
114. Saliminejad K, Khorram Khorshid HR, Soleymani Fard S, Ghaffari SH. An overview of microRNAs: Biology, functions, therapeutics, and analysis methods. J Cell Physiol. 2019;234(5):5451–65.
115. Shah MY, Ferrajoli A, Sood AK, Lopez-Berestein G, Calin GA. microRNA Therapeutics in Cancer—An Emerging Concept. EBioMedicine. 2016;12:34–42.
116. Chakraborty C, Sharma AR, Sharma G, Lee SS. Therapeutic advances of miRNAs: A preclinical and clinical update. J Adv Res. 2021;28:127–38.
117. Liu Y, Liu X, Yang S. MicroRNA-221 Upregulates the Expression of P-gp and Bcl-2 by Activating the Stat3 Pathway to Promote Doxorubicin Resistance in Osteosarcoma Cells. Biol Pharm Bull. 2021;44(6):861–8.

118. Wang Y, Chen G, Dai F, Zhang L, Yuan M, Yang D, et al. miR-21 Induces Chemoresistance in Ovarian Cancer Cells via Mediating the Expression and Interaction of CD44v6 and P-gp. Onco Targets Ther. 2021;14:325–36.
119. Hong L, Han Y, Zhang Y, Zhang H, Zhao Q, Wu K, Fan D. MicroRNA-21: a therapeutic target for reversing drug resistance in cancer. Expert Opin Ther Targets. 2013;17(9):1073–80.
120. Zhou H, Lin C, Zhang Y, Zhang X, Zhang C, Zhang P, et al. miR-506 enhances the sensitivity of human colorectal cancer cells to oxaliplatin by suppressing MDR1/P-gp expression. Cell Prolif. 2017;50(3): e12341.
121. Lu X, Liu R, Wang M, Kumar AK, Pan F, He L, et al. MicroRNA-140 impedes DNA repair by targeting FEN1 and enhances chemotherapeutic response in breast cancer. Oncogene. 2020;39(1):234–47.
122. Li M, Gao M, Xie X, Zhang Y, Ning J, Liu P, Gu K. MicroRNA-200c reverses drug resistance of human gastric cancer cells by targeting regulation of the NER-ERCC3/4 pathway. Oncol Lett. 2019;18(1): 145–52.
123. Tao L, Shu-Ling W, Jing-Bo H, Ying Z, Rong H, Xiang-Qun L, et al. MiR-451a attenuates doxorubicin resistance in lung cancer via suppressing epithelialmesenchymal transition (EMT) through targeting c-Myc. Biomed Pharmacother. 2020;125:109962.
124. Wang LQ, Yu P, Li B, Guo YH, Liang ZR, Zheng LL, et al. miR-372 and miR-373 enhance the stemness of colorectal cancer cells by repressing differentiation signaling pathways. Mol Oncol. 2018;12(11):1949–64.
125. Zhou S, Ye W, Zhang Y, Yu D, Shao Q, Liang J, Zhang M. miR-144 reverses chemoresistance of hepatocellular carcinoma cell lines by targeting Nrf2-dependent antioxidant pathway. Am J Transl Res. 2016;8(7):2992–3002.
126. Sun DM, Tang BF, Li ZX, Guo HB, Cheng JL, Song PP, Zhao X. MiR-29c reduces the cisplatin resistance of non-small cell lung cancer cells by negatively regulating the PI3K/Akt pathway. Sci Rep. 2018;8(1):8007.
127. Si W, Shen J, Zheng H, Fan W. The role and mechanisms of action of microRNAs in cancer drug resistance. Clin Epigenetics. 2019;11(1):25.
128. Mohammadzadeh I, Qujeq D, Yousefi T, Ferns GA, Maniati M, Vaghari-Tabari M. CRISPR/Cas9 gene editing: A new therapeutic

approach in the treatment of infection and autoimmunity. IUBMB Life. 2020;72(8):1603–21.

129. Yang Y, Qiu JG, Li Y, Di JM, Zhang WJ, Jiang QW, et al. Targeting ABCB1-mediated tumor multidrug resistance by CRISPR/Cas9-based genome editing. Am J Transl Res. 2016;8(9):3986–94.

130. Ha JS, Byun J, Ahn DR. Overcoming doxorubicin resistance of cancer cells by Cas9-mediated gene disruption. Sci Rep. 2016;6:22847.

131. Norouzi-Barough L, Sarookhani M, Salehi R, Sharifi M, Moghbelinejad S. CRISPR/Cas9, a new approach to successful knockdown of ABCB1/P-glycoprotein and reversal of chemosensitivity in human epithelial ovarian cancer cell line. Iran J Basic Med Sci. 2018;21(2):181–7.

132. Liu T, Li Z, Zhang Q, De Amorim Bernstein K, Lozano-Calderon S, Choy E, et al. Targeting ABCB1 (MDR1) in multi-drug resistant osteosarcoma cells using the CRISPR-Cas9 system to reverse drug resistance. Oncotarget. 2016;7(50):83502–13.

133. Vaghari-Tabari M, Majidinia M, Moein S, Qujeq D, Asemi Z, Alemi F, et al. MicroRNAs and colorectal cancer chemoresistance: New solution for old problem. Life Sci. 2020;259:118255.

134. Johnson N, Shapiro GI. Cyclin-dependent kinases (cdks) and the DNA damage response: rationale for cdk inhibitor-chemotherapy combinations as an anticancer strategy for solid tumors. Expert Opin Ther Targets. 2010;14(11):1199–212.

135. Malumbres M, Barbacid M. Cell cycle, CDKs and cancer: a changing paradigm. Nat Rev Cancer. 2009;9(3):153–66.

136. Sherr CJ, Beach D, Shapiro GI. Targeting CDK4 and CDK6: From Discovery to Therapy. Cancer Discov. 2016;6(4):353–67.

137. Cornell L, Wander SA, Visal T, Wagle N, Shapiro GI. MicroRNA-Mediated Suppression of the TGF-β Pathway Confers Transmissible and Reversible CDK4/6 Inhibitor Resistance. Cell Rep. 2019;26(10):2667–80.e7.

138. Liu X, Gao Y, Shen J, Yang W, Choy E, Mankin H, et al. Cyclin-Dependent Kinase 11 (CDK11) Is Required for Ovarian Cancer Cell Growth In Vitro and In Vivo, and Its Inhibition Causes Apoptosis and Sensitizes Cells to Paclitaxel. Mol Cancer Ther. 2016; 15(7):1691–701.

139. Feng Y, Sassi S, Shen JK, Yang X, Gao Y, Osaka E, et al. Targeting CDK11 in osteosarcoma cells using the CRISPR-Cas9 system. J Orthop Res. 2015;33(2):199–207.

140. Wu J, Lu LY, Yu X. The role of BRCA1 in DNA damage response. Protein Cell. 2010;1(2):117–23.
141. Balmaña J, Díez O, Rubio IT, Cardoso F. BRCA in breast cancer: ESMO Clinical Practice Guidelines. Ann Oncol. 2011;22 Suppl 6:vi31–4.
142. Kennedy RD, Quinn JE, Mullan PB, Johnston PG, Harkin DP. The role of BRCA1 in the cellular response to chemotherapy. J Natl Cancer Inst. 2004;96(22):1659–68.
143. Taron M, Rosell R, Felip E, Mendez P, Souglakos J, Ronco MS, et al. BRCA1 mRNA expression levels as an indicator of chemoresistance in lung cancer. Hum Mol Genet. 2004;13(20):2443–9.
144. Mintz RL, Lao YH, Chi CW, He S, Li M, Quek CH, et al. CRISPR/Cas9-mediated mutagenesis to validate the synergy between PARP1 inhibition and chemotherapy in BRCA1-mutated breast cancer cells. Bioeng Transl Med. 2020;5(1):e10152.
145. Wang H, Sun W. CRISPR-mediated targeting of HER2 inhibits cell proliferation through a dominant negative mutation. Cancer Lett. 2017;385:137–43.
146. Król SK, Kaczmarczyk A, Wojnicki K, Wojtas B, Gielniewski B, Grajkowska W, et al. Aberrantly Expressed RECQL4 Helicase Supports Proliferation and Drug Resistance of Human Glioma Cells and Glioma Stem Cells. Cancers (Basel). 2020;12(10):2919.
147. Mo D, Fang H, Niu K, Liu J, Wu M, Li S, et al. Human Helicase RECQL4 Drives Cisplatin Resistance in Gastric Cancer by Activating an AKT-YB1-MDR1 Signaling Pathway. Cancer Res. 2016;76(10):3057–66.
148. Hientz K, Mohr A, Bhakta-Guha D, Efferth T. The role of p53 in cancer drug resistance and targeted chemotherapy. Oncotarget. 2017;8(5):8921–46.
149. Sampath J, Sun D, Kidd VJ, Grenet J, Gandhi A, Shapiro LH, et al. Mutant p53 cooperates with ETS and selectively up-regulates human MDR1 not MRP1. J Biol Chem. 2001;276(42):39359–67.
150. Sui H, Fan ZZ, Li Q. Signal transduction pathways and transcriptional mechanisms of ABCB1/Pgp-mediated multiple drug resistance in human cancer cells. J Int Med Res. 2012;40(2):426–35.
151. Liu P, Wang Y, Li X. Targeting the untargetable KRAS in cancer therapy. Acta Pharm Sin B. 2019;9(5):871–9.
152. Siddiqui AD, Piperdi B. KRAS mutation in colon cancer: a marker of resistance to EGFR-I therapy. Ann Surg Oncol. 2010;17(4):1168–76.

153. Messersmith WA, Ahnen DJ. Targeting EGFR in colorectal cancer. N Engl J Med. 2008;359(17):1834–6.
154. Cao X, Hou J, An Q, Assaraf YG, Wang X. Towards the overcoming of anticancer drug resistance mediated by p53 mutations. Drug Resist Updat. 2020;49:100671.
155. Tang F, Min L, Seebacher NA, Li X, Zhou Y, Hornicek FJ, et al. Targeting mutant TP53 as a potential therapeutic strategy for the treatment of osteosarcoma. J Orthop Res. 2019;37(3):789–98.
156. Sigismund S, Avanzato D, Lanzetti L. Emerging functions of the EGFR in cancer. Mol Oncol. 2018;12(1):3–20.
157. Zheng HC. The molecular mechanisms of chemoresistance in cancers. Oncotarget. 2017;8(35):59950–64.
158. Tomasello C, Baldessari C, Napolitano M, Orsi G, Grizzi G, Bertolini F, et al. Resistance to EGFR inhibitors in non-small cell lung cancer: Clinical management and future perspectives. Crit Rev Oncol Hematol. 2018;123:149–61.
159. Koo T, Yoon AR, Cho HY, Bae S, Yun CO, Kim JS. Selective disruption of an oncogenic mutant allele by CRISPR/Cas9 induces efficient tumor regression. Nucleic Acids Res. 2017;45(13):7897–908.
160. Liu B, Diaz Arguello OA, Chen D, Chen S, Saber A, Haisma HJ. CRISPR-mediated ablation of overexpressed EGFR in combination with sunitinib significantly suppresses renal cell carcinoma proliferation. PLoS One. 2020;15(5):e0232985.
161. Rizzo M, Porta C. Sunitinib in the treatment of renal cell carcinoma: an update on recent evidence. Ther Adv Urol. 2017;9(8):195–207.
162. Gonias SL, Hu J. Urokinase receptor and resistance to targeted anticancer agents. Front Pharmacol. 2015;6:154.
163. Li Santi A, Napolitano F, Montuori N, Ragno P. The Urokinase Receptor: A Multifunctional Receptor in Cancer Cell Biology. Therapeutic Implications. Int J Mol Sci. 2021;22(8):4111.
164. Wang K, Xing ZH, Jiang QW, Yang Y, Huang JR, Yuan ML, et al. Targeting uPAR by CRISPR/Cas9 System Attenuates Cancer Malignancy and Multidrug Resistance. Front Oncol. 2019;9:80.
165. Reynolds IS, Fichtner M, McNamara DA, Kay EW, Prehn JHM, Burke JP. Mucin glycoproteins block apoptosis; promote invasion, proliferation, and migration; and cause chemoresistance through diverse pathways in epithelial cancers. Cancer Metastasis Rev. 2019;38(1–2):237–57.

166. Skrypek N, Duchêne B, Hebbar M, Leteurtre E, van Seuningen I, Jonckheere N. The MUC4 mucin mediates gemcitabine resistance of human pancreatic cancer cells via the Concentrative Nucleoside Transporter family. Oncogene. 2013;32(13):1714–23.
167. Sagar S, Leiphrakpam PD, Thomas D, McAndrews KL, Caffrey TC, Swanson BJ, et al. MUC4 enhances gemcitabine resistance and malignant behaviour in pancreatic cancer cells expressing cancer-associated short O-glycans. Cancer Lett. 2021;503:91–102.
168. Elton TS, Ozer HG, Yalowich JC. Effects of DNA topoisomerase IIα splice variants on acquired drug resistance. Cancer Drug Resist. 2020;3(2):161–70.
169. Hernandez VA, Carvajal-Moreno J, Papa JL, Shkolnikov N, Li J, Ozer HG, et al. CRISPR/Cas9 Genome Editing of the Human Topoisomerase IIα Intron 19 5′ Splice Site Circumvents Etoposide Resistance in Human Leukemia K562 Cells. Mol Pharmacol. 2021;99(3):226–41.
170. Luo Z, Gao M, Huang N, Wang X, Yang Z, Yang H, et al. Efficient disruption of bcr-abl gene by CRISPR RNA-guided FokI nucleases depresses the oncogenesis of chronic myeloid leukemia cells. J Exp Clin Cancer Res. 2019;38(1):224.
171. Dhadve AC, Hari K, Rekhi B, Jolly MK, De A, Ray P. Decoding molecular interplay between RUNX1 and FOXO3a underlying the pulsatile IGF1R expression during acquirement of chemoresistance. Biochim Biophys Acta Mol Basis Dis. 2020;1866(6):165754.
172. Xiao L, Peng Z, Zhu A, Xue R, Lu R, Mi J, et al. Inhibition of RUNX1 promotes cisplatin-induced apoptosis in ovarian cancer cells. Biochem Pharmacol. 2020;180:114116.
173. Dong C, Wu J, Chen Y, Nie J, Chen C. Activation of PI3K/AKT/mTOR Pathway Causes Drug Resistance in Breast Cancer. Front Pharmacol. 2021;12:628690.
174. Zhang L, Li Y, Wang Q, Chen Z, Li X, Wu Z, et al. The PI3K subunits, P110α and P110β are potential targets for overcoming P-gp and BCRP-mediated MDR in cancer. Mol Cancer. 2020;19(1):10.
175. Liao Y, Chen L, Feng Y, Shen J, Gao Y, Cote G, et al. Targeting programmed cell death ligand 1 by CRISPR/Cas9 in osteosarcoma cells. Oncotarget. 2017;8(18):30276–87.
176. Zhang P, Ma Y, Lv C, Huang M, Li M, Dong B, et al. Upregulation of programmed cell death ligand 1 promotes resistance response in

non-small-cell lung cancer patients treated with neo-adjuvant chemotherapy. Cancer Sci. 2016;107(11):1563–71.

177. Bialk P, Wang Y, Banas K, Kmiec EB. Functional Gene Knockout of NRF2 Increases Chemosensitivity of Human Lung Cancer A549 Cells In Vitro and in a Xenograft Mouse Model. Mol Ther Oncolytics. 2018;11:75–89.
178. Kawamura N, Nimura K, Nagano H, Yamaguchi S, Nonomura N, Kaneda Y. CRISPR/Cas9-mediated gene knockout of NANOG and NANOGP8 decreases the malignant potential of prostate cancer cells. Oncotarget. 2015;6(26):22361–74.
179. Cain JW, Hauptschein RS, Stewart JK, Bagci T, Sahagian GG, Jay DG. Identification of CD44 as a surface biomarker for drug resistance by surface proteome signature technology. Mol Cancer Res. 2011;9(5):637–47.
180. Gao Y, Foster R, Yang X, Feng Y, Shen JK, Mankin HJ, et al. Up-regulation of CD44 in the development of metastasis, recurrence and drug resistance of ovarian cancer. Oncotarget. 2015;6(11):9313–26.
181. Ravindranath AK, Kaur S, Wernyj RP, Kumaran MN, Miletti-Gonzalez KE, Chan R, et al. CD44 promotes multi-drug resistance by protecting P-glycoprotein from FBXO21-mediated ubiquitination. Oncotarget. 2015;6(28):26308–21.
182. Tamada M, Nagano O, Tateyama S, Ohmura M, Yae T, Ishimoto T, et al. Modulation of glucose metabolism by CD44 contributes to antioxidant status and drug resistance in cancer cells. Cancer Res. 2012;72(6):1438–48.
183. Asai R, Tsuchiya H, Amisaki M, Makimoto K, Takenaga A, Sakabe T, et al. CD44 standard isoform is involved in maintenance of cancer stem cells of a hepatocellular carcinoma cell line. Cancer Med. 2019;8(2):773–82.
184. Liu T, Yan Z, Liu Y, Choy E, Hornicek FJ, Mankin H, Duan Z. CRISPR-Cas9-Mediated Silencing of CD44 in Human Highly Metastatic Osteosarcoma Cells. Cell Physiol Biochem. 2018;46(3):1218–30.
185. Lin SC, Wu HL, Yeh LY, Yang CC, Kao SY, Chang KW. Activation of the miR-371/372/373 miRNA Cluster Enhances Oncogenicity and Drug Resistance in Oral Carcinoma Cells. Int J Mol Sci. 2020;21(24):9442.
186. Huo W, Zhao G, Yin J, Ouyang X, Wang Y, Yang C, et al. Lentiviral CRISPR/Cas9 vector mediated miR-21 gene editing inhibits the epithelial to mesenchymal transition in ovarian cancer cells. J Cancer. 2017;8(1):57–64.

187. Shaath H, Vishnubalaji R, Elango R, Khattak S, Alajez NM. Single-cell long noncoding RNA (lncRNA) transcriptome implicates MALAT1 in triple-negative breast cancer (TNBC) resistance to neo-adjuvant chemotherapy. Cell Death Discov. 2021;7(1):23.
188. Malla R, Kamal MA. E6 and E7 Oncoproteins: Potential Targets of Cervical Cancer. Curr Med Chem. 2021;28(39):8163–81.
189. Vishnoi K, Mahata S, Tyagi A, Pandey A, Verma G, Jadli M, et al. Human papillomavirus oncoproteins differentially modulate epithelial-mesenchymal transition in 5-FU-resistant cervical cancer cells. Tumour Biol. 2016;37(10):13137–54.
190. Hu Z, Yu L, Zhu D, Ding W, Wang X, Zhang C, et al. Disruption of HPV16-E7 by CRISPR/Cas system induces apoptosis and growth inhibition in HPV16 positive human cervical cancer cells. Biomed Res Int. 2014;2014:612823.
191. Zhen S, Lu JJ, Wang LJ, Sun XM, Zhang JQ, Li X, et al. In Vitro and In Vivo Synergistic Therapeutic Effect of Cisplatin with Human Papillomavirus16 E6/E7 CRISPR/Cas9 on Cervical Cancer Cell Line. Transl Oncol. 2016;9(6):498–504.
192. Pirouzfar M, Amiri F, Dianatpour M, Takhshid MA. CRISPR/Cas9-mediated knockout of MLL5 enhances apoptotic effect of cisplatin in HeLa cells in vitro. Excli J. 2020;19:170–82.
193. Ryu J-Y, Choi YJ, Won E-J, Hui E, Kim H-S, Cho Y-S, Yoon T-J. Gene editing particle system as a therapeutic approach for drug-resistant colorectal cancer. Nano Research. 2020;13(6):1576–85.
194. Xiao Z, Wan J, Nur AA, Dou P, Mankin H, Liu T, Ouyang Z. Targeting CD44 by CRISPR-Cas9 in Multi-Drug Resistant Osteosarcoma Cells. Cell Physiol Biochem. 2018;51(4):1879–93.
195. Saber A, Liu B, Ebrahimi P, Haisma HJ. CRISPR/Cas9 for overcoming drug resistance in solid tumors. Daru. 2020;28(1):295–304.
196. Coleman N, Zhang B, Byers LA, Yap TA. The role of Schlafen 11 (SLFN11) as a predictive biomarker for targeting the DNA damage response. Br J Cancer. 2021;124(5):857–9.
197. Murai J, Thomas A, Miettinen M, Pommier Y. Schlafen 11 (SLFN11), a restriction factor for replicative stress induced by DNA-targeting anti-cancer therapies. Pharmacol Ther. 2019;201:94–102.
198. Lok BH, Gardner EE, Schneeberger VE, Ni A, Desmeules P, Rekhtman N, et al. PARP Inhibitor Activity Correlates with SLFN11 Expression and Demonstrates Synergy with Temozolomide in Small Cell Lung Cancer. Clin Cancer Res. 2017;23(2):523–35.

199. Murai J, Feng Y, Yu GK, Ru Y, Tang SW, Shen Y, Pommier Y. Resistance to PARP inhibitors by SLFN11 inactivation can be overcome by ATR inhibition. Oncotarget. 2016;7(47):76534–50.
200. Chen T, Liu C, Lu H, Yin M, Shao C, Hu X, et al. The expression of APE1 in triple-negative breast cancer and its effect on drug sensitivity of olaparib. Tumour Biol. 2017;39(10):1010428317713390.
201. Cai G, Yang Q, Sun W. RSF1 in cancer: interactions and functions. Cancer Cell Int. 2021;21(1):315.
202. Chen X, Sun X, Guan J, Gai J, Xing J, Fu L, et al. Rsf-1 Influences the Sensitivity of Non-Small Cell Lung Cancer to Paclitaxel by Regulating NF-κB Pathway and Its Downstream Proteins. Cell Physiol Biochem. 2017;44(6):2322–36.
203. Pozo K, Bibb JA. The Emerging Role of Cdk5 in Cancer. Trends Cancer. 2016;2(10):606–18.
204. Dhavan R, Tsai LH. A decade of CDK5. Nat Rev Mol Cell Biol. 2001;2(10):749–59.
205. Ardelt MA, Fröhlich T, Martini E, Müller M, Kanitz V, Atzberger C, et al. Inhibition of Cyclin-Dependent Kinase 5: A Strategy to Improve Sorafenib Response in Hepatocellular Carcinoma Therapy. Hepatology. 2019;69(1):376–93.
206. Blivet-Van Eggelpoël MJ, Chettouh H, Fartoux L, Aoudjehane L, Barbu V, Rey C, et al. Epidermal growth factor receptor and HER-3 restrict cell response to sorafenib in hepatocellular carcinoma cells. J Hepatol. 2012;57(1):108–15.
207. Wang H, Tang Z, Li T, Liu M, Li Y, Xing B. CRISPR/Cas9-Mediated Gene Knockout of ARID1A Promotes Primary Progesterone Resistance by Downregulating Progesterone Receptor B in Endometrial Cancer Cells. Oncol Res. 2019;27(9):1051–60.
208. Yu J, Zhou J, Xu F, Bai W, Zhang W. High expression of Aurora-B is correlated with poor prognosis and drug resistance in non-small cell lung cancer. Int J Biol Markers. 2018;33(2):215–21.
209. Han B, Cai J, Gao W, Meng X, Gao F, Wu P, et al. Loss of ATRX suppresses ATM dependent DNA damage repair by modulating H3K9me3 to enhance temozolomide sensitivity in glioma. Cancer Lett. 2018;419:280–90.
210. Wong LH, McGhie JD, Sim M, Anderson MA, Ahn S, Hannan RD, et al. ATRX interacts with H3.3 in maintaining telomere structural integrity in pluripotent embryonic stem cells. Genome Res. 2010;20(3):351–60.

211. Khan Z, Khan AA, Yadav H, Prasad G, Bisen PS. Survivin, a molecular target for therapeutic interventions in squamous cell carcinoma. Cell Mol Biol Lett. 2017;22:8.
212. Zhao G, Wang Q, Gu Q, Qiang W, Wei JJ, Dong P, et al. Lentiviral CRISPR/Cas9 nickase vector mediated BIRC5 editing inhibits epithelial to mesenchymal transition in ovarian cancer cells. Oncotarget. 2017;8(55):94666–80.
213. Schuster A, Erasimus H, Fritah S, Nazarov PV, van Dyck E, Niclou SP, Golebiewska A. RNAi/CRISPR Screens: from a Pool to a Valid Hit. Trends Biotechnol. 2019;37(1):38–55.
214. Shalem O, Sanjana NE, Hartenian E, Shi X, Scott DA, Mikkelson T, et al. Genome-scale CRISPR-Cas9 knockout screening in human cells. Science. 2014;343(6166):84–7.
215. Hodges C, Kirkland JG, Crabtree GR. The Many Roles of BAF (mSWI/SNF) and PBAF Complexes in Cancer. Cold Spring Harb Perspect Med. 2016;6(8):a026930.
216. Liao S, Davoli T, Leng Y, Li MZ, Xu Q, Elledge SJ. A genetic interaction analysis identifies cancer drivers that modify EGFR dependency. Genes Dev. 2017;31(2):184–96.
217. Iwaizumi M, Shinmura K, Mori H, Yamada H, Suzuki M, Kitayama Y, et al. Human Sgo1 downregulation leads to chromosomal instability in colorectal cancer. Gut. 2009;58(2):249–60.
218. Sun W, He B, Yang B, Hu W, Cheng S, Xiao H, et al. Genome-wide CRISPR screen reveals SGOL1 as a druggable target of sorafenib-treated hepatocellular carcinoma. Lab Invest. 2018;98(6):734–44.
219. Rushworth LK, Harle V, Repiscak P, Clark W, Shaw R, Hall H, et al. In vivo CRISPR/Cas9 knockout screen: TCEAL1 silencing enhances docetaxel efficacy in prostate cancer. Life Sci Alliance. 2020;3(12):e202000770.
220. Wei W, He Y, Wu YM. Identification of genes associated with SiHa cell sensitivity to paclitaxel by CRISPR-Cas9 knockout screening. Int J Clin Exp Pathol. 2018;11(4):1972–8.
221. Goodspeed A, Jean A, Costello JC. A whole-genome CRISPR screen identifies a role of MSH2 in cisplatin-mediated cell death in muscle-invasive bladder cancer. European Urology. 2019;75(2):242–50.
222. Xu S, Zhan M, Jiang C, He M, Yang L, Shen H, et al. Genome-wide CRISPR screen identifies ELP5 as a determinant of gemcitabine sensitivity in gallbladder cancer. Nat Commun. 2019;10(1):5492.
223. Makhov P, Sohn JA, Serebriiskii IG, Fazliyeva R, Khazak V, Boumber Y, et al. CRISPR/Cas9 genome-wide loss-of-function screening

identifies druggable cellular factors involved in sunitinib resistance in renal cell carcinoma. Br J Cancer. 2020;123(12):1749–56.

224. Nagler A, Vredevoogd DW, Alon M, Cheng PF, Trabish S, Kalaora S, et al. A genome-wide CRISPR screen identifies FBXO42 involvement in resistance toward MEK inhibition in NRAS-mutant melanoma. Pigment Cell Melanoma Res. 2020;33(2):334–44.
225. Damnernsawad A, Bottomly D, Kurtz SE, Eide CA, McWeeney SK, Tyner JW, Nechiporuk T. Genome-wide CRISPR screen identifies regulators of MAPK and MTOR pathways mediating sorafenib resistance in acute myeloid leukemia. Haematologica. 2022;107(1): 77–85.
226. Barghout SH, Aman A, Nouri K, Blatman Z, Arevalo K, Thomas GE, et al. A genome-wide CRISPR/Cas9 screen in acute myeloid leukemia cells identifies regulators of TAK-243 sensitivity. JCI Insight. 2021;6(5):e141518.
227. Jung HR, Oh Y, Na D, Min S, Kang J, Jang D, et al. CRISPR screens identify a novel combination treatment targeting BCL-X(L) and WNT signaling for KRAS/BRAF-mutated colorectal cancers. Oncogene. 2021;40(18):3287–302.
228. Rocha CRR, Reily Rocha A, Molina Silva M, Rodrigues Gomes L, Teatin Latancia M, Andrade Tomaz M, et al. Revealing Temozolomide Resistance Mechanisms via Genome-Wide CRISPR Libraries. Cells. 2020;9(12):2573.
229. Zhang XH, Tee LY, Wang XG, Huang QS, Yang SH. Off-target Effects in CRISPR/Cas9-mediated Genome Engineering. Mol Ther Nucleic Acids. 2015;4(11):e264.
230. Han HA, Pang JKS, Soh BS. Mitigating off-target effects in CRISPR/Cas9-mediated in vivo gene editing. J Mol Med (Berl). 2020;98(5): 615–32.
231. Uddin F, Rudin CM, Sen T. CRISPR Gene Therapy: Applications, Limitations, and Implications for the Future. Front Oncol. 2020;10:1387.
232. Charlesworth CT, Deshpande PS, Dever DP, Camarena J, Lemgart VT, Cromer MK, et al. Identification of preexisting adaptive immunity to Cas9 proteins in humans. Nat Med. 2019;25(2):249–54.
233. Lino CA, Harper JC, Carney JP, Timlin JA. Delivering CRISPR: a review of the challenges and approaches. Drug Deliv. 2018;25(1): 1234–57.

https://doi.org/10.1142/9789819826759_0014

CHAPTER 14

Nanoparticles for the Delivery of CRISPR/Cas9 System in Cancer Therapy

Mehrdad Hashemi[1,2], *Alireza Khosravinejad*[1,3], *Mina Alimohammadi*[4], *Reza Mohajer Shirazi*[1,3], *Behdokht Jamali*[5], *Kimia Sadat Esfahani*[1,3], *Ali Shirazi*[1,3], *Rojin Ghannad Zadeh*[1,6], *Faranak Jamshidian*[1,7], *Neda Zali*[3], *Najma Farahani*[1,*], *Afshin Taheriazam*[1,8,*], *Payman Rahimzadeh*[9,*], *Maliheh Entezari*[1,2,*]

[1]Farhikhtegan Medical Convergent Sciences Research Center, Farhikhtegan Hospital, Faculty of Medicine, TeMs. C., Islamic Azad University, Tehran, Iran
[2]Department of Genetics, Faculty of Advanced Sciences and Technology, TeMs. C, Islamic Azad University, Tehran, Iran
[3]Basic and Molecular Epidemiology of Gastrointestinal Disorders Research Center, Research Institute for Gastroenterology and Liver Diseases, Shahid Beheshti University of Medical Sciences, Tehran, Iran
[4]Department of Immunology, School of Medicine, Shahid Beheshti University of Medical Sciences, Tehran, Iran
[5]Department of Microbiology and Genetics, Kherad Institute of Higher Education, Bushehr, Iran

---

**Corresponding authors:* Najmafarahani@gmail.com (N.F.); a.taheriazam@iautmu.ac.ir (A.T.); P.rahimzadeh76@gmail.com (P.R.); mentezari@iautmu.ac.ir (M.E.)

[6]Department of Art & Sciences, Faculty of Biology, University of North Florida, Jacksonville, Florida, USA
[7]Department of Biology, ET.C., Islamic Azad University, Tehran, Iran
[8]Department of Orthopedics, Faculty of Medicine, TeMs. C, Islamic Azad University, Tehran, Iran
[9]Surgical Research Society (SRS), Students' Scientific Research Center, Tehran University of Medical Sciences, Tehran, Iran

Abstract

CRISPR/Cas9 delivered by nanoparticles is emerging as a convergent strategy to translate precise genome editing into practical cancer therapies by solving the core challenge of safe, efficient, and tumor-selective delivery. By packaging Cas9 and guide RNAs into engineered nanocarriers, such as lipid and polymer nanoparticles, mesoporous silica, porous silicon, and metal-organic frameworks, this approach improves protection from degradation, enhances cellular uptake and endosomal escape, and enables targeted accumulation within tumors. These design features can raise on-target editing while reducing systemic exposure and immunogenicity relative to conventional physical or viral delivery, thereby widening the therapeutic window for *in vivo* gene editing. Within oncology, nanoparticle-enabled CRISPR/Cas9 has been applied to disrupt oncogenic drivers, repair or silence pathogenic variants, remodel tumor-immune interactions, and sensitize malignant cells to existing therapies. Importantly, tunable particle attributes — size, charge, surface chemistry, and ligand functionalization — allow tailored delivery of diverse CRISPR formats (plasmid DNA, mRNA/sgRNA, or ribonucleoprotein complexes) to distinct tumor contexts and anatomical compartments, supporting both gene editing and immunotherapeutic applications. This chapter synthesizes the rationale and strategies for nanotechnology-facilitated CRISPR/Cas9 delivery, highlights representative materials and targeting paradigms, and outlines translational considerations for moving from preclinical efficacy to clinical benefit.

Keywords: CRISPR/Cas9; nanotechnology; lipid nanoparticles; polymer nanoparticles; mesoporous silica; metal–organic frameworks; targeted delivery; ribonucleoprotein; extracellular vesicles

14.1 Introduction

Despite advancements in traditional treatment methods including surgery, chemotherapy, and radiation therapy, cancer remains a major health concern with substantial mortality rates [1, 2]. The continuous development of drug resistance and cancer recurrence necessitates the exploration of alternative therapeutic approaches. Research has documented over 600 mutations in the cancer somatic abnormality database, emphasizing how genetic and epigenetic modifications contribute to cancer development and progression, suggesting that targeted gene editing could serve as a viable treatment strategy [3, 4].

Scientists have transformed the CRISPR-Cas9 technology into a versatile and powerful genomic modification tool capable of making specific DNA changes. This technique utilizes single-guide (sgRNA) to direct Cas9 nuclease activity to specific DNA sequences, enabling targeted genetic modifications through DNA cutting and subsequent repair mechanisms [5, 6]. The CRISPR-Cas9 platform demonstrates superior versatility, effectiveness, and accuracy compared to earlier gene-editing technologies like transcription activator-like effector nucleases and zinc finger nucleases, making it particularly suitable for therapeutic use [5, 7, 8]. Following its first application in mammalian cells during 2013, CRISPR-Cas9 has quickly become prominent in various fields, particularly cancer research. Researchers have shown great enthusiasm for its potential in modifying cancer-related genes, enhancing cancer immunotherapy, creating disease models, and complementing conventional cancer treatments [9, 10].

The successful clinical application of CRISPR-Cas9 technology relies heavily on delivering its key components — Cas9 protein and sgRNA — efficiently to target cell nuclei. While researchers have explored both viral and physical delivery methods, these approaches often face challenges including insufficient delivery rates, immune system responses, limited cargo capacity, and unintended genetic modifications [11–13]. Nanotechnology presents a promising alternative, employing nano-scale materials with distinct physicochemical properties that can effectively protect and transport CRISPR/Cas9 components while facilitating targeted delivery and cellular absorption. Researchers have investigated various nanomaterials for this purpose, including polymeric compounds, lipid-based carriers, porous silicon structures, mesoporous silica particles, and metal-organic framework systems. This section explores how combining CRISPR/Cas9 with nanotechnology could advance cancer treatment, examining various therapeutic applications in genetic modification and immune system-based therapies [12, 14–17].

This portion focuses on analyzing effective CRISPR-Cas9 delivery systems and their cancer treatment applications. The discussion covers its role in improving distribution within living organisms, enhancing CRISPR-Cas9 performance, and supporting cancer immunotherapy approaches. The ongoing advancements in nanodelivery systems show considerable promise for maximizing CRISPR-Cas9's therapeutic potential and addressing complex challenges in cancer treatment.

14.2 Types of Nanoparticles for CRISPR/Cas9 Delivery

14.2.1 *Lipid-based Nanoparticles*

Lipid nanoparticles (LNP) have emerged as promising carriers for delivering nucleic acids, particularly in CRISPR/Cas9 gene editing applications. These particles function through the fundamental principle of charge-based interactions, where positively charged lipids interact with the negative phosphate groups in DNA. This interaction facilitates DNA plasmid encapsulation within the LNP's core while promoting cellular uptake through interactions with the cell's negatively charged membrane. Scientists have developed numerous LNP formulations specifically designed for CRISPR/Cas9 plasmid delivery through extensive research efforts.

In a significant study, Wang and colleagues [18] engineered an advanced LNP system to deliver Cas9-containing plasmids targeting the MutT homolog 1 (MTH1) gene in non-small cell lung cancer. Their innovative approach involved first compacting the plasmid using protamine, a protein carrying positive charges and a nuclear localization sequence (NLS), before incorporating it into a cationic liposome structure. The researchers enhanced the nanocarrier's tumor-targeting ability by adding DSPE-PEG-HA modifications, which significantly improved both cellular uptake and nuclear targeting. This optimized delivery system successfully disrupted the MTH1 gene, effectively inhibiting progression [18].

Scientists have modified LNP formulations to achieve various therapeutic objectives, including specific targeting, prolonged circulation time, better transfection rates, reduced toxicity, and enhanced stability. In a notable study, Liu and collaborators [19] engineered cationic lipid-assisted polymeric nanoparticles, combining BHEM-Chol (a cationic lipid) with PEG-PLGA polymer, to deliver Cas9 plasmids targeting the BCR-ABL fusion gene in chronic myeloid leukemia cells. Their system achieved precise gene editing of BCR-ABL, resulting in prolonged survival and decreased leukemia burden in mouse models [19].

Chen and colleagues [20] advanced this approach by developing a sophisticated cationic LNP system (DOX-CB@lipo-pDNA-iRGD) that simultaneously delivered a CD47-targeting Cas9 plasmid and a boron compound. Their design incorporated doxorubicin for nuclear targeting and iRGD peptide for tumor specificity. This combined approach, integrating CRISPR/Cas9-mediated CD47 knockout with boron neutron capture therapy, demonstrated improved anti-tumor effects and enhanced survival rates in experimental models.

Recent innovations include the development of ionizable LNPs with superior endosomal escape capabilities. Li et al. [21] reported a formulation (iLP181) that effectively delivered PLK1-targeting Cas9 plasmids to hepatoma carcinoma cells. This system showed better endosomal escape and gene editing efficiency compared to standard lipofectamine 2000, leading to significant tumor suppression in living organisms.

14.2.2 *Polymeric Nanoparticles*

Polymer-based nanocarriers represent an effective delivery system for CRISPR/Cas9 ribonucleoprotein (RNP) complexes, offering advantages including stability in colloidal systems, compatibility with biological systems, and adaptability for specific targeting and cellular entry. While traditional carriers like polyethyleneimine (PEI) remain relevant, researchers have developed new approaches involving chemically modified RNP systems that demonstrate enhanced stability and more efficient gene editing capabilities. Scientists are also investigating DNA nanostructures, which can encapsulate RNPs through specific sequence recognition, providing better protection and controlled release to target cells.

A breakthrough study by Ruan and colleagues [22] demonstrated the effectiveness of a novel polymer system modified with angiopep-2 and coated with guanidinium and fluorine groups for targeted RNP delivery to brain tissue. Their nanocarrier successfully penetrated the blood-brain barrier, achieving significant gene knockout and protein reduction in glioblastoma models. In parallel developments, researchers have created DNA nanoflower systems incorporating MUC1 aptamers and miR-21-sensitive sequences, enabling tumor-specific delivery and responsive gene editing capabilities. These innovative approaches represent significant advances in polymer-based delivery strategies, combining targeted delivery mechanisms with immune checkpoint modification.

14.2.3 *Inorganic Nanoparticles*

Alongside polymer-based nanocarriers, inorganic nanomaterials have shown promise for plasmid Cas9 (pCas9) delivery, with their unique properties facilitating cellular uptake and endosomal escape. Metal-organic frameworks (MOFs), consisting of metal ions or clusters linked with organic ligands to form porous structures with tunable properties, have garnered particular attention in biological applications [23].

While MOF research for pCas9 delivery remains nascent, initial results appear promising. A recent investigation demonstrated the potential of polymer-modified NH2-UiO-66 MOF for simultaneous delivery of doxorubicin and pCas9. Though transfection efficiency was moderate, this study highlights MOFs' potential as CRISPR/Cas9 component carriers [24].

Zeolitic imidazole frameworks (ZIFs), a MOF subclass, show particular promise for delivering biological macromolecules. ZIF-8 has been extensively studied for gene delivery applications. Pyreddy and colleagues [25] developed an innovative ZIF-based system (ZIF-C) that achieved significant gene editing efficiency in prostate cancer cells. Additionally, Poddar et al. [26] demonstrated successful Paxillin knock-in through homology-directed repair using a pCas9-ZIF-8 system, showcasing ZIFs' versatility in complex gene editing applications.

Gold nanoparticles represent another effective approach for pCas9 delivery. Chen and team [27] extensively studied how gold nanorod (AuNR) aspect ratios influence pCas9 delivery and editing efficiency. Their findings revealed that high-aspect-ratio AuNRs, modified with cationic polymers like PEI, demonstrated superior DNA binding, cellular uptake, and endosomal escape, leading to effective gene editing. The researchers further developed supramolecular cationic AuNRs combining NIR-II light-activated hyperthermia with CRISPR/Cas9 delivery, enhancing both gene editing efficiency and immunogenic cell death [28].

Hollow mesoporous silica nanoparticles (HMSNs) constitute a unique class of inorganic nanomaterials particularly suited for gene delivery due to their distinctive hollow mesoporous structure, which enables efficient encapsulation of both therapeutic agents and gene editing components. Recent research demonstrated successful co-delivery of sorafenib and pCas9 using polyamidoamine-aptamer-coated HMSNs, achieving effective gene suppression and enhanced therapeutic effects in liver cancer cells [29].

The ability of cationic polymers to compress and encapsulate negatively charged DNA has made them essential in developing pCas9 delivery systems. These polymers form complexes with plasmid DNA through electrostatic interactions, improving packaging and cellular delivery. He and colleagues [30] developed a sophisticated delivery system using protamine, a natural cationic protein, combined with calcium carbonate to create a pCas9-containing core targeting β-catenin. They enhanced this system by adding hyaluronic acid modified with TAT-NLS peptide and AS1411 aptamer, improving cellular uptake and nuclear targeting. This comprehensive approach achieved effective β-catenin suppression through combined protamine-mediated DNA condensation and targeted delivery. In a related development, Tao et al. [31] pioneered protamine-capped gold nanoclusters for pCas9 delivery, combining protamine's cationic properties with gold's biocompatibility and cellular uptake advantages.

Chitosan, a natural amino-rich polysaccharide, shows significant potential for pCas9 delivery, with its adaptability and biological compatibility driving the development of various chitosan-based carriers [32]. Researchers developed a sophisticated platform using folic acid and 2-(diisopropylamino) ethyl methacrylate double-grafted trimethyl chitosan for simultaneous delivery of survivin-targeting plasmid DNA and doxorubicin. This system effectively protected and condensed plasmid DNA, enabling successful gene editing and improved anti-cancer effects both in laboratory and living systems [33].

Dendrimers offer unique advantages for gene delivery through their highly organized branching structure and abundant surface functional groups [34]. Zhao et al. developed an innovative system using fluorinated G5 PAMAM dendrimer to deliver HSP70-promoter-driven pCas9 targeting PD-L1 along with photosensitizer Ce6. This combined approach merged photodynamic therapy with CRISPR/Cas9 gene editing for enhanced anti-tumor effects. The HSP70 promoter provided spatial control over Cas9 expression, minimizing potential off-target effects [35].

Poly(β-amino ester) [PBAE], a versatile cationic polymer, has been extensively studied for gene delivery. Recent polymer engineering advances have produced sophisticated linear-branched and hyperbranched PBAEs that outperform traditional agents like PEI in gene transfection and silencing. Zhang and colleagues [36] created an innovative internally and externally engineered exosome system by incorporating a PBAE/CRISPRi/dCas9 nanocomplex within

CRV-expressing exosome membranes. This system achieved precise delivery to tumor-associated macrophages, successfully converting them from M2 to M1 phenotype and inhibiting tumor growth.

Poly (disulfide) has emerged as a promising carrier due to its ability to facilitate intracellular cargo transport through disulfide exchange mechanisms, avoiding endosomal entrapment. Recent studies by Xu et al. [37] demonstrated successful plasmid delivery using PEG-modified poly(disulfide), while others utilized poly-(disulfide)for liver-targeted delivery of Cas-editing plasmids.

Table 14.1 and **Figure 14.1** represent a comprehensive summary on nanoparticle technology used for CRISPR/Cas9 delivery.

14.2.4 *mRNA-based Delivery*

RNA-based CRISPR/Cas9 systems using Cas9 mRNA and sgRNA present compelling advantages over plasmid-based approaches, offering transient expression, reduced off-target effects, and lower immunogenicity. However, effective mRNA delivery remains challenging due to its inherent instability and limited cell penetration capabilities.

While mRNA translation occurs in the cytoplasm, eliminating nuclear entry requirements, the large size and degradation susceptibility of Cas9 mRNA create delivery challenges. Additionally, successful gene editing requires simultaneous delivery of both Cas9 mRNA and sgRNA to target cells.

Liu and colleagues [40] developed innovative bioreducible LNPs using BAMEA-O16B cationic lipid for co-delivery of Cas9 mRNA and sgRNA. These particles effectively protected and released mRNA cargo in response to reductive conditions, achieving rapid and efficient gene editing in both laboratory and living systems. Rosenblum et al. [41] created amino ionizable lipid libraries for delivering modified Cas9 mRNA and sgRNA, demonstrating significant tumor suppression in glioma models through single intracerebral administration.

To address endosomal escape challenges, Siegwart's team developed innovative phospholipids that form conical structures

Table 14.1 Nanoparticle delivery systems for pCas9.

Nanoparticle Type	Material or System	Application or Target	Key Findings	Reference
Metal-organic frameworks	Polymer-functionalized NH_2-UiO-66 MOF	Co-delivery of doxorubicin and pCas9	Moderate transfection efficiency, potential as CRISPR/Cas9 carriers	[24]
Zeolitic imidazole frameworks	ZIF-C (ZIF-based platform)	Delivery of pCas9 in prostate cancer cells	Notable gene editing efficacy	[25]
Zeolitic imidazole frameworks	pCas9-ZIF-8 system	Paxillin knockin via homology-directed repair	Adaptability for intricate gene editing	[26]
Gold nanoparticles	High-aspect-ratio AuNRs with PEI	pCas9 delivery and gene editing	Enhanced DNA binding, cellular uptake, and endosomal escape	[27]
Gold nanoparticles	Supramolecular cationic AuNRs	NIR-II light-activated CRISPR/Cas9 delivery	Improved gene editing and immunogenic cell death	[28]
Hollow mesoporous silica nanoparticles	Polyamidoamine-aptamer-coated HMSNs	Co-delivery of sorafenib and pCas9	Effective gene knockdown in liver cancer	[29]
Cationic proteins	Protamine + $CaCO_3$ core with hyaluronic acid/TAT-NLS/AS1411	β-catenin knockdown	Effective knockdown via DNA condensation and targeted delivery	[30]
Cationic polymers	Protamine-capped gold nanoclusters	pCas9 delivery vehicle	Leverages protamine cationic characteristics and gold nanocluster biocompatibility	[31]
Poly(β-amino ester)	PBAE/CRISPRi/dCas9 nanocomplex	Delivery to tumor-associated macrophages	Repolarizes tumor-associated macrophages from M2 to M1 phenotype, suppresses tumor growth	[38, 39]

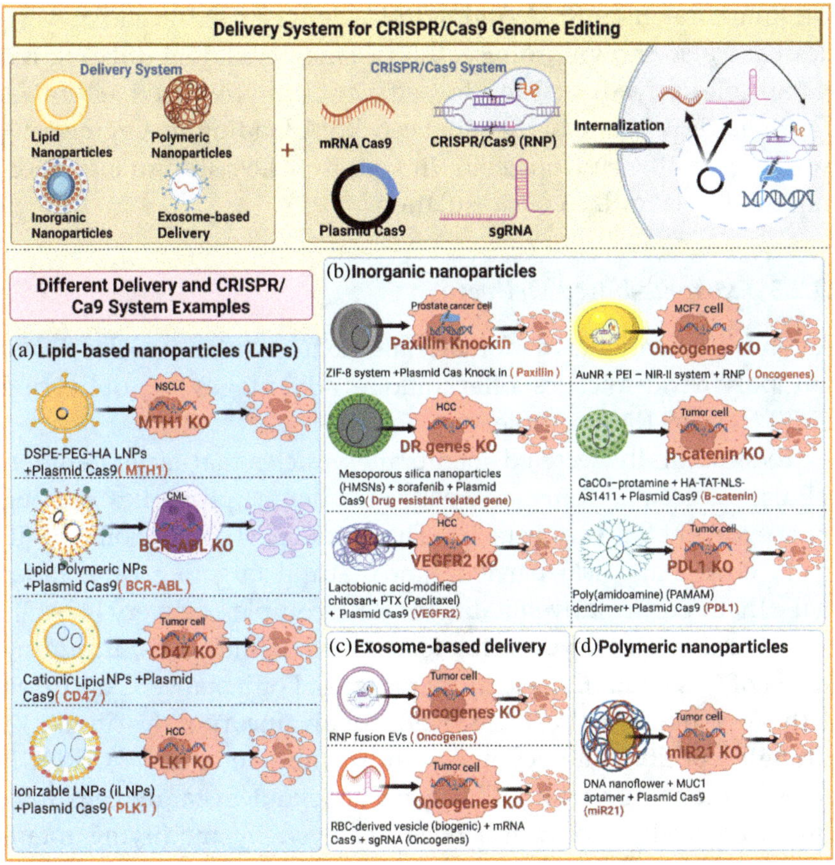

Figure 14.1 Nano-delivery systems for CRISPR/Cas9 genome editing in cancer therapy.

in acidic endosomal environments, facilitating membrane disruption and cargo release. Farbiak et al. [42] advanced the field by creating dendrimer-based LNPs for delivering complete CRISPR/Cas9 components, achieving exceptional homology-directed repair efficiency. Zhang et al. [2022] [43] further enhanced this approach by combining FAK-targeting siRNA with Cas9 mRNA and sgRNA delivery, improving tumor targeting and gene editing outcomes.

Beyond LNPs, researchers have explored alternative delivery systems. Abbasi et al. [44] developed PEGylated polyplex micelles for simultaneous mRNA and sgRNA delivery. Extracellular vesicles have also shown promise, with Usman et al. [45] utilizing red blood cell-derived vesicles for efficient mRNA-based CRISPR/Cas9 delivery. Li et al. [46] enhanced RNA loading by engineering exosomes with HuR protein linked to CD9, improving ARE-modified Cas9 mRNA encapsulation.

14.2.5 *Exosome-based Delivery*

Beyond conventional nanomaterials, extracellular vesicles (EVs) and polymeric micelles offer unique advantages for delivering CRISPR/Cas9 RNP complexes.

EVs, naturally secreted membrane vesicles that facilitate intercellular molecular transport, possess inherent properties making them excellent delivery vehicles. Their biological compatibility, ability to cross biological barriers, and natural targeting capabilities make them particularly suitable for RNP complex delivery [47–49].

Several strategies exist for loading RNPs into EVs, including fusion of Cas9 with EV structural proteins. For instance, Cas9 fused with WW domain (WW-Cas9) effectively incorporates into EVs through specific interactions with membrane-bound ARRDC1, demonstrating successful GFP gene knockout in target cells [50]. Enhanced RNP loading has been achieved by modifying membrane proteins to improve cargo recognition and encapsulation, leading to more effective gene knockout results.

Scientists have developed methods to enhance EV targeting specificity for RNP delivery by incorporating DNA aptamers and precisely controlled tetrahedral DNA nanostructures. These modifications improve tumor-specific EV accumulation and gene editing efficiency, resulting in significant tumor growth inhibition.

Polymeric micelles, self-assembling nanostructures formed from amphiphilic polymers, offer advantages including easy functionalization, improved stability, and biological compatibility. Zhang and colleagues [51] developed an innovative mesoporous nanoflower platform [Cas9-NF] by linking Cas9 RNP with Pluronic 127 micelles using reduction-responsive bonds. This system achieved effective intracellular delivery and controlled RNP release, leading to significant gene editing and tumor growth suppression. Additionally, Cas9-NF nanoflowers can serve as versatile carriers for both hydrophilic and hydrophobic drugs, enabling combined gene therapy and conventional treatment approaches.

14.2.6 *Plasmid-based Delivery*

Research has established that nanocarriers loaded with pCas9 facilitate the entry of the CRISPR/Cas9 system into cells through two main pathways. The primary route involves endocytic uptake followed by endosomal escape, allowing the plasmid to reach the cytoplasm. Alternatively, certain nanocarriers enable direct cellular entry of plasmids via non-endocytic mechanisms, effectively bypassing lysosomal compartments and thereby protecting the cargo from degradation [52, 53].

Once inside the cell, the plasmid is released from its nanocarrier and transported to the nucleus, where transcription occurs to produce mRNA and sgRNA. The mRNA then migrates to the cytoplasm, where it is translated into Cas9 protein. This protein subsequently binds to the sgRNA to form the RNP complex, which must re-enter the nucleus to execute genome editing.

Given pCas9's large molecular size and strong negative charge, most delivery strategies rely on positively charged materials to condense the plasmid into smaller complexes via electrostatic interactions. Commonly used materials for this purpose include cationic lipids, PEI-based polymers, inorganic compounds, chitosan, protamine sulfate, and dendrimers. These positively charged carriers are essential for condensing and protecting plasmid DNA while enhancing cellular uptake and delivery efficiency.

14.3 Nanoparticle-Mediated CRISPR/Cas9 Delivery in the Clinical Setting

Recent advances in gene-editing technology, particularly CRISPR/Cas9, have shown remarkable progress in cancer treatment research.

Clinical studies are exploring how modifying key immune system genes like PD-1, TCR, CISH, and TRAC can enhance T cell therapy outcomes for both solid tumors and blood cancers. One significant strategy involves deactivating the PD-1 gene to strengthen anti-cancer immune responses. Currently, researchers are testing PD-1-modified T cells in several contexts, including various solid tumors (NCT03545815), treatment-resistant prostate cancer (NCT02867345), and lung cancer (NCT02793856). Studies have shown that techniques like electroporation can significantly improve gene modification success rates. These approaches aim to overcome cancer's immune evasion mechanisms, as demonstrated in ongoing trials of mesothelin-targeting CAR-T therapy (NCT03747965).

Research in enhanced CAR-T cell treatments has made significant strides, particularly in treating B-cell disorders. A notable example is CTX110, which uses CRISPR to modify TRAC and β2M genes, currently showing promising results in B cell cancer trials (NCT04035434). Another innovative treatment, CTX130, targets CD70 and is being evaluated for both T cell lymphoma (NCT04502446) and kidney cancer (NCT04438083), utilizing electroporation for cellular gene modification. These innovative approaches offer new possibilities for patients whose cancers have not responded to conventional treatments.

Scientists are also investigating CRISPR technology's role in treating virus-linked cancers. Research includes targeting human papillomavirus's E6/E7 genes in associated cancers (NCT03057912) and using Cas9 plasmids to modify T cells for treating Epstein-Barr virus-related malignancies (NCT03044743). These studies highlight CRISPR's versatility across different cancer types and viral origins, suggesting broader potential applications in cancer immunotherapy.

Blood cancers, including acute lymphocytic leukemia and acute myeloid leukemia, are prime candidates for CRISPR/Cas9 therapeutic interventions. Scientists are currently evaluating CD33-modified hematopoietic stem and progenitor cells as a treatment approach for acute myeloid leukemia (NCT05662904). Other investigations focus on novel treatments like CTX112 for B cell lymphoma (NCT05643742) and CB-011, which targets BCMA in treatment-resistant multiple myeloma (NCT05722418).

These approaches commonly employ external cell modification to create enhanced T cells or blood-forming cells capable of mounting stronger anti-cancer responses. Research is underway on universal CAR-T cells targeting multiple proteins (CD19, CD20, CD22) for blood cancers, using advanced Cas9 techniques (NCT03398967). This donor-derived approach could potentially address the limitations of patient-specific CAR-T treatments.

Despite promising potential, CRISPR therapy faces several obstacles. Several clinical trials have been discontinued due to complications, including studies of WT1 using Cas9 RNP (NCT05066165) and PD-1-modified T cells for metastatic kidney cancer (NCT02867332). These challenges emphasize the importance of enhancing gene-editing methods, including better delivery systems, minimizing unintended modifications, and ensuring long-term patient safety.

The broad spectrum of CRISPR/Cas9 clinical trials demonstrates its expanding role in cancer therapy. These studies target various genetic elements, including PD-1, TCR, β2M, and CD33, across different cancer types. Various delivery methods have proven effective, with many trials progressing to advanced stages, suggesting both safety and initial effectiveness. As research continues, CRISPR/Cas9 therapies show promise in revolutionizing cancer treatment, particularly for difficult-to-treat cases. Current research highlights the potential of gene editing to enhance immunotherapy, with numerous innovative approaches being developed to improve treatment precision and durability.

The combination of CRISPR/Cas9 technology and nanoscience represents a revolutionary advancement in cancer treatment approaches. While laboratory studies show promising results, implementing these findings in clinical settings remains challenging. Present clinical studies primarily focus on external cell modification, where immune cells or stem cells undergo genetic alterations outside the body before reintroduction to patients. This approach, while innovative, has certain limitations. Direct genetic modification within the body offers distinct advantages, including the ability to target multiple tissues simultaneously and reduce operational costs.

The successful clinical implementation of direct genetic modification faces several technical challenges related to delivery methods. Therapeutic success requires nanomaterials that can efficiently transport CRISPR/Cas9 components into cells, facilitate their escape from lysosomes, and ensure they reach the nucleus. Another crucial consideration is the need to reduce the size of Cas proteins to improve their incorporation into nanocarriers. Clinical implementation heavily emphasizes safety considerations. Key requirements include developing systems for temporary CRISPR/Cas9 expression and using compatible nanomaterials. Minimizing unintended genetic modifications is crucial, with potential solutions including tissue-specific gene activation and specialized nanoparticles that enable controlled delivery and targeted distribution. For clinical approval of nanocarriers, adherence to CGMP standards is essential.

14.4 Challenges and Limitations of Nanoparticle-based Delivery

Despite the potential of CRISPR therapies, significant obstacles persist. Several clinical studies have been discontinued due to unexpected issues, including trials examining WT1 with Cas9 RNP (NCT05066165) and PD-1-modified T cells for metastatic kidney cancer (NCT02867332). These challenges highlight the necessity for improved gene-editing methods, enhanced delivery mechanisms, reduced unintended effects, and confirmed safety profiles.

The integration of CRISPR/Cas9 technology with advanced nanotechnology represents a crucial development in cancer treatment. Although laboratory research demonstrates significant promise, transferring these findings to patient care remains challenging. Most current clinical research focuses on external cell modification, where genetic alterations occur outside the patient's body. While this method shows promise, it has specific drawbacks. Direct genetic modification within the body offers unique benefits, such as targeting multiple tissue types and reducing operational expenses.

The successful implementation of direct CRISPR/Cas9 modification faces significant delivery challenges. Effective treatment requires nanomaterials that can successfully transport genetic components into cells, avoid lysosomal degradation, and reach the cell nucleus. A critical technical challenge involves reducing Cas protein dimensions to improve their incorporation into nanocarriers.

Managing unintended genetic modifications is crucial for clinical applications. These unwanted effects can lead to various complications, including genetic toxicity, unexpected gene insertions, or abnormal gene activity patterns. Addressing these concerns is essential for safe and effective treatment development.

Various approaches exist to improve targeting accuracy. These include the use of modified Cas9 variants such as SpCas9-HF1 and eSpCas9, enhanced gRNA designs, shortened sgRNAs, alternative Cas systems, and specialized nanoparticles that enable controlled delivery and precise targeting, thereby minimizing widespread exposure. The implementation of RNP delivery methods, which allow for transient Cas9 expression, naturally reduces the likelihood of off-target modifications compared to plasmid or viral delivery systems. Advances in computational prediction tools for identifying potential off-target sites, along with robust molecular testing techniques such as CIRCLE-seq, GUIDE-seq, and Digenome-seq, are essential for thorough pre-clinical validation.

Safety considerations for nanocarriers must encompass both immediate and long-term effects. In terms of breakdown and elimination, nanocarriers must be biologically compatible and degradable to avoid tissue accumulation, as long-term retention can lead to chronic inflammation, toxicity, and organ dysfunction. Regarding immune system response, although nanoparticles generally elicit lower immune reactions than viral vectors, they can still provoke immune responses. Therefore, comprehensive testing must assess both immediate and delayed immune reactions, including cytokine release, complement system activation, and antibody formation.

Safety assessment requires detailed pre-clinical studies to evaluate dose-dependent toxicity effects on organs such as the liver and kidneys, as well as inflammatory responses. It is also critical to assess the safety of breakdown products from biodegradable carriers. Finally, component safety and expression control demand rigorous safety verification of all carrier constituents, and the use of transient expression systems like mRNA or RNP further enhances safety by limiting the duration of gene editing activity and reducing unintended effects.

Following CGMP guidelines is crucial for translating nanocarrier-based treatments into clinical applications, as they ensure consistent product quality and safety throughout the development and manufacturing process. Ongoing clinical studies highlight the transformative potential of gene-editing technologies in immune-based therapies, with researchers actively exploring innovative strategies to enhance treatment precision and durability.

Despite existing challenges, continuous advancements in nanocarrier design, coupled with a deeper understanding of CRISPR/Cas9 mechanisms and rigorous safety evaluations, indicate that these technologies could fundamentally reshape cancer therapy. This progress brings renewed hope to patients battling hard-to-treat cancers.

The successful clinical implementation of CRISPR/Cas9-based cancer treatments hinges on the development of reliable and safe delivery systems. Researchers have engineered a variety of nanocarrier platforms, each offering unique advantages and limitations for transporting different CRISPR/Cas9 components, including plasmid DNA, mRNA, and RNP complexes. Comparative analysis of these delivery strategies provides critical insights for guiding future innovations in nanocarrier design tailored to specific cancer contexts.

Achieving success in this field will require striking the optimal balance between therapeutic efficacy and safety, conducting extensive long-term studies to assess outcomes and risks, and refining nanoparticle-based CRISPR/Cas9 delivery systems for targeted cancer treatment. This integrated and methodical approach is essential to unlock the full therapeutic potential of CRISPR/Cas9 technologies in oncology.

14.5 Future Perspectives

Nanotechnology-enhanced CRISPR/Cas9 delivery mechanisms show remarkable promise for cancer treatment, though significant obstacles remain that require continued research and innovation [54]. A central focus is the development of advanced nanocarriers with tailored biological and physicochemical properties designed to overcome both organ-specific and tumor-specific barriers.

In the case of brain cancers such as glioblastoma, addressing the blood-brain barrier (BBB) necessitates a multifaceted strategy. This includes the creation of biomimetic nanocarriers equipped with BBB-crossing peptides like angiopep-2 or receptor-specific antibodies such as anti-TfR and anti-LDLR, which exploit endogenous transport systems. Another approach involves controlled BBB disruption using magnetic resonance imaging-guided focused ultrasound in combination with gas-containing nanovesicles. Additionally, nasal delivery systems incorporating adhesive polymers and trigeminal nerve-targeting compounds offer a non-invasive route to bypass the BBB [55]. These delivery strategies must be integrated with tumor-penetrating designs that leverage the abnormal vasculature of tumors while evading immune system clearance.

Recent studies have demonstrated successful targeted gene-editing delivery for both brain and pancreatic cancers. Notably, the use of focused ultrasound with microbubbles has proven effective in transiently opening the BBB, facilitating CRISPR/Cas9 delivery with minimal damage to surrounding healthy neural tissue.

Pancreatic ductal adenocarcinoma presents unique challenges that demand specialized solutions. Research priorities include the development of stroma-targeting nanocarriers containing enzymes such as PEGylated hyaluronidase and collagenase, or CRISPR systems directed at TGF-β and SHH signaling pathways. Dual-targeting mechanisms that first engage the tumor stroma before addressing cancer cells are also critical. Furthermore, designing nanoparticles with optimal physical properties — specifically an elastic modulus between 10–50 kPa — can enhance tissue penetration and therapeutic efficacy.

For metastatic cancers, future research should focus on delivery systems capable of targeting multiple organs. This can be achieved through environment-responsive coatings that adapt to the specific conditions of each organ site, improving localization and minimizing off-target effects.

Additional innovations include olive oil-based nanocapsules with CD44-targeting capabilities for cancer stem cells, lipid-coated silica nanoparticles for enhanced drug delivery, and exosome-based CRISPR/Cas9 systems targeting KRAS^G12D mutations. These advancements point toward the potential of artificial intelligence-designed, stimulus-responsive nanocarriers integrated with sophisticated delivery technologies to enable precise genetic modification in some of the most challenging cancer types.

The integration of artificial intelligence with nanomedicine marks a revolutionary leap forward in cancer therapy, demanding rigorous analysis and multidisciplinary collaboration. Machine learning models — especially graph neural networks and transformer architectures — are capable of processing complex multi-omic datasets to uncover correlations between fundamental nanocarrier properties (such as size, electrical charge, and PEG concentration), their interactions with biological systems (including protein binding profiles and cellular uptake rates), and therapeutic outcomes like gene modification efficiency and tumor response.

Reinforcement learning offers powerful tools for optimizing competing design goals, such as enhancing tumor specificity while minimizing off-target accumulation in organs like the liver. Simultaneously, generative artificial intelligence models can propose novel biomaterials with tailored degradation profiles, accelerating the discovery of safer and more effective delivery systems. Realizing these capabilities hinges on the establishment of standardized testing protocols and the development of comprehensive databases that integrate data from laboratory experiments, animal models, and human clinical trials. Unlocking the full potential of nano-enabled CRISPR/Cas9 systems for resistant cancers will require a coordinated effort across basic science, translational research, and clinical development. By embracing a systematic and collaborative approach, the medical community can move closer to realizing the transformative promise of these advanced therapeutic technologies in overcoming some of the most challenging forms of cancer.

14.6 Conclusion

Nanoparticle delivery is central to realizing the therapeutic promise of CRISPR/Cas9 in cancer because it couples molecular precision with pharmacologic control — shielding and ferrying editors to tumors, timing intracellular release, and restricting activity to malignant tissue. By enabling format-flexible delivery and tumor-selective targeting, nanocarriers can increase editing efficiency, reduce off-target and immune liabilities, and support combination strategies that augment chemotherapy, radiotherapy, and immunotherapy. Continued progress will depend on rational material design for deep-tumor penetration and endosomal escape, validated targeting ligands and release mechanisms, and manufacturable, reproducible platforms that meet clinical quality standards. As these delivery innovations mature alongside safer editors and biomarker-guided patient selection, nanoparticles can turn CRISPR/Cas9 from a powerful experimental tool into a clinically actionable modality for durable, mechanism-based cancer therapy.

References

1. Anand U, Dey A, Chandel AKS, Sanyal R, Mishra A, Pandey DK, et al. Cancer chemotherapy and beyond: Current status, drug candidates, associated risks and progress in targeted therapeutics. Genes Dis. 2023;10(4):1367–401.

2. Leng G, Duan B, Liu J, Li S, Zhao W, Wang S, et al. The advancements and prospective developments in anti-tumor targeted therapy. Neoplasia. 2024;56:101024.
3. Casotti MC, Meira DD, Zetum ASS, Campanharo CV, da Silva DRC, Giacinti GM, et al. Integrating frontiers: a holistic, quantum and evolutionary approach to conquering cancer through systems biology and multidisciplinary synergy. Front Oncol. 2024;14:1419599.
4. Pandey M, Shah SK, Gromiha MM. Databases and computational algorithms for identifying cancer hotspot residues and mutations in proteins. In Protein Mutations: Consequences on Structure, Functions, and Diseases: World Scientific; 2025. p. 229–59.
5. Aljabali AA, El-Tanani M, Tambuwala MM. Principles of CRISPR-Cas9 technology: Advancements in genome editing and emerging trends in drug delivery. J Drug Deliv Sci Technol. 2024;92:105338.
6. Li H, Yang Y, Hong W, Huang M, Wu M, Zhao X. Applications of genome editing technology in the targeted therapy of human diseases: mechanisms, advances and prospects. Signal Transduct Target Ther. 2020;5(1):1.
7. Gupta D, Bhattacharjee O, Mandal D, Sen MK, Dey D, Dasgupta A, et al. CRISPR-Cas9 system: A new-fangled dawn in gene editing. Life Sci. 2019;232:116636.
8. Li T, Li S, Kang Y, Zhou J, Yi M. Harnessing the evolving CRISPR/Cas9 for precision oncology. J Transl Med. 2024;22(1):749.
9. Liu Z, Shi M, Ren Y, Xu H, Weng S, Ning W, et al. Recent advances and applications of CRISPR-Cas9 in cancer immunotherapy. Mol Cancer. 2023;22(1):35.
10. Wang L, Chen Y, Liu X, Li Z, Dai X. The Application of CRISPR/Cas9 Technology for Cancer Immunotherapy: Current Status and Problems. Front Oncol. 2021;11:704999.
11. Karimian A, Azizian K, Parsian H, Rafieian S, Shafiei-Irannejad V, Kheyrollah M, et al. CRISPR/Cas9 technology as a potent molecular tool for gene therapy. J Cell Physiol. 2019;234(8):12267–77.
12. Liu C, Zhang L, Liu H, Cheng K. Delivery strategies of the CRISPR-Cas9 gene-editing system for therapeutic applications. J Control Release. 2017;266:17–26.
13. Xu X, Wan T, Xin H, Li D, Pan H, Wu J, Ping Y. Delivery of CRISPR/Cas9 for therapeutic genome editing. J Gene Med. 2019;21(7):e3107.
14. Aghamiri S, Talaei S, Ghavidel AA, Zandsalimi F, Masoumi S, Hafshejani NH, Jajarmi V. Nanoparticles-mediated CRISPR/Cas9

delivery: recent advances in cancer treatment. J Drug Deliv Sci Technol. 2020;56:101533.

15. Chen K, Jiang S, Hong Y, Li Z, Wu Y-L, Wu C. Cationic polymeric nanoformulation: Recent advances in material design for CRISPR/Cas9 gene therapy. Prog Nat Sci Mater Int. 2019;29(6):617–27.
16. Rahimi H, Salehiabar M, Charmi J, Barsbay M, Ghaffarlou M, Razlighi MR, et al. Harnessing nanoparticles for the efficient delivery of the CRISPR/Cas9 system. Nano Today. 2020;34:100895.
17. Xu X, Liu C, Wang Y, Koivisto O, Zhou J, Shu Y, Zhang H. Nanotechnology-based delivery of CRISPR/Cas9 for cancer treatment. Adv Drug Deliv Rev. 2021;176:113891.
18. Wang Y, Tang Y, Zhao XM, Huang G, Gong JH, Yang SD, et al. A multifunctional non-viral vector for the delivery of MTH1-targeted CRISPR/Cas9 system for non-small cell lung cancer therapy. Acta Biomater. 2022;153:481–93.
19. Liu Y, Zhao G, Xu CF, Luo YL, Lu ZD, Wang J. Systemic delivery of CRISPR/Cas9 with PEG-PLGA nanoparticles for chronic myeloid leukemia targeted therapy. Biomater Sci. 2018;6(6):1592–603.
20. Chen J, Dai Q, Yang Q, Bao X, Zhou Y, Zhong H, et al. Therapeutic nucleus-access BNCT drug combined CD47-targeting gene editing in glioblastoma. J Nanobiotechnol. 2022;20(1):102.
21. Li C, Yang T, Weng Y, Zhang M, Zhao D, Guo S, et al. Ionizable lipid-assisted efficient hepatic delivery of gene editing elements for oncotherapy. Bioact Mater. 2022;9:590–601.
22. Ruan W, Jiao M, Xu S, Ismail M, Xie X, An Y, et al. Brain-targeted CRISPR/Cas9 nanomedicine for effective glioblastoma therapy. J Control Release. 2022;351:739–51.
23. Wuttke S, Braig S, Preiß T, Zimpel A, Sicklinger J, Bellomo C, et al. MOF nanoparticles coated by lipid bilayers and their uptake by cancer cells. Chem Commun (Camb). 2015;51(87):15752–5.
24. Rabiee N, Bagherzadeh M, Heidarian Haris M, Ghadiri AM, Matloubi Moghaddam F, Fatahi Y, et al. Polymer-Coated NH(2)-UiO-66 for the Codelivery of DOX/pCRISPR. ACS Appl Mater Interfaces. 2021;13(9):10796–811.
25. Pyreddy S, Poddar A, Carraro F, Polash SA, Dekiwadia C, Murdoch B, et al. Targeting telomerase utilizing zeolitic imidazole frameworks as non-viral gene delivery agents across different cancer cell types. Biomater Adv. 2023;149:213420.

26. Poddar A, Conesa JJ, Liang K, Dhakal S, Reineck P, Bryant G, et al. Encapsulation, Visualization and Expression of Genes with Biomimetically Mineralized Zeolitic Imidazolate Framework-8 (ZIF-8). Small. 2019;15(36):e1902268.
27. Chen Y, Chen X, Wu D, Xin H, Chen D, Li D, et al. Delivery of CRISPR/Cas9 plasmids by cationic gold nanorods: impact of the aspect ratio on genome editing and treatment of hepatic fibrosis. Chemistry of Materials. 2020;33(1):81–91.
28. Tang H, Xu X, Chen Y, Xin H, Wan T, Li B, et al. Reprogramming the Tumor Microenvironment through Second-Near-Infrared-Window Photothermal Genome Editing of PD-L1 Mediated by Supramolecular Gold Nanorods for Enhanced Cancer Immunotherapy. Adv Mater. 2021;33(12):e2006003.
29. Zhang BC, Luo BY, Zou JJ, Wu PY, Jiang JL, Le JQ, et al. Co-delivery of Sorafenib and CRISPR/Cas9 Based on Targeted Core-Shell Hollow Mesoporous Organosilica Nanoparticles for Synergistic HCC Therapy. ACS Appl Mater Interfaces. 2020;12(51):57362–72.
30. He XY, Liu BY, Peng Y, Zhuo RX, Cheng SX. Multifunctional Vector for Delivery of Genome Editing Plasmid Targeting β-Catenin to Remodulate Cancer Cell Properties. ACS Appl Mater Interfaces. 2019;11(1):226–37.
31. Tao Y, Yi K, Hu H, Shao D, Li M. Coassembly of nucleus-targeting gold nanoclusters with CRISPR/Cas9 for simultaneous bioimaging and therapeutic genome editing. J Mater Chem B. 2021;9(1):94–100.
32. Caprifico AE, Foot PJS, Polycarpou E, Calabrese G. Advances in Chitosan-Based CRISPR/Cas9 Delivery Systems. Pharmaceutics. 2022;14(9):1840.
33. Li Q, Lv X, Tang C, Yin C. Co-delivery of doxorubicin and CRISPR/Cas9 or RNAi-expressing plasmid by chitosan-based nanoparticle for cancer therapy. Carbohydr Polym. 2022;287:119315.
34. Menjoge AR, Kannan RM, Tomalia DA. Dendrimer-based drug and imaging conjugates: design considerations for nanomedical applications. Drug Discov Today. 2010;15(5–6):171–85.
35. Zhao L, Li D, Zhang Y, Huang Q, Zhang Z, Chen C, et al. HSP70-Promoter-Driven CRISPR/Cas9 System Activated by Reactive Oxygen Species for Multifaceted Anticancer Immune Response and Potentiated Immunotherapy. ACS Nano. 2022;16(9):13821–33.
36. Zhang L, Lin Y, Li S, Guan X, Jiang X. In Situ Reprogramming of Tumor-Associated Macrophages with Internally and Externally

Engineered Exosomes. Angew Chem Int Ed Engl. 2023;62(11): e202217089.
37. Xu X, Tang H, Guo J, Xin H, Ping Y. A dual-specific CRISPR-Cas nanosystem for precision therapeutic editing of liver disorders. Signal Transduct Target Ther. 2022;7(1):269.
38. Cordeiro RA, Serra A, Coelho JFJ, Faneca H. Poly(β-amino ester)-based gene delivery systems: From discovery to therapeutic applications. J Control Release. 2019;310:155–87.
39. Zhou D, Cutlar L, Gao Y, Wang W, O'Keeffe-Ahern J, McMahon S, et al. The transition from linear to highly branched poly(β-amino ester)s: Branching matters for gene delivery. Sci Adv. 2016;2(6): e1600102.
40. Liu J, Chang J, Jiang Y, Meng X, Sun T, Mao L, et al. Fast and Efficient CRISPR/Cas9 Genome Editing In Vivo Enabled by Bioreducible Lipid and Messenger RNA Nanoparticles. Adv Mater. 2019;31(33): e1902575.
41. Rosenblum D, Gutkin A, Kedmi R, Ramishetti S, Veiga N, Jacobi AM, et al. CRISPR-Cas9 genome editing using targeted lipid nanoparticles for cancer therapy. Sci Adv. 2020;6(47):eabc9450.
42. Farbiak L, Cheng Q, Wei T, Álvarez-Benedicto E, Johnson LT, Lee S, Siegwart DJ. All-In-One Dendrimer-Based Lipid Nanoparticles Enable Precise HDR-Mediated Gene Editing In Vivo. Adv Mater. 2021;33(30): e2006619.
43. Zhang D, Wang G, Yu X, Wei T, Farbiak L, Johnson LT, et al. Enhancing CRISPR/Cas gene editing through modulating cellular mechanical properties for cancer therapy. Nat Nanotechnol. 2022;17(7):777–87.
44. Abbasi S, Uchida S, Toh K, Tockary TA, Dirisala A, Hayashi K, et al. Co-encapsulation of Cas9 mRNA and guide RNA in polyplex micelles enables genome editing in mouse brain. J Control Release. 2021;332: 260–8.
45. Usman WM, Pham TC, Kwok YY, Vu LT, Ma V, Peng B, et al. Efficient RNA drug delivery using red blood cell extracellular vesicles. Nat Commun. 2018;9(1):2359.
46. Li Z, Zhou X, Wei M, Gao X, Zhao L, Shi R, et al. In Vitro and in Vivo RNA Inhibition by CD9-HuR Functionalized Exosomes Encapsulated with miRNA or CRISPR/dCas9. Nano Lett. 2019;19(1):19–28.
47. Brezgin S, Danilik O, Yudaeva A, Kachanov A, Kostyusheva A, Karandashov I, et al. Basic Guide for Approaching Drug Delivery with Extracellular Vesicles. Int J Mol Sci. 2024;25(19):10401.

48. Le Saux S, Aubert-Pouëssel A, Mohamed KE, Martineau P, Guglielmi L, Devoisselle JM, et al. Interest of extracellular vesicles in regards to lipid nanoparticle based systems for intracellular protein delivery. Adv Drug Deliv Rev. 2021;176:113837.
49. Wang X, Chen Y, Zhao Z, Meng Q, Yu Y, Sun J, et al. Engineered Exosomes With Ischemic Myocardium-Targeting Peptide for Targeted Therapy in Myocardial Infarction. J Am Heart Assoc. 2018;7(15):e008737.
50. Lu Y, Godbout K, Lamothe G, Tremblay JP. CRISPR-Cas9 delivery strategies with engineered extracellular vesicles. Mol Ther Nucleic Acids. 2023;34:102040.
51. Zhang C, Ren H, Liu G, Li J, Wang X, Zhang Y. Effective Genome Editing Using CRISPR-Cas9 Nanoflowers. Adv Healthc Mater. 2022;11(10):e2102365.
52. Guo J, Wan T, Li B, Pan Q, Xin H, Qiu Y, Ping Y. Rational Design of Poly(disulfide)s as a Universal Platform for Delivery of CRISPR-Cas9 Machineries toward Therapeutic Genome Editing. ACS Cent Sci. 2021;7(6):990–1000.
53. Zhu Y, Lin M, Hu W, Wang J, Zhang ZG, Zhang K, et al. Controllable Disulfide Exchange Polymerization of Polyguanidine for Effective Biomedical Applications by Thiol-Mediated Uptake. Angew Chem Int Ed Engl. 2022;61(23):e202200535.
54. Rauf MA, Rao A, Sivasoorian SS, Iyer AK. Nanotechnology-Based Delivery of CRISPR/Cas9 for Cancer Treatment: A Comprehensive Review. Cells. 2025;14(15):1136.
55. Kofoed RH, Aubert I. Focused ultrasound gene delivery for the treatment of neurological disorders. Trends Mol Med. 2024;30(3):263–77.